Antidepressants for
Elderly People

Antidepressants for Elderly People

Edited by
KARABI GHOSE

Honorary Consultant in Geriatric Medicine
University of Wales College of Medicine

 Springer-Science+Business Media, B.V.

©1989 Springer Science+Business Media Dordrecht

Originally published by Chapman and Hall Ltd in 1989.
Softcover reprint of the hardcover 1st edition 1989

Typeset in 10/12 Palatino by Photoprint, Torquay, Devon

ISBN 978-0-412-32460-4   ISBN 978-1-4899-3436-9 (eBook)
DOI 10.1007/978-1-4899-3436-9

British Library Cataloguing in Publication Data

Antidepressants for elderly people.
 1. Antidepressant drugs
 I. Ghose, K. (Karabi), *1941–*
 615'.78

Contents

Contents

Contributors

George W. Ashcroft MBChB, DRCOG, DSc, DPM, FRCPE, FRSE, FRCPsych, Professor, Department of Mental Health, University of Aberdeen.

Anthony J. Bayer Lecturer, University Department of Geriatric Medicine, University of Wales, College of Medicine, Cardiff Royal Infirmary.

Diana Cody MB, BA, MRCPsych, Senior Registrar, Department of Psychological Medicine, Hammersmith Hospital, London.

John R.M. Copeland MA, MD, FRCP, FRCPsych, DPM, Professor of Psychiatry, and Director Institute of Human Ageing, University of Liverpool.

Alec Coppen MD, DSc, FRCP, FRCPsych, Medical Research Council, Neuropsychiatry Research Laboratory, West Park Hospital, Epsom, Surrey.

Peter Crome MD, FRCP Edin., Consultant Physician in Geriatric Medicine, Orpington Hospital, Kent, and Clinical Associate Professor, Department of Medicine, University of Saskatchewan, Canada.

Jila Dana-Haeri MD, PhD, Charterhouse Clinical Research Unit Ltd., London.

Sheila Dawling BSc, PhD, Principal Biochemist, Poisons Unit, New Cross Hospital, London.

Klaus P. Ebmeier Ger. Med. State Exam. MRCPsych, Lecturer, Department of Mental Health, University of Aberdeen.

Karabi Ghose PhD, MRCP, Senior Lecturer and Honorary Consultant in Geriatric Medicine, University of Wales College of Medicine, Cardiff.

Cosmo Hallstrom MB, BCh, MRCP, MRCPsych, Consultant Psychiatrist, Charing Cross Hospital, London.

Cornelius L.E. Katona MA(Cantab), MB, BCh, MRCPsych, Senior Lecturer and Honorary Consultant in Psychiatry with Special Interest in the Elderly, University College and Middlesex School of Medicine and Whittington Hospital, London.

Contributors

John H. Lazarus MD, FRCP, Senior Lecturer, Department of Medicine, University of Wales College of Medicine, Cardiff.

Katy Malcolm Senior Registrar in Psychiatry, Northern General Hospital, Sheffield.

Ian McKeith MB, BS, MRCPsych, Senior Lecturer and Consultant Psychiatrist, Department of Psychiatry, University of Newcastle-upon-Tyne.

Isabel C.A. Moyes* Senior Lecturer and Honorary Consultant in Psychiatry with Special Interest in the Elderly, The London Hospital.

M.S. John Pathy Professor of Geriatric Medicine, University of Wales College of Medicine, Cardiff.

Malcolm Peet Consultant Psychiatrist, Northern General Hospital, Sheffield.

Vimal K. Sharma MB, BS, MD, MRCPsych, Consultant Psychiatrist, Walton Hospital, Liverpool and Honorary Research Fellow, Department of Psychiatry, University of Liverpool.

David M. Shaw FRCP, PhD, FRCPsych, Senior Lecturer and Honorary Consultant Psychiatrist, University of Wales College of Medicine, Cardiff.

Hilary Standish-Barry MRCPsych, Consultant Psychiatrist, Epsom District Hospital, Surrey.

Steve J. Warrington MA, MD, MRCP, Charterhouse Clinical Research Unit Ltd, London.

*Sadly, Isabel Moyes died before this book was published (Editor's note).

Preface

Depression is one of the commonest problems in old age. Yet until recently, old people were systematically excluded from participating in drug trials and similar investigations. As a result, knowledge regarding incidence, natural history and management of depression in the elderly are somewhat limited.

It is now well-established that old people are sensitive to most psychotropic drugs and they tend to suffer from adverse effects and side effects of antidepressant drugs more frequently than any other age group. These are considered to be due to age-related physiological changes. In addition, because of the frequent association with multiple pathology, the elderly are likely to receive polypharmacy which further complicates the management of antidepressant drug therapy.

The aim of this book is to provide a comprehensive guidance on the drug therapy of depression for the clinicians involved in the health care of the elderly. In the first section, epidemiology, presentations and assessment of depression in old age and neuroendocrine abnormalities observed in patients with depression are briefly discussed. However, it mainly deals with the problems of antidepressant drug therapy, such as which antidepressant to prescribe, how to monitor efficacy and side effects, what is the adequate dose, how long to treat a single episode of depression and who requires long term medication. Information regarding pharmacology, side effects, adverse effects, drug interaction and pharmacokinetics of most currently available drugs are provided. Special emphasis has been given on continuation therapy and the choice of an antidepressant drug and their long term safety.

The elderly should not be deprived of a medication for fear of side effects. Quality of their life can be improved by prescribing a prophylactic drug, such as lithium, but close supervision is required in this population.

The safety and efficacy of electroconvulsive therapy are summarized in chapter 14. The factors influencing the outcome of depression and the management of treatment resistant depression are also discussed.

In dealing with a book of this kind involving multiple authors from multidisciplinary backgrounds, some degree of overlapping of contents are inevitable. It is also intended to include as many different opinions as possible on various controversial aspects of clinical management of depression in old age.

I would like to express my gratitude to the authors for their valuable contribution and support. I also gratefully acknowledge the help and assistance provided by the editorial staff of Chapman and Hall publishers.

KARABI GHOSE

ONE

The Nature and Presentation of Depression

Chapter One

Presentation and assessment of depression in old age

VIMAL K. SHARMA and JOHN R. M. COPELAND

CONTENTS

1.1 INTRODUCTION

Depression is the most common psychiatric disorder in old age. Recent UK (Copeland *et al.*, 1987; Williamson, 1978) as well as US (Blazer and Williams 1980; Gurland *et al.*, 1980) population studies have reported that 10–15% of the elderly population over the age of 65 suffer from significant depressive symptoms. Despite the high prevalence, only a small proportion of the depressed elderly seek or receive psychiatric help. Williamson *et al.* (1964) reported that 71% of depressed patients were unknown to their GPs. Gurland *et al.* (1983) reported that only 3% of depressed subjects in New York and 14% in London were receiving antidepressant medication. In our study, in Liverpool, only 4% of the depressed subjects were on some kind of antidepressants prescribed by their GP (Sharma *et al.*, 1989). MacDonald in his recent study (1986) found that the GPs had no difficulty in recognizing depressed states in elderly people who attended surgery, but the recognition was unaccompanied by treatment with antidepressants or psychiatric referral. The

3

possible reasons for lack of recognition or inadequate management of old age depressive disorder are:

1. That elderly persons complain less about their depressed state.
2. Depressive symptoms are considered to be 'understandable' in terms of their physical condition or psychosocial background.
3. Some of the depressive symptoms are accepted as part of a normal ageing process.

1.2 PRESENTATION OF OLD AGE DEPRESSION

Beck (1967) has given an elaborate account of depressive symptomatology. He categorized depressive symptoms into emotional, cognitive, motivational, vegetative and physical.

The emotional manifestations include dysphoric mood, negative feelings towards self, crying spells, loss of gratification and joy. The patients may express their dejected mood by using adjectives like: 'I feel miserable' or hopeless, blue, sad, downhearted, humiliated, useless, guilty. Sometimes the feeling is expressed in somatic terms e.g. 'empty feeling in my stomach', 'heavy feeling in my chest'. Freeling *et al.* (1985) found that the depressed subjects unrecognized by their GPs often complained of 'feeling empty inside' or 'feeling cold inside'. Loss of interest in the social environment is characteristic of old age depression. Irritability, worry and the impulse to cry are other frequent symptoms (Blazer, 1980). The chief complaint made by the depressed older person frequently does not indicate depressive feelings as expressed by younger age groups. The complaint may be a physical symptom, difficulty in social relationships or dissatisfaction with financial circumstances. Skilful questioning, however usually brings out the core depressive feelings that underlie the chief complaint. A feeling of emptiness is a frequently reported symptom in depressed elderly persons (Goldfarb, 1974). Quite often, feelings of boredom and loneliness may be due to social withdrawal resulting from depression in old age.

The cognitive manifestations of depression include low self evaluation, negative expectations, self blame and self criticism, indecisiveness and distortion of body image (Beck, 1967). In older depressives, ruminations about present and past problems are common. These ruminations may be accompanied by frank delusions of uselessness (Blazer, 1980). Post (1972) described psychotic symptoms in 37% of 92 consecutively admitted depressed patients over the age of 60. Most of them communicated severe depression as well as delusional ideas of disease, poverty or guilt. Nihilistic delusions were voiced by only a very small number of patients. Many investigators have reported that guilt is a less common symptom in the depressed elderly compared to younger age groups (Winoker, Behar and Schlesser, 1980; Blazer, 1982; Kay *et al.*, 1985; Sharma *et al.*, 1989b). Because of increasing health problems, feelings of worthlessness and hopelessness about the future may have a different meaning for older individuals (Raskin, 1981; Kay *et al.*, 1985). These symptoms sometimes accompany ageing and may therefore lose some of their diagnostic significance (Raskin, 1981). Post (1972) points out that para-noid symptoms are not uncommon in elderly depressives, when de-pressive mood is apparently replaced by hostile feelings. Traditionally the severe depression of old age, with a constellation of depressive affect, agitation and persecutory ideas has been called involutional melancholia, a concept which has recently declined in popularity (Post and Schulman, 1985).

The relationship between hypochondriacal symptoms and old age depression has been emphasized by various investigators (Gurland 1976, Goldfarb, 1974; Steuer *et al.*, 1980). The gastro-intestinal tract is the most frequent target of complaints. Other common complaints of physical symptoms include headache, tinnitus and those associated with the urogenital system (Salzman and Shader, 1979). Localized pain can be an occasional manifestation of depression in elderly people (Williamson, 1978). At times the symptoms associated with long-standing physical illness seem exaggerated in patients suffering from an underlying depressive disorder (Williamson, 1974). When depression 'hides' behind somatic symptoms including tiredness, fatigue, lack of energy, chronic pain and hypochondriacal preoccupation, it is some-times referred to as 'masked depression'. Occasionally, the first appear-ance of alcohol dependence in late life is associated with depressive disorder (Williamson, 1978). It is not clear how much somatic complaints in older individuals are associated with significant health problems and how much with normal ageing (Raskin, 1979). For example, early morning wakening and loss of libido are accepted in younger age groups as important biological symptoms of depressive illness but the same symptoms may not be of great diagnostic value in old age depression. (Raskin, 1981).

Beck (1967) described a 'paralysis of will' as an important symptom of depression, but such motivational difficulties may be common in elderly people due to a variety of causes. Older persons with depression tend to withdraw from social activities (Fassler and Gavirin, 1978) and memory difficulties are often reported (Kahn *et al.*, 1975; Albert, 1984). In fact, depression in old age sometimes presents with symptoms of forgetfulness, apathy, listlessness and self neglect, a condition often described as 'depressive pseudodementia' (Epstein, 1976). Roth and Myers (1969) and Wells (1980) have reviewed the differentiating features

5

between depressive pseudodementia and true dementia. Acute onset with impairment of sleep, appetite and energy; sustained depressed affect; patchy, inconsistent cognitive impairment; past history of depressive illness and response to treatment are said to be distinguishing features.

1.2.1 Suicide

Suicidal ideas occur fairly frequently in elderly depressed patients and the risk of suicide tends to be greater than for younger depressed persons; four times greater in depressed elderly men than depressed elderly women. Barraclough (1972) in his study of elderly suicide victims found that they tended also to be suffering from a physical illness at the time, as well as tending to live alone and to commit suicide on the anniversaries of important bereavements. Two-thirds of the victims in his study had been depressed for less than a year before death and 90% had seen their GP within three months of committing suicide.

1.3 FREQUENCY OF DEPRESSIVE SYMPTOMS IN COMMUNITY POPULATIONS

Blazer (1980) found worry, feelings of uselessness, sadness, pessimism, fatigue, inability to sleep and volutional difficulties to be common symptoms in the elderly population. In our study using a semi-structured interview schedule, the Geriatric Mental State (GMS), community version (GMSA) Copeland *et al.*, 1976; McWilliam *et al.*, 1988, elderly subjects, identified as cases of depression by psychiatrists, frequently reported symptoms of depressed mood, sleep disturbance,

Table 1.1 The most common symptoms of depressive illness (pyschiatrists' diagnosis) assessed using the GMS–AGECAT Package on a random sample (*n* = 81) from 1070 subjects living in the community in Liverpool

Symptom	Number	Percentage of sample
Depressed mood	74	91.4
Sleep disturbance	58	71.6
Worries	55	67.9
Loss of energy	53	65.4
Loneliness	52	64.2
Crying spells	46	57
Pessimism	43	53.1
Tension	42	52

worries and loss of energy (Table 1.1). Nearly a quarter of them admitted to suicidal thoughts (Sharma *et al.*, 1989b). Feelings of guilt were reported by only 12%. While assessing an elderly person for depressive disorder, it is worth remembering that there are many circumstances which can produce depressive symptoms in this age group (Copeland, 1987). The association of physical illness such as malignant disease and endocrine disorders with depression is well recognized. Depression is also a common symptom in organic brain disease, including dementia. Chronic disabling illnesses causing restricted mobility and pain may be a cause of unhappiness sometimes amounting to illness (Murphy, 1982), while depressive symptoms are occasionally the side effects of drugs used for the treatment of physical conditions. The relationship between physical illness and depression has been reviewed by Rodin and Voshart (1986). As in younger age groups, psychological and social factors contribute to depressive symptoms in old age, for example bereavement, poor social support and financial difficulties.

1.4 ASSESSMENT OF OLD AGE DEPRESSION

Assessment of depression includes determining the presence, frequency and severity of typical symptoms. Clinicians should, but rarely do, use the operational criteria described in various diagnostic and classificatory systems, such as the World Health Organisation Glossary of Mental Disorders, or more recently the descriptions and criteria of ICD10. The Diagnostic and Statistical Manual (DSM-III) produced by the American Psychiatric Association (1980) classifies depressive disorders into major depressive episode, dysthymic disorder and atypical depression. The diagnostic criteria for each are clearly set out. The residual category for individuals with depressive symptoms who cannot be diagnosed as having a major or other specific or adjustment disorder is called an atypical depression. The classificatory system applies to all age groups including the elderly.

In recent years various standardized assessment tools (rating scales and interview schedules) have been used in different epidemiological studies. Assessment of depression can be made by using self rating scales, by observer ratings and by using standardized interview schedules. The first standardized rating scale was developed by Hamilton (1960). Hamilton's rating scale for depression includes 23 items and the rating is based on the interview by a trained rater. It has been used extensively in young populations. However, its value in the elderly population is doubtful because of its emphasis on the biological symptoms of depression e.g. late insomnia.

Beck's Depressive Inventory (Beck *et al.*, 1961) and Zung's Depressive

Scales (Zung, 1965) are widely used. Neither of these scales was specifically devised for the particular depressive symptomatology encountered in the elderly (Bird *et al.*, 1987). Myers and Weisman (1980) criticized the use of depression scales because they measure depressive symptoms quantitatively without distinguishing different syndromes. Self Care D (Bird *et al.*, 1987), and the Geriatric Depression Scale (Brink *et al.*, 1982) are self rating scales devised exclusively for elderly populations. These scales have proved useful in large epidemiological studies as screening instruments.

The Geriatric Mental State (GMS)–AGECAT Package which was developed by Copeland *et al.* (1976, 1986, 1988) has been widely used. It consists of several semi-structured interview schedules to assess mental state, onset and course of the illness, family history and possible aetiological factors in elderly populations. It has been translated into twelve languages. The computer assisted diagnostic system (AGECAT) (Copeland *et al.*, 1986, 1988; Dewey, Copeland and Griffiths-Jones, 1986) is based on the GMS and the History and Aetiology Schedule ratings. The agreement between the AGECAT diagnosis and psychiatrists' diagnosis of cases of depression is good. Kappa values in excess of 0.80 are obtained for subjects in psychiatric in-patient facilities and for random community samples (Copeland *et al.*, 1986, 1988). AGECAT also provides different levels of diagnostic confidence equating with severity (Copeland *et al.*, 1989b) and caseness, records levels of co-morbid states as well as provides scores for depression. The latter can be employed

Table 1.2 Scales/schedules used to measure depression in the elderly

Scale/schedule	Reference
Self rating scales:	
Zung Depression Scale (20 items)	*Zung (1965)
Beck Depression Inventory (21 items)	*Beck *et al.* (1961)
Geriatric Rating Scale (30 items)	Brink *et al.* (1982)
Self Care D (12 items)	Bird *et al.* (1987)
Depression scales based on interview	
The Older American Resources and Services (OARS) Depression Scale	Blazer (1980)
Hamilton Rating Scale for Depression	*Hamilton (1960)
Interview schedules	
The Geriatric Mental State Schedule (GMS)	Copeland *et al.* (1976)
Comprehensive Assessment and Referral Evaluation Schedule (CARE)	Gurland *et al.* (1983)

*Not specifically developed for elderly subjects.

for screening populations for 'syndrome cases' of depression. Mc-William *et al.* (1988) have demonstrated a sensitivity of 79% and a specificity of 92% applying a Dementia Depression Index (DDI) to these GMS scores using a split half, community design. The DDI can be applied in the field and subsequently checked by its computer programme. It seems to discriminate reasonably well between cases of dementia and depression.

The Comprehensive Assessment and Referral Evaluation interview (CARE) by Gurland *et al.* (1983) is a detailed semi-structured interview schedule covering over 1500 items of information concerning the health and social problems of older individuals including a number of indicator scales of depression. The CARE schedule is very comprehensive and suitable for those studies wishing to collect substantial information about their subjects, in addition to identifying a range of mental illness.

Common rating scales or interview schedules for the assessment of depression are listed in Table 1.2.

REFERENCES

Albert, M. (1984) Assessment of cognitive function in the elderly. *Psychosomatics*, **25**, 310–17.

American Psychiatric Association (1980) *Diagnostic and Statistical Manual of Mental Disorders (DSM-III)*, 3rd edn., American Psychiatric Association, Washington D.C.

Barraclough, B. (1972) Suicide in the elderly. *Br. J. Psychiat.* (Special Publication **6**), 87.

Beck, A.T., Ward, C.H., Mendelson, M. *et al.* (1961) An inventory for measuring depression. *Arch. Gen. Psychiat.*, **4**, 561–71.

Beck, A.T. (1967) Symptomatology of Depression. In: *Depression: Clinical, Experimental and Theoretical Aspects* (ed. A.T. Beck), Staples Press, London, pp. 10–43.

Bird, A.S., MacDonald, A.J.D., Mann, A.H. and Philpot, M.P. (1987) Preliminary experience with the Self Care D: a self-rating depression questionnaire for use in elderly, non-institutionalized subjects. *Int. J. Ger. Psych.*, **2**, 31–8.

Blazer, D.G. (1980) The diagnosis of depression in the elderly. *J. Am. Geriat. Soc.* **28**, (2), 52–8.

Blazer, D. and Williams, C.D. (1980) Epidemiology of dysphoria and depression in an elderly population. *Am. J. Psychiat.*, **137**, 439–44.

Blazer, D.G. (1982) Symptoms and signs. In: *Depression in Late Life* (ed. K. Berger), The CV Mosby Company, St. Louis, pp. 19–31.

Brink, T.A., Yesavage, J.A., Lum, O. *et al.* (1982) Screening tests for geriatric depression in *Clin. Gerontologist*, **1**, 37–44.

Copeland, J.R.M., Kelleher, M.J., Kellett, J.M. *et al.* (1976) A semi-structured clinical interview for the assessment of diagnosis and mental state in the elderly. The Geriatric Mental State schedule. 1. development and reliability. *Psychol. Med.*, **6**, 439–49.

Copeland, J.R.M., Dewey, M.E. and Griffiths-Jones, H.M. (1986) Computerised psychiatric diagnostic system and case nomenclature for elderly subjects: GMS and AGECAT. *Psychol. Med.*, **16**, 89–99.

Copeland, J.R.M., Dewey, M.E., Wood, N. *et al.* (1987) Range of mental illness among the elderly in the community. *Br. J. Psychiat.*, **150**, 815–23.

Copeland, J.R.M. (1987) Prevalence of depressive illness in the elderly community. In: *The Presentation of Depression: Current Approaches* (eds. P. Freeling, L.J. Downey and J.C. Malkin), The Royal College of General Practitioners, London, Occasional Paper 36, pp. 5–8.

Copeland, J.R.M., Dewey, M.E., Henderson, A.S. *et al.* (1988) The Geriatric Mental State (GMS) used in the community: replication studies of the computerized diagnosis AGECAT. *Psychol. Med.*, **17** (in press).

Copeland, J.R.M. and Dewey, M.E. (1989) Depression amongst the elderly in the community: the clinical picture of major and minor depressive illness assessed by AGECAT. (in prep.).

Dewey, M.E., Copeland, J.R.M. and Griffiths-Jones H.M. (1986) The computerization of AGECAT. In: *Psychiatric Disorders in the Elderly* (eds. P.E. Bebbington and R. Jacoby), Mental Health Foundation, London.

Epstein, L.J. (1976) Depression in the elderly. *J. Gerontol.*, **31**, 278–82.

Fassler, L.B. and Gavirin, M. (1978) Depression in old age. *J. Am. Geriat. Soc.*, **26**, (10), 471–5.

Freeling, P., Rao, B.M., Paykel, E.S. *et al.* (1985) Unrecognized depression in General Practice. *Br. Med. J.*, **290**, 1880–3.

Goldfarb, A.I. (1974) Masked depression in the elderly. In: *Masked Depression* (ed. S. Lesse), Jason Aronson, New York, pp. 236–49.

Gurland, B.J., Fleiss, J.L., Goldberg, K. *et al.* (1976) A semi-structured clinical interview for the assessment of diagnosis and mental state in the elderly. The geriatric mental state schedule 2. A factor analysis. *Psychol. Med.*, **6**, 451–9.

Gurland, B.J., Copeland, J.R.M., Kelleher, M.J. *et al.*, (1983) *The Mind and Mood of Ageing: The Mental Health Problems of the Community Elderly in New York and London*, Haworth Press, New York.

Gurland, B., Dean, L., Gross, P. and Golden, R. (1980) Epidemiology of depression and dementia in the elderly. In: *Psychopathology in the Aged* (eds. J.O. Cole and J.E. Barrett) Raven Press, New York, pp. 37–62.

Hamilton, M. (1960) A rating scale for depression. *Journal of Neurology, Neurosurgery and Psychiatry*, **23**, 56–62.

Kahn, R.L., Zarit, S.H., Hilbert, H.M. and Niederche, O. (1975) Memory complaint and impairment in the aged. *Arch. Gen. Psychiat.*, **32**, 1569–73.

Kay, D.W.K., Henderson, A.S., Scott, R. *et al.* (1985) Dementia and depression among the elderly living in the Hobart community: the effect of the diagnostic criteria on the prevalence rates. *Psychol. Med.*, **15**, 771–88.

MacDonald, A.J.D. (1986) Do General Practitioners 'miss' depression in elderly patients? *Br. Med. J.*, **292**, 1365–7.

McWilliam, C., Copeland, J.R.M., Dewey, M.E. and Wood, N. (1988) The

Geriatric Mental State examination. As a case-finding instrument in the community. *Br. J. Psychiat.* (in press).

Murphy, E. (1982) Social origins of depression in old age. *Br. J. Psychiat.*, **141**, 135–42.

Myers, J.K. and Weismann, M.M. (1980) Use of a self report symptom scale to detect depression in a community sample in *Am. J. Psychiatry*, **137**, (9), 1081–3.

Post, F. (1972) The management and nature of depressive illness in late life: a follow-through study. *Br. J. Psychiat.*, **121**, 393–404.

Post, F. and Shulman, K. (1985) New views on old age affective disorders. In: *Recent Advances in Psychogeriatrics No. 1* (ed. T. Arie), Churchill Livingstone, London, pp. 119–40.

Raskin, A., (1979) Signs and symptoms of psychopathology in the elderly. In: *Psychiatric Symptoms and Cognitive Loss in the Elderly* (eds. A. Raskin and L.F. Jarvik) John Wiley, New York, pp. 3–18.

Raskin, A. (1981) Special considerations in the assessment of psychopathology in the elderly. *Psychopharmacol. Bull.*, **17**, 104–7.

Rodin, G. and Voshart, K. (1986) Depression in the medically ill: an overview. *Am. J. Psychiat.*, **143**, (6), 696–705.

Roth, M. and Myers, D.H. (1969) The diagnosis of dementia. *Br. J. Hosp. Med.*, **1**, 705–17.

Salzman, C. and Shader, R.I. (1979) Clinical evaluation of depression in the elderly. In: *Psychiatric Symptoms and Cognitive Loss in the Elderly* (eds. A. Raskin and L.F. Jarvik), John Wiley, New York, pp. 39–72.

Sharma, V.K., Copeland, J.R.M., Davidson, I.A. and Dewey, M.E. (1989) The 3 year outcome of depressive illness in a random community sample of persons aged over 65 living in Liverpool. (GMS–AGECAT) (in prep.).

Sharma, V.K., Copeland, J.R.M., Dewey, M.E. *et al.* (1989b) Prevalence of depressive symptoms in the elderly population: findings of the Liverpool community study. (GMS–AGECAT) (in prep.).

Steuer, J., Bank, L., Osten, E.J. and Jarvik, L.F. (1980) Depression, physical health and somatic complaints in the elderly. A study of the Zung Self-Rating Depression Scale. *J. Gerontol.*, **35**, 683–8.

Wells, C.E. (1980) The differential diagnosis of psychiatric disorders in the elderly. In: *Psychopathology in the Aged* (eds. J.O. Cole and J.E. Barrett), Raven Press, New York, pp. 19–36.

Williamson, J., Stockhoe, I.H., Gray, S. *et al.* (1964) Old People at home, their unreported needs. *Lancet*, i, 1117–22.

Williamson, J. (1974) Depression. In: *Geriatric Medicine* (eds. W.F. Anderson and T.G. Judge) Academic Press, London.

Williamson, J. (1978) Depression in the elderly. *Age and Ageing*, (**Supp. 7**) 35–40.

Winoker, G., Behar, D. and Schlesser, M. (1980) Clinical and biological aspect of depression in the elderly. In: *Psychopathology in the Aged* (eds. J.O. Cole and J.E. Barrett), Raven Press, New York, pp. 145–56.

Zung, W.W.K. (1965) A self rating depression scale *Arch. Gen. Psychiat.*, **12**, 63–70.

Chapter Two

Identification of depression in geriatric medical patients

ANTHONY J. BAYER and M.S. JOHN PATHY

CONTENTS

2.1 INTRODUCTION

The strong association in elderly subjects between depression and physical ill health has been long recognized, though clear evidence regarding a causal relationship in either direction is generally lacking (Levenson and Hall, 1981; Eastwood and Corbin, 1986). That either condition can influence the development and course of the other, however, is well known. Depressive illness predisposes to physical ill health (Wigdor and Morris, 1977) and good mental health appears to be protective (Valliant, 1979). Improved physical state correlates with reduced psychiatric morbidity (Shephard, 1983) and, similarly, physical

Table 2.1 Published studies reporting prevalence of depression in elderly medical patients

Author	Country	Number of patients	Source	Age (Yrs)	% Male	Criteria for diagnosis	% Depressed
Bergmann and Eastham (1974)	UK	100	General medical inpatients	65+	45	Psychiatric interview, Glossary of Mental Disorders	19 (5% endogenous, 14% neurotic)
Schuckit et al. (1975)	USA	50	Medical/surgical in-patients, without admission psychiatric diagnosis	65+	100	Unipolar depression (Feighner et al., 1972)	6
Pitt and Silver (1980)	UK	289	Geriatric/ psychogeriatric assessment unit	65+	44	Discharge diagnosis of depression	10
Kitchell et al. (1982)	USA	42	In-patients, Veteran's Hospital	60+ (mean 68)	95	DSM-III	45

Study	Country	N	Population	Age	%	Diagnostic criteria	Prevalence %
Okimato et al. (1982)	USA	55	Out-patients, Veteran's Hospital	60+ (mean 69)	98	DSM-III	31
Schnieder and Plopper (1984)	USA	75	Medical/surgical in-patients	60+	Not stated	Not stated	23
Magni et al. (1985)	Italy	406	Geriatric medical in-patients	mean 76	44	SDS 50 / SDS 60	42 / 12
Borson et al. (1986)	USA	406	Out-patients, Veteran's Hospital	60+	95	SDS ≥60 / Estimated DSM-III	24 / 10
Norris et al. (1987)	USA	31	Out-patients, Veteran's Hospital	60–95 (mean 78)	96	DSM-III	30 (10% dysthymia, 20% major depression)
Feldman (1987)	UK	133	General medical in-patients	70–98	44	PSE ID5+ (Index of Definition 5 and above)	7

DSM-III Diagnostic and Statistical Manual of Mental Disorders, 3rd edn (American Psychiatric Association, 1980)
SDS Zung Self Rating Depression Scale (Zung, 1965)
PSE Present State Examination (Wing et al., 1974)

illness is more common in depressed patients with a poor psychiatric outcome than in those who recover and remain well (Murphy, 1983). Studies in young subjects suggest that severity of medical illness in hospitalized patients is related to the presence of depression (Stewart, Drake and Winokur, 1965; Moffic and Paykel, 1975); and in geriatric medical patients with multiple pathology, the number of medical problems as well as their severity often appears to be a determining factor in the development of depression.

2.2 PREVALENCE OF DEPRESSION IN GERIATRIC MEDICAL PATIENTS

With such a close interrelationship between medical illness and depression, there is inevitably a high prevalence of depressive illness among patients in medical wards and out-patient clinics. Table 2.1 lists the published studies which have assessed the prevalence of depression in elderly hospital patients. Identifying cases purely by self-rating scales will include some false positives and thus studies using a structured psychiatric interview tend to be more conservative in their estimates. As female sex may be a predictive factor for depression (Magni, deLeo and Schifano, 1985), it is unfortunate that so many of the studies were carried out within the predominantly male patient populations attending Veterans' Administration Hospitals. Furthermore, these cannot include a comparative group of younger hospital patients.

The two recent studies which have compared rates in young and old patients came to very different conclusions, possibly because of the different diagnostic criteria used or because of the different range of medical conditions in the age groups studied. Feldman *et al.* (1987) found a prevalence of affective disorder of 16% in general medical patients aged under 70 years and 7% in those older, whereas the study from Italy (Magni, deLeo and Schifano, 1985) identified depressive symptoms in 20% of younger adults and 42% of the elderly. Using stricter diagnostic criteria, however, depressive illness was considered to be present in only 12% of the older patients. Despite the varied patient populations in each study and the major differences in diagnostic criteria, both these studies confirm a significantly greater prevalence of depressive symptoms than is found in studies of the elderly at home.

2.3 DEPRESSION ASSOCIATED WITH SPECIFIC MEDICAL ILLNESSES

Some medical conditions seem particularly prone to causing depression.

2.3.1 Neurological disease

Following acute stroke, about 30% of patients are depressed and the prevalence remains high for at least two years (Robinson *et al.*, 1983; Wade, Legh-Smith and Hewer, 1987). It has been suggested that symptoms may be specifically associated with injury to the left frontal lobe (Robinson *et al.*, 1984) and more frequent in those with aphasia (Benson, 1973). Other workers, however, have questioned whether depression is any more common after stroke than in other disabling conditions (Robins, 1976; House, 1987). Certainly depression is a recognized symptom of Parkinson's disease and appears to be not only reactive to the disability but also biochemically related to the disease (Assnis, 1977; Gotham, Brown and Marsden, 1986). It is common in patients with cerebral tumours (Strub, 1985), following head injury (Lishman, 1973) and during the early stages of a dementing illness when it may delay accurate diagnosis (Liston, 1978; Reifler *et al.*, 1986).

2.3.2 Malignancy

In hospitalized patients with cancer, at least a third of patients meet DSM-III criteria for major depression (Bukberg, Penman and Holland, 1984), though the prevalence among out-patients is much lower than this (Derogatis *et al.*, 1983). Sometimes depression develops before the diagnosis of cancer has been made (Hughes, 1985). Certain neoplasms would seem particularly related to the development of mood change: the prevalence of psychiatric symptoms in patients with carcinoma of the pancreas, for example, being four times that found in patients with colonic cancer (Fras, Litin and Pearson, 1967).

2.3.3 Cardiorespiratory disease

Depression associated with cardiac disease is most common in elderly patients (Schuckit, 1977), and may develop acutely, following myocardial infarction (Lloyd and Cawley, 1983) or more insidiously in patients with chronic heart failure (Levenson and Friedel, 1985). In many of these patients, particularly those with previous psychiatric history, symptoms often persist for many months (Stern, Pascale and Ackerman, 1977; Pathy and Peach, 1980). In chronic obstructive pulmonary disease in the elderly, depression may be the presenting feature; the increasing isolation and decreasing physical activity result in the patient not exercising enough to be dyspnoeic and being too apathetic to volunteer symptoms of recurrent infections (Hall, 1981).

2.3.4 Endocrine and rheumatological disorders

Endocrine abnormalities in older patients, notably hypothyroidism (Gold, Pottash and Extein, 1982; Sinaikin and Gold, 1987), but also hyperthyroidism (Ronnov-Jessen and Kirkegaard, 1973) may present as a major depressive episode and metabolic disturbances (Surridge *et al.*, 1984) and renal disease (Hong *et al.*, 1982) may often be associated with significant changes in mood. Systematic diseases such as polymyalgia rheumatica and temporal arteritis (Cochran, Fox and Kelly, 1978), rheumatoid arthritis and fibromyalgia (Mindham *et al.*, 1981; Hudson *et al.*, 1985) and other conditions associated with chronic pain (Blumer and Heilbronn, 1987) may all be associated with significant depressive symptomatology. Osteoarthritis with resultant pain and immobility is particularly common in depressed geriatric patients.

2.4 DEPRESSION ASSOCIATED WITH DRUGS

Depression has been reported to be a potentially serious adverse effect for over 100 commonly prescribed drugs (Zelnik, 1987) and the disproportionate use of medication by the elderly and their greater susceptibility to side-effects results in significant levels of drug-induced depression in geriatric medical patients (Davie, 1983).

Often, however, evidence for a causal relationship between a particular drug and the development of depression does not stand up to scrutiny and the distinction between the presence of subjective depressive symptoms, such as lethargy, weakness, anorexia, poor concentration or sleep disturbance, and true depressive illness is rarely attempted in published reports. Nevertheless, depression is a well recognized, if infrequent complication of treatment with certain drugs, particularly antihypertensives and centrally acting agents. Those patients with previous histories of depressive episodes or a family history seem most at risk.

The antihypertensive drug, reserpine, now no longer widely prescribed, was one of the earliest recognized to induce depression, in up to 20% of patients (Goodwin, Ebert and Bunney, 1971). The onset of symptoms may be delayed and appears to be dose related. The mechanism is assumed to be the depletion of catecholamines in the brain. Clonidine and methyldopa are also said to precipitate depression in susceptible patients and, more recently, diuretics (Okada, 1985) and betablockers (Salem and Stewart, 1984) have been implicated, although a causal relationship has generally not been proven. Sedative drugs, such as the benzodiazepines, may induce or aggravate depressive symptoms in short-term use (Hall and Joffe, 1972) and in the longer term (Nathan *et al.*, 1985). Anti-Parkinsonian drugs, particularly Levodopa (Goodwin *et al.*, 1972), may precipitate or exacerbate depression in some patients, though significant improvement in mood may also occur (O'Brien *et al.*, 1971). Other commonly used drugs which may result in depressive symptoms or illness include corticosteroids (Ling, Perry and Tsuang, 1981), cimetidine (Johnson and Bailey, 1979), digoxin (Wamboldt, Jefferson and Wamboldt, 1986) and indomethacin (Robinson, 1965).

2.5 RECOGNIZING THE DEPRESSED PATIENT

As with other common medical conditions in the geriatric medical patient, the diagnosis of depression may be delayed or missed because of atypical presentation. Somatic symptoms tend to be prominent in the elderly (Lipscombe and Katon, 1987) and most patients, and many of their physicians, find a physical explanation for their problems more acceptable than a possible psychiatric diagnosis. Complaints are often taken at face value, without an adequate search for associated symptoms and the inevitable minor abnormalities of laboratory and radiological tests which are found serve only to detract further from a careful appraisal of the patient's mental state. Compared to psychiatrists, physicians tend to base a diagnosis of depression on their general impression of the patient, rather than specific cues such as feelings of guilt, hopelessness or risk of suicide (Fisch, Hammond and Joyce, 1982). Often the diagnosis is considered only as one of exclusion (Goldberg, 1984), yet a full history will enable each complaint to be put into context and an overall depressive profile of symptoms and responses may be more apparent (Paykel and Norton, 1982).

A previous history of admission to a psychiatric hospital or of 'nervous breakdown' should be noted. Questioning patients about psychological symptoms is difficult in the middle of a busy ward with many ears ready to listen to any conversation and constant distractions from other patients and staff, and an effort should always be made to talk in private. The tendency to dismiss any symptom considered understandable in the light of the patient's other medical and social problems needs to be controlled. Thus apathy, fatigue and cognitive difficulties are sometimes mistakenly attributed to old age. Change of appetite and disturbed bowel function are assumed to be a consequence of general ill health. Disturbed sleep and early morning waking are accepted as secondary to hospital ward routine. Even open expressions of despondency, hopelessness and frustration are sometimes regarded as an understandable and therefore unimportant response to the patient's situation. Whilst the significance of any one symptom is impossible to interpret in isolation, taken together a pattern may emerge. The final distinction between normal and abnormal psychological reactions will always be largely arbitrary but it is probably safer to overdiagnose rather than risk the possibility of missing significant depressive illness.

2.6 FREQUENCY OF MISSED DIAGNOSIS

Despite the weight of evidence suggesting a high prevalence of serious depressive illness among geriatric medical patients, many clinicians still show a high threshold of suspicion for the diagnosis. Thus, in up to 50% of patients, the diagnosis is overlooked (Burville, 1971; Nielsen and Williams, 1980) or the severity of emotional disturbance underestimated (Feldman *et al.*, 1987). Missed diagnosis is especially common in those admitted from institutional care rather than from home, the very elderly and those widowed, single or divorced (Kidd, 1962). A past history of psychiatric illness is, not surprisingly, also frequently present but generally unrecorded in the current medical notes (Schuckit, Miller and Hahlbohm, 1975), though readily available from general practitioner letters, previous notes and nursing records (Feldman *et al.*, 1987).

2.7 AIDS TO DIAGNOSIS – DEPRESSION RATING SCALES

It is sometimes argued that routinely identifying depressive illness is not possible on busy non-psychiatric wards by doctors who are not appropriately trained and are anyhow too hard pressed to carry out lengthy enquiries. Bergmann and Eastham (1974) observed that elderly patients presenting with functional disorders were often seen on general wards as merely 'different' and advocated the routine use of short screening tests to help identify patients with affective disorders who might benefit from treatment. Certainly accurate diagnosis will always necessitate a careful interview but simple rating scales deserve wider use as screening measures to alert clinicians to the possibility of depressive symptomatology and to help monitor change. For use with geriatric medical patients, such measures must be brief and acceptable, of proven validity in the elderly and in those with physical illness, and with a cut-off score which identifies as many cases as possible, without too many errors. Few scales are available which meet these criteria adequately and, in particular, the inclusion of many somatic items (e.g. constipation, insomnia) presents difficulties in interpreting responses.

The GDS, the Geriatric Depression Scale (Yesavage and Brink, 1983) has the advantage of having been specifically designed for use with the elderly and is not heavily weighted towards health concerns. It has a simple yes/no response format and can be administered aurally. There is preliminary evidence of its validity with the physically ill (Norris *et al.*, 1987) as well as in subjects with mild to moderate cognitive impairment, though not the severely demented (Brink, 1984). A short 15-item version has recently been developed which may be especially useful for patients with physical illness who are likely to feel fatigued and are often limited in their ability to concentrate for any length of time (Sheikh and Yesavage, 1986). Our own experience of both the long and short forms of the Geriatric Depression Scale as a screening device for measuring depression among geriatric in-patients has confirmed its general acceptability with both patients and staff and we advocate its routine use, particularly among convalescent and rehabilitating patients. Patients scoring above the cut-off (greater than 11 on the GDS) may be followed up by more detailed interview, with assessment of the mental state and the depressive symptoms being put into their medical and social context. Experience suggests that about two-thirds of these patients will fulfil criteria for a clinically significant depressive illness.

2.8 PLANNING MANAGEMENT

Recognizing depression among patients on geriatric medical wards or attending out-patient clinics serves little purpose unless followed by appropriate referral or intervention. It is neither necessary nor practical for all such patients to be seen by a psychiatrist. Indeed, many patients and relatives may resent an implication that at least some of their problems may be emotional rather than medical and therefore compliance with psychiatric referral and treatment may be poor. It is important, however, that a specific plan of management is made and followed through. All patients should be listened to and helped to regain a sense of hope and an interest in the future. Many will require the addition of antidepressant drugs and, if symptoms persist, referral for electroconvulsant therapy should not be delayed. An active approach to both identification and management of depression will then be as rewarding to the clinician as to the patient and carers.

REFERENCES

American Psychiatric Association (1980) *Diagnostic and Statistical Manual of Mental Disorders*, 3rd edn, American Psychiatric Association, Washington, DC.

Assnis, G. (1977) Parkinson's disease, depression and ECT: a review and care study. *Am. J. Psychiat.*, **134**, 191–9.

Benson, D.F. (1973), Psychiatric aspects of aphasia. *Br. J. Psychiat.*, **123**, 555–66.

Bergmann, K. and Eastham, E.J. (1974) Psychogeriatric ascertainment and assessment for treatment in an acute medical ward setting. *Age Ageing*, **3**, 174–8.

Blumer, D. and Heilbronn, M. (1987) Depression and chronic pain. In: *Presen-*

tations of Depression, ed. O.G. Cameron, John Wiley and Sons, New York, pp. 215–36.

Borson, S., Barnes, R.A., Kukull, W.A. *et al.* (1986) Symptomatic depression in elderly medical out-patients. *J. Am. Geriatr. Soc.*, **34**, 341–7.

Brink, T.L. (1984) Limitations of the GDS in cases of pseudodementia. *Clin. Gerontol.*, **2**, 60–1.

Bukberg, J., Penman, D. and Holland, J.C. (1984) Depression in hospitalized cancer patients. *Psychosom. Med.*, **46**, 199–212.

Burville, P. (1971) Consecutive psychogeriatric admissions to psychiatric and geriatric hospitals. *Geriatrics*, **26**, 156–68.

Cochran, J.W., Fox, J.H. and Kelly, M.P. (1978) Reversible mental symptoms in temporal arteritis. *J. Nerv. Ment. Dis.*, **166**, 466–8.

Davie, J.W. (1983) Depression in old age: a geriatrician's view. In: *Advanced Geriatric Medicine 3* (eds. F.I. Caird and J. Grimley Evans) Pitman Books, London, pp. 99–104.

Derogatis, L.R., Morrow, G.R., Fetting, J. *et al.* (1983) The prevalence of psychiatric disorders among cancer patients. *J. Am. Med. Assoc.*, **249**, 751–7.

Eastwood, M.R. and Corbin, S.L. (1986) The relationship between physical illness and depression in old age. In: *Affective Disorders in the Elderly* (ed. E. Murphy) Churchill Livingstone, London, pp. 177–86.

Feighner, J.P., Robins, E., Guze, S.B. *et al.* (1972) Diagnostic criteria for use in psychiatric research. *Arch. Gen. Psychiat.*, **26**, 57–63.

Feldman, E., Mayou, R., Hawtonk, K. *et al.* (1987) Psychiatric disorder in medical in-patients. *Q. J. Med.*, **241**, 405–12.

Fisch, H.U., Hammond, K.R. and Joyce, C.R.B. (1982) On evaluating the severity of depression: an experimental study of psychiatrists. *Br. J. Psychiat.*, **140**, 378–83.

Fras, I., Litin, E.M. and Pearson, J.S. (1967) Comparison of psychiatric symptoms in carcinoma of the pancreas with those in some other intra-abdominal neoplasms. *Am. J. Psychiat.*, **123**, 1553–62.

Gold, M.S., Pottash, A.C. and Extein, I. (1982) Symptomless autoimmune thyroiditis in depression. *Psychiat. Res.*, **6**, 261–9.

Goldberg, D. (1984) The recognition of psychiatric illness by non-psychiatrists. *Aust. NZ. J. Psychiat.* **18**, 123–8.

Goodwin, F.K., Ebert, M.H. and Bunney, W.E. (1971) Depression following reserpine: a re-evaluation. *Seminars in Psychiatry*, **3**, 435–48.

Goodwin, F.K., Murphy, D.O., Brodie, K.H. and Bunney, W.E. (1972) Levodopa: alterations in behaviour. *Clin. Pharmacol. Ther.*, **12**, 383–96.

Gotham, A.M., Brown, R.G. and Marsden, C.D. (1986) Depression in Parkinson's disease: a quantitative and qualitative analysis. *J. Neurol. Neurosurg. Psychiat.*, **49**, 381–9.

Hall, W.J. (1981) Psychiatric problems in the elderly related to organic pulmonary disease. In: *Neuropsychiatric Manifestations of Physical Disease in the Elderly* (eds. A.J. Levenson and R.C.W. Hall) Raven Press, New York, pp. 41–8.

Hall, R.C.W. and Joffe, J.R. (1972) Aberrant response to diazepam: a new syndrome. *Am. J. Psychiat.*, **129**, 114–18.

Hong, B.A., Smith, M.D., Valerius, T.J. and Robson, A.M. (1982) Pre-treatment depression in end-state renal disease. *Lancet*, **i**, 104–5.

House, A. (1987) Depression after stroke. *Br. Med. J.*, **294**, 76–8.

Hudson, J.L., Hudson, M.S., Pliner, L.F. *et al.* (1985) Fibromyalgia and affective disorder: a controlled phenomenology and family history study. *Am. J. Psychiat.*, **142**, 441–6.

Hughes, J.E. (1985) Depressive illness and lung cancer I: depression before diagnosis. *Eur. J. Surg. Oncol.*, **11**, 15–20.

Johnson, J. and Bailey, S. (1979) Cimetidine and psychiatric complications. *Br. J. Psychiat.*, **134**, 315–16.

Kidd, C. (1962) Criteria for admission of the elderly to geriatric and psychiatric units. *J. Ment. Sci.*, **108**, 68–74.

Kitchell, M.A., Barnes, R.F., Veith, R.C. *et al.* (1982) Screening for depression in hospitalized geriatric medical patients. *J. Am. Geriatr. Soc.*, **30**, 174–7.

Levenson, A.J. and Hall, R.C.W. (eds.) (1981) *Neuropsychiatric Manifestations of Physical Disease in the Elderly*. Raven Press, New York.

Levenson, J.L. and Friedel, R.O. (1985) Major depression in patients with cardiac disease: diagnosis and somatic treatment. *Psychosomatics*, **26**, 91–102.

Ling, M.H.M., Perry, P.J. and Tsuang, M.T. (1981) Side effects of corticosteroid therapy: psychiatric aspects. *Arch. Gen. Psychiat.*, **38**, 471–7.

Lipscombe, P.A. and Katon, W. (1987) Depression and somatization. In: *Presentations of Depression* (ed. O.G Cameron), John Wiley and Sons, New York, pp. 185–212.

Lishman, W.A. (1973) The psychiatric sequelae of head injury: a review. *Psychol. Med.*, **3**, 304–18.

Liston, E.H. (1978) Diagnostic delay in presenile dementia. *J. Clin. Psychiat.*, **3**, 599–609.

Lloyd, G.G. and Cawley, R.H. (1983) Distress or illness: a study of psychological symptoms after myocardial infarction. *Br. J. Psychiat.*, **142**, 120–5.

Magni, G., deLeo, D. and Schifano, F. (1985) Depression in geriatric and adult medicine in-patients. *J. Clin. Psychol.*, **41**, 337–44.

Mindham, R.H.S., Bagshaw, C., James, S.A. and Swannell, A.J. (1981) Factors associated with the appearance of psychiatric symptoms in rheumatoid arthritis. *J. Psychosom. Res.*, **25**, 429–35.

Moffic, H.S. and Paykel, E.S. (1975) Depression in medical in-patients. *Br. J. Psychiat.*, **126**, 346–53.

Murphy, E. (1983) The prognosis of depression in old age. *Br. J. Psychiat.*, **142**, 111–19.

Nathan, R.G., Robinson, D., Cherek, D.R. *et al.* (1985) Long-term benzodiazepine use and depression. *Am. J. Psychiat.*, **142**, 144–5.

Nielsen, A.C. and Williams, T.A. (1980) Depression in ambulatory medical patients: prevalence by self-report questionnaire and recognition by non-psychiatric physicians. *Arch. Gen. Psychiat.*, **37**, 999–1004.

Norris, J.T., Gallagher, D., Wilson, A. and Wihograd, C.H. (1987) Assessment of depression in geriatric medical out-patients: the validity of two screening measures. *J. Am. Geriatr. Soc.*, **35**, 989–95.

O'Brien, C.P., DiGiacomo, J.N., Fahn, S. and Schwartz, G.A. (1971) Mental effects of high-dosage levodopa. *Arch. Gen. Psychiat.*, **24**, 61–4.

Okada, F. (1985) Depression after treatment with thiazide diuretics for hypertension. *Am. J. Psychiat.*, **142**, 1101–2.

Okimato, M.A., Barnes, R.F., Veith, R.C. *et al.* (1982) Screening for depression in geriatric medical patients. *Am. J. Psychiat.*, **139**, 799–802.

Pathy, M.S.J. and Peach, H. (1980) Disability among the elderly after myocardial infarction: a 3 year follow-up. *J. R. Coll. Physicians. Lond.*, **14**, 221–3.

Paykel, E.S. and Norton, K.R.W. (1982) Masked depression. *Br. J. Hosp. Med.*, **25**, 151–7.

Pitt, B. and Silver, C.P. (1980) The combined approach to geriatrics and psychiatry: evaluation of a joint unit in a teaching hospital district. *Age Ageing*, **9**, 33–7.

Reifler, B.V., Larsone, E., Teri, L. and Pulsen, M. (1986) Dementia of the Alzheimer's type and depression. *J. Am. Geriatr. Soc.*, **34**, 855–9.

Robins, A.H. (1976) Are stroke patients more depressed than other disabled subjects? *J. Chronic. Dis.*, **29**, 479–82.

Robinson, K.L., Starr, L.B., Rao, K. and Price, T.R. (1984) Mood changes in stroke patients: Importance of location of lesion. *Brain*, **107**, 81–93.

Robinson, R.G. (1965) Indomethacin in rheumatic disease: a clinical assessment. *Med. J. Aust.*, **1**, 266–9.

Robinson, R.G., Tarr, L.B., Kubos, K.L. and Price, T.R. (1983) A two year longitudinal study of post-stroke mood disorders: findings during the initial evaluation. *Stroke*, **14**, 736–41.

Ronnov-Jessen, V. and Kirkegaard, C. (1973) Hyperthyroidism a disease of old age? *Br. Med. J.*, **1**, 41–3.

Salem, R.B. and Stewart, R.B. (1984) Depression from beta-adrenergic blocking drugs. *Drug. Intell. Clin. Pharm.*, **18**, 741–2.

Schneider, L. and Plopper, M. (1984) Geropsychiatry and Consultation – Liaison Services. *Am. J. Psychiat.*, **141**, 721–2.

Schuckit, M.A., Miller, P.L. and Hahlbohm, D. (1975) Unrecognised psychiatric illness in elderly medical-surgical patients. *J. Gerontol.*, **30**, 655–60.

Schuckit, M.A. (1977) The high rate of psychiatric disorders in elderly cardiac patients. *Angiology*, **28**, 235–47.

Sheikh, J.I. and Yesavage, J.A. (1986) Geriatric Depression Scale (GDS): recent evidence and development of a shorter version. *Clin. Gerontol.*, **5**, 165–74.

Shephard, R.J. (1983) Physical activity and the healthy mind. *Can. Med. Assoc. J.*, **128**, 525–30.

Sinaikin, P. and Gold, M.S. (1987) Endocrinology and depression II: thyroid function. In: *Presentations of depression* (ed. O.G. Cameron), John Wiley and Sons, New York, pp. 275–90.

Stewart, M.A., Drake, F. and Winokur, G. (1965) Depression among medically ill patients. *Dis. Nerv. System*, **26**, 479–85.

Stern, M.H., Pascale, L. and Ackerman, A. (1977) Life adjustment post-myocardial infarction: determining predictive variables. *Arch. Intern. Med.*, **137**, 1680–5.

Strub, R.L. (1985) Mental disorders in brain disease. In: *Handbook of Clinical*

Neurology (eds. P.J. Vinken and G.W. Bruyen), Elsevier, New York, pp. 413–42.

Surridge, D.C.H., Erdahl, D.L., Lawson, J.S. *et al.* (1984) Psychiatric aspects of diabetes mellitus. *Brit. J. Psychiat.*, **145**, 269–76.

Valliant, G.E. (1979) Natural history of male psychologic health: Effects of mental health on physical health. *New. Eng. J. Med.*, **301**, I, 1249–54.

Wade, D.T., Legh-Smith, J. and Hewer, R.A. (1987) Depressed mood after stroke: a community study of its frequency. *Br. J. Psychiat.*, **151**, 200–205.

Wamboldt, F.S., Jefferson, J.W. and Wamboldt, M.Z. (1986) Digitalis intoxication misdiagnosed as depression by primary care physicians. *Am. J. Psychiat.*, **143**, (2), 219–21.

Wigdor, B.T. and Morris, G. (1977) A comparison of twenty year medical histories of individuals with depressive and paranoid states. *J. Gerontol.*, **32**, 160.

Wing, J.K., Cooper, J. and Sartorius, N. (1974) *The measurement and classification of psychiatric illness.* Cambridge University Press, Cambridge.

Yesavage, J. and Brink, T.L. (1983) Development and validation of a geriatric depression screening scale: A preliminary report. *J. Psychiatr. Res.*, **17**, 37–49.

Zelnik, T. (1987) Depressive effects of drugs. In: *Presentations of Depression* (ed. O.G. Cameron), John Wiley and Sons, New York, pp. 355–400.

Zung, W.W.K. (1965) A self-rating depression scale. *Arch. Gen. Psychiat.*, **12**, 63–75.

Chapter Three

The epidemiology and natural history of depression in old age

CORNELIUS L.E. KATONA

CONTENTS

3.1 Introduction

3.2 Epidemiology

3.3 Suicide and attempted suicide in the elderly

3.4 The natural history of depression in old age

3.5 Conclusion

References

3.1 INTRODUCTION

Depressive symptoms are very common in the elderly. There are, however, considerable methodological problems in estimating the prevalence of depressive symptoms in an elderly population and in deciding on the circumstances in which they may be said to constitute a full blown depressive illness. This chapter concentrates on British and North American studies and is intended to be representative rather than comprehensive. Available data on the age-related prevalence of depression is reviewed, with particular reference to the problems of diagnosis; the epidemiology of suicide and attempted suicide in old age;

and the prognosis of, including the impact of treatment on, depression in the elderly.

3.2 EPIDEMIOLOGY

3.2.1 Methodological problems

Estimates of the prevalence of depression in the elderly vary widely (Post and Shulman, 1985). Discrepancies result from a number of methodological problems that have only recently been adequately addressed. The first of these problems is in the selection of subjects to be studied. This area is well reviewed by Kay and Bergmann (1980). In their view, the ideal method is to trace a cohort identified at birth to a specified age and then to identify all past and present episodes of depressive illness. This approach is unpractical in all but the most geographically isolated communities with excellent record keeping and little population movement. A 'census' approach, studying a defined population over a short period is the most widely used alternative. Censuses may be taken not only of geographically defined community samples, but also of more restricted populations such as those in hospitals or in residential care. This approach relies on good information on demographic characteristics of the population with adequate care taken to select an unbiased sample.

The second problem is that of defining and detecting depression within the population being studied. The most widely used techniques are questionnaires, semi-structured interviews and unstructured psychiatric interviews. The elderly may have particular difficulties in reading, understanding and responding appropriately to questionnaires and the results of interviews may be influenced considerably by the training and personality of the interviewer. An elderly population is likely to fall prey to a variety of physical illnesses; the presence of pain, legitimate preoccupation with physical health, and changes in sleep pattern secondary to either normal ageing or to physical illness, may lead to over-detection of depression.

A further issue relevant to all psychiatric research as well as to epidemiology is that of defining 'What is a case'. Copeland, Dewey and Griffiths-Jones (1986) who have made a considerable contribution to the understanding of this issue, point out that level of agreement between raters for most unstructured psychiatric diagnoses is low. Criteria for individual symptoms need to be operationalized, and the interview techniques for detecting them standardized, as preliminaries to the rigorous definition of criteria for caseness. They advocate the use of a semi-structured interview linked to a computerized hierarchical diag-

Table 3.1 Affective disorder: admission rates and outcome

Hospital	n	Percentage of total admissions	Six-month outcome (%)			Two-year outcome (%)		
			Discharged	In-patient	Dead	Discharged	In-patient	Dead
Graylingwell*	43	30	53	35	12	42	19	39
Crighton Royal†	64	24	75	9	16	70	6	24
St Nicholas‡	87	27	81	15	4	62	21	17

* Roth (1955(
† Christie (1982)
‡ Blessed and Wilson (1982)

nostic procedure which has the advantage of consistency, can take a wide range of unusual combinations of symptoms into account and can provide symptom profiles and scale scores as well as diagnoses.

Even in a clinical situation where the possibility of depression is raised, its diagnosis may present particular difficulties in the elderly. Many elderly subjects complain of hypochondriacal symptoms or sleep disturbance rather than of depressed mood. This problem can be minimized by the inclusion of separate 'somatic symptoms' rating scale, as incorporated in the diagnostic schedules of Copeland, Dewey and Griffiths-Jones (1986). A further problem may be the clinical distinction between depression and dementia (Katona and Aldridge, 1985). Although the syndrome of depressive pseudodementia (in which cognitive dysfunction is a prominent feature of a depressive illness in old age) is well recognized (Bulbena and Berrios, 1986), it is likely that many such patients turn out on follow-up to have dementing illnesses. In a recent study, Kral (1983) found this to be the case in 20 of 22 subjects. The danger of demented subjects contaminating a survey sample of elderly depressives is thus considerable.

3.2.2 Epidemiological studies

Studies of the prevalence of depression in the elderly can usefully be divided into hospital, residential and community samples.

(a) Hospital samples
Two recent hospital census studies by Christie (1982) and Blessed and Wilson (1982) replicated the methodology of the much earlier study by Roth (1955) and enabled a comparison to be made between hospital admission rates for depression in the elderly in two modern British psychogeriatric services, as well as contrasting those practices with admission rates preceding the introduction of antidepressant drugs. The studies all used Roth's classification of mental illness in old age: affective psychoses; late paraphrenias; acute confusional states; arteriosclerotic dementias, and senile psychoses (which correspond with a modern clinical diagnosis of Alzheimer's disease). Though the category of affective phychosis in these studies includes a small proportion of subjects with mania, it is likely that the overall figures for depression alone would not be significantly different. The proportion of patients with affective psychoses is remarkably similar in the three studies (Table 3.1), and suggests that among the psychiatric illnesses in the elderly that are sufficiently severe to warrant hospitalization, between one quarter and one third of patients suffer from depression. It must be emphasized that all these studies are retrospective and based on case notes. The lack

of operational definitions for Roth's diagnostic categories and the frequently poor quality of case notes means that such diagnostic data lacks the rigour embodied in the diagnostic procedures recommended by Copeland, Dewey and Griffiths-Jones (1986a).

(b) Residential care samples

As an adjunct to a more general community study of the prevalence of depression and dementia in the elderly, MacDonald and Dunn (1982) studied a non-random sample of subjects attending old people's homes, in-patient wards, day hospitals and day centres. It was possible to obtain interview and informant data on 397 out of 633 subjects. Most of the rest were too severely demented to be interviewed meaningfully. Of the subjects studied, 76 (19.1%) were classified as depressed. Mann, Graham and Ashby (1984) used the same interview schedule, the Brief Assessment Schedule, as MacDonald and Dunn (1982) and attempted to assess all the residents of the old people's homes in the London Borough of Camden. It was possible to assess the presence of depression in approximately two-thirds of the residents studied and of these, using a severity criterion for depression somewhat less strict than MacDonald and Dunn (1982) but which was shown to correspond well with psychiatric clinical judgement, a depression prevalence rate of 38% was recorded. Depression was found to be associated with incontinence, visual handicap, minority religious grouping and intermediate length of stay in residential care (between two and eight years).

(c) Community samples

Many studies of depression within geographically defined communities have used rating scale questionnaires as case finding instruments. Raymond, Michals and Steer (1980) attempted to administer the Wakefield Self Assessment Depression Inventory to 576 randomly selected residents aged 60 and over from census defined areas of south Philadelphia. Five hundred and two completed the inventory and 34.5% were classified as depressed. Depression was more frequent in females, in the housebound and in those with physical illness. Studies such as this, several of which have been well reviewed by Kay and Bergmann (1980) make no attempt to make formal psychiatric diagnoses. Gianturco and Busse (1978) studied 264 volunteers aged 60 and over who were willing to complete interviews and clinical examinations lasting two days as part of a longitudinal study of ageing. They do not give any detail on the procedures used to identify depressives and, although they attempted to make their sample demographically representative of the local population in Durham, North Carolina, the sample is likely to be biased by the self-selection of volunteers for such detailed interviews. Depression was recorded in 55 subjects (21%); there was no significant difference in prevalence of depression with increasing age.

Though published more than 20 years ago the Newcastle study of Kay, Beamish and Roth (1964) remains representative of the potential and the difficulties in carrying out surveys of mental illness in old age. A total of 505 subjects aged 65 and over were studied; the majority were selected by random sampling from an electoral register and the remainder were a deliberate oversampling from institutional care. A detailed medical and psychiatric inventory was performed by a psychiatrist and a total prevalence of 'affective disorders and neuroses' of 26% was found (29.4% in women, 20.9% in men). The authors found it impossible to make a satisfactory distinction between affective disorders and neuroses but they found that relatively mild disorders were present in 8.7% of men and 20.6% of women and moderate to severe disorders in 12.2% of men and 8.8% of women. Almost all these subjects were living at home and not receiving any form of psychiatric care. Depression was apparently rare in subjects in residential care – in marked contrast to the more recent studies cited above.

The importance of diagnostic subtyping in subjects with significant depressive symptomatology is emphasized by Blazer and Williams (1980). Using a detailed questionnaire they were able to make DSM-III (American Psychiatric Association, 1980) diagnoses on a random sample of subjects aged 65 and over from Durham, North Carolina. One hundred and forty-seven (14.7%) had significant depressive symptoms. Of these, 65 (44%) had depressions related to physical illness and 37 (25%) had major depressive illnesses, half of the latter were secondary to cognitive dysfunction and/or thought disorder. Forty-five (30%) were considered simply 'dysphoric'; they had substantial depressive symptoms but did not meet the criteria for depressive illness. Major depressive disorder was twice as common in women as in men, and was associated

Table 3.2 Prevalence of AGECAT diagnostic depression syndrome

	New York* (n = 445)	London* (n = 396)	(%)	Liverpool† (n = 235)	Hobart‡ (n = 274)
Male	13.0	13.1		7.6	
Female	18.3	22.8		13.5	
Total	16.2	19.6		11.2	14.2
Total Psychotic	1.8	3.3		2.9	

* Copeland *et al.* (1987a).
† Copeland *et al.* (1987).
‡ Kay *et al.* (1985): subjects aged over 70.

with widowhood, poverty and social isolation. Simple dysphoria on the other hand was associated with excessive use of analgesia.

Three very recent studies of randomly selected community samples have all used the Geriatric Mental State Schedule (GMS) of Copeland, Dewey and Griffiths-Jones (1986) and have reported prevalence rates for depression in subjects aged 65 and over in New York and London (Copeland *et al.*, 1987a), Liverpool (Copeland *et al.*, 1987b) and in subjects aged 70 and over in Hobart, Tasmania (Kay *et al.*, 1985). Prevalence rates in studies using the AGECAT computer-based diagnostic syndrome case level for depression are summarized in Table 3.2. The prevalence of psychotic illness is very low and depression is significantly commoner in women than in men. Copeland *et al.* (1987b) and Kay *et al.* (1985) demonstrate that the AGECAT diagnoses are broadly comparable to those of DSM-III. The Hobart study reports a DSM-III major depression rate of 10.7%, which is considerably higher than that reported by Blazer and Williams (1980) and also much higher than that reported in a recent study (Myers *et al.*, 1984) in which DSM-III diagnoses were made in a general adult community sample in the United States using the Diagnostic Interview Schedule (DIS) which is specifically designed for the purpose. In this study the prevalence of major depressive disorder in subjects aged 65 and over was 3.3% and of all affective disorders (including dysthymia) 6.0%. Rates both for major depression and dysthymia were twice as high in women as in men.

A recent study by MacDonald (1986a) examined elderly subjects attending GP surgeries and used the same interview schedule, closely related to the GMS, and depression rating scale as MacDonald and Dunn (1982) and Mann, Graham and Ashby (1984). In this group, which might be expected to contain a higher proportion of depressives than a random community sample, he found prevalence rates for depression of 19.3% in men and 36.8% in women, using a cut-off point for depression intermediate between those of the other studies cited.

The reported prevalence of depression depends both on the sampling technique used and on the criteria for depressive caseness. The clearest conclusions to be drawn from the studies cited are, however, that depression, especially if relatively mild, is commonest in elderly women; and that physical ill-health is the variable most consistently associated with the presence of depression.

3.3 SUICIDE AND ATTEMPTED SUICIDE IN THE ELDERLY

The misconception that successful suicide is rare in old age is widely held both in lay and medical circles. Shulman (1978) points out that in

1961 the suicide rate in men aged 65 and over was 350 per million, more than seven times the rate in the 15–24 age group. By 1974 this ratio had fallen to about 3:1, probably as a result of the introduction of natural gas for domestic supply to replace coal gas, which used to be the favourite medium for suicide in the elderly. Since then however, as is shown in Fig. 3.1 (adapted from McClure, 1984), not only has the overall suicide rate in Britain been rising both for males and for females but the rise has been particularly prominent in the elderly. The rates for elderly men are approximately twice those for women. Stenback (1980) points out

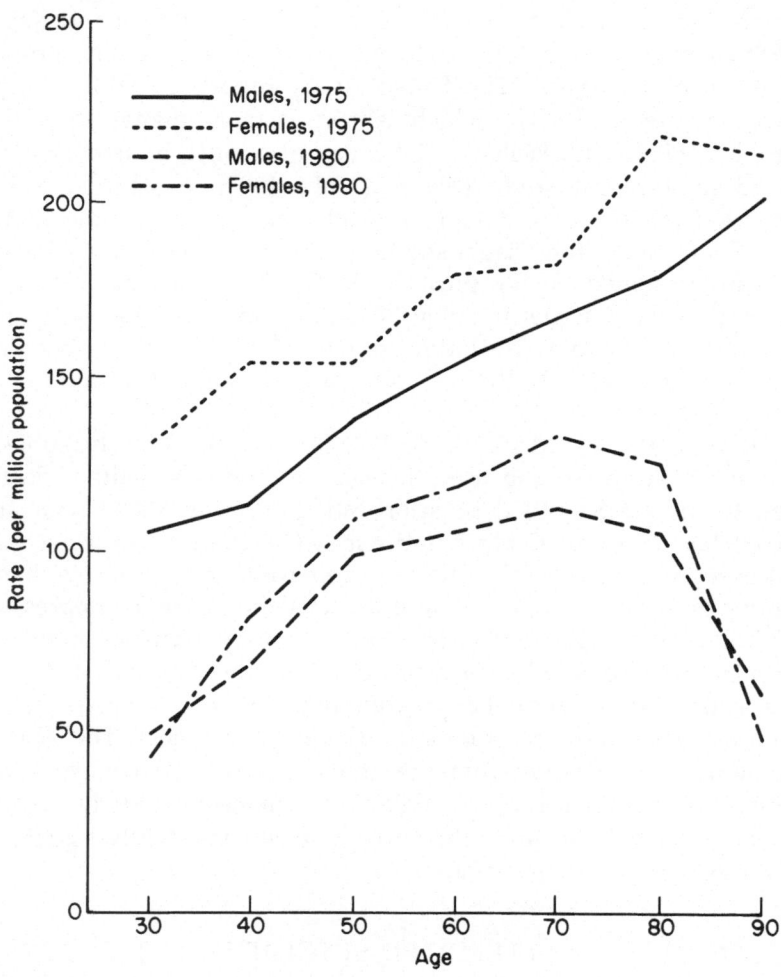

Fig. 3.1 Suicide rates in England and Wales, 1975–1980. (Adapted from McClure, 1984.)

that both absolute suicide rates and age-related rates vary widely between countries, although broadly there are three patterns: steady increases with age (as in Austria, Hungary and the USA), a peak at ages around 50–60 with a subsequent decline (as in Canada, Norway and Poland); and a peak between 50–60 with a subsequent fall and second peak at age 75 and over (as in Denmark, Sweden and Switzerland).

Recent evidence from the USA (Murphy and Wetzel, 1980), using a birth cohort analytical method to compare suicide rates at the same age for cohorts of subjects at five-year birth intervals, suggests that not only do successive cohorts start with higher suicide rates but that the increases are maintained through follow-up. Murphy, Lindesay and Grundy (1986) have demonstrated that the reverse has been true in Britain in the past 60 years, with steady falls in the suicide rates of successive elderly cohorts. They also failed to find a consistent relationship between early and late suicide rates within cohorts, thus casting doubt on the underlying assumption justifying cohort studies as predictors. This study makes little, however, of the apparent reversal of previously falling suicide rates between 1975 and 1980.

Whether or not still further increases in suicide rate in old age are to be predicted, it is clear that, as Shulman (1978) points out, although less than 15% of the population of most Western countries is aged 65 and over, up to 30% of suicides occur in the over 65s. A number of studies have investigated retrospectively the characteristics of elderly successful suicides. Barraclough (1971) found that 26 out of 30 elderly suicides were clearly mentally ill. All had depressive illnesses, though in seven the depression was associated with terminal physical illness, alcoholism or acute confusion. None were demented. In contrast, an earlier study by Sainsbury (1955) reported that between 15 and 20% of suicides over the age of 60 showed signs of dementia. A number of specific symptoms were common in Barraclough's (1971) depressed suicides: notably insomnia (90%), weight loss (75%) and hypochondriasis (50%). Two-thirds had been depressed for less than a year. Half had consulted their GPs within the week before their deaths and 90% within three months. Physical illness was also an important association; 17 of the 30 suicides as compared with 9 out of 30 matched 'accidental death' controls had significant physical disorder.

Social factors have also been implicated in the etiology of suicide in old age. Particular factors such as recent house moves (Sainsbury, 1973), recent bereavement (Stenbeck, 1980) and living alone (Sainsbury, 1955) have been implicated and as Shulman (1978) points out, a pattern of recently increased social isolation is frequently found in elderly suicides, corresponding with Durkheim's (1951) model of anomic suicide. However, Whitlock (1973) has shown that unfavourable social factors are considerably less important in elderly suicides than in younger groups with the exception of loneliness in elderly men.

Attempted suicide in the elderly has been studied by Krietman (1976) who investigated a one year cohort of 822 patients attempting suicide and admitted to the Edinburgh Royal Infirmary. Subjects were divided into 15–34, 35–54 and over 55 age groups. The older subjects showed a higher proportion of subjects who were widowed and had chronic physical illnesses and a relative under-representation of alcoholics, those with personality disorders and Roman Catholics. Fifty-eight percent of the older subjects were women and the proportion did not differ significantly from that in younger groups. Nearly two-thirds of the older subjects had clear depressive illnesses and fewer than 10% had organic syndromes. Eight percent of the older males and 3% of the older females had successfully committed suicide within a three year follow-up period; a figure considerably higher than that in younger subjects. An earlier study by Parkin and Stengel (1965) had found that in Sheffield over a two year period, the ratio of suicide attempts to completed suicides was 4:1 in the over 60s and 20:1 in the 20–40s. Among the over 60s, 66% of the attempters but only 31% of the suicides were female.

It seems clear that suicide in the elderly is not only common but that a number of psychiatric and social factors have been shown to be clearly associated with it. In particular, the profile of elderly attempted suicides is more similar to that of completed suicides than in younger groups, and attempted suicide in the elderly is much more often succeeded by completed suicide. Shulman (1978) has identified a high-risk profile for elderly suicide and attempted suicide. He suggests that subjects at particular risk are older white males with depressive illness associated with hypochondriasis and sleep disturbance who live alone, have concomitant physical illness, have recently been bereaved, and who have made recent previous suicide attempts. The importance of recognizing subjects with some or all of these factors cannot be over emphasized.

3.4 THE NATURAL HISTORY OF DEPRESSION IN OLD AGE

There have been surprisingly few 'naturalistic' follow-up studies of depressive subjects in whom the results have not been significantly distorted by initial entry criteria. These can conveniently be divided into hospital and community studies.

3.4.1 Hospital studies

The papers by Christie (1982) and by Blessed and Wilson (1982), summarized in Table 3.1, present six month and two year follow-up figures on subjects admitted as in-patients to Crighton Royal Hospital between 1974–76 and St Nicholas Hospital during 1976. Both studies found that approximately three-quarters of the subjects with affective psychoses were living in the community at six months and about two-thirds were in the community at two years. Only a small proportion had died within six months but about one-fifth were dead by two years. Discharge rate at both intervals is considerably higher than that reported by Roth (1955) from Graylingwell Hospital but the paper by Blessed and Wilson (1982) emphasizes that in their study one in five of the patients with affective psychoses had either not been discharged or been re-admitted by two years. Blessed and Wilson conclude that affective illness in old age is associated with considerable persisting morbidity. Post (1972) provides a much more detailed follow-up study of depression in patients admitted under his own consultant care between 1965 and 1967 as well as comparison with his own previous study of patients admitted 16 years earlier. Post emphasizes that the more recent series probably consisted of patients with more severe or resistant illnesses since a much higher proportion (60.9% vs. 14.8%) had been given treatment for their depression and had failed to respond prior to admission. The main findings of the study were that although duration of initial in-patient stay had decreased, the overall outcome between the two series was largely unchanged. In the more recent study, in which the follow-up period was three years, about one-quarter of the patients had made a lasting recovery, one-third had had one or more relapses but were recovered at the time of follow-up and one-third had persisting symptoms of depression. One-third of the latter had been continuously ill for the three year period of follow-up. The incidence of dementia at follow-up (6.5%) was no higher than could be expected in a non-depressed population of that age. The factors most clearly associated with a poor prognosis were age over 70 and duration of unrelieved depression for more than two years before admission.

The recent study by Murphy (1983) presents the findings of a one year follow-up study of a sample of 124 depressed patients referred over the course of the year to the psychogeriatric services at the London Hospital and Goodmayes Hospital, suffering from a first episode of depression in old age and meeting research criteria for primary depression. At one year 35% were well, 19% had relapsed, 29% remained ill throughout the year, 3% had developed dementia and 14% were dead. Significant predictors of poor outcome were severity of illness, physical ill-health, duration of illness and number of life events during the follow-up year. Interestingly only one in ten of those subjects with depressive delusions had a good outcome whereas 70% of those with psychotic depressions without delusions did well. Although direct comparison with Post's (1972) study cannot be made because the follow-up period is different, Murphy's (1983) sample appears if anything to have fared somewhat worse. It is noteworthy that Murphy's sample consisted of out-patients as well as in-patients and that fewer than one in five received ECT as compared with slightly over half in Post's study.

Another recent study by Baldwin and Jolley (1986) reported a somewhat more favourable prognosis in a follow up study of one hundred elderly patients aged 65 and over who had been admitted with severe, non-neurotic depressive states over a 42 to 104 months period. In the study 79% fitted Murphy's criterion of a 'new' case i.e. no previous episode of depression since the age of 60, although 46% of the whole group had a history of depression and 35% had been in-patients. An interim appraisal at one year was made to allow comparison with the findings of Murphy (1983). It was found that 58% of the whole sample (65% of 'new' cases) were well, 15% had relapsed but had been well for a substantial part of the year, and 18% had continuing symptoms. Only 8% had died. At the end of the follow up period 60% had either remained well throughout or had further episodes followed by complete recovery. Only 7% suffered continuous depressive symptoms. Male sex and poor physical health, whether at presentation or developing subsequently, were associated with a poorer prognosis, a finding consistent with a number of previous studies, but there was no relationship between initial presentation with deluions and subsequent outcome.

Jacoby, Levy and Bird (1981), in a study of 41 elderly depressed subjects who underwent research computed tomography and were followed up for two years, found that mortality at two years was significantly associated with ventricular enlargement at the time of initial admission. Ventricular enlargement did not otherwise seem associated with poor clinical course and in particular was not associated with significantly longer original admission. The deaths in this study were all from natural causes, six out of nine being non-cerebral. Although systematic comparisons are not possible the overall prognosis of the subjects in this study is broadly similar to that in the studies reported above and it seems possible that ventricular enlargement, like physical illness, may be an adverse prognostic sign in depression in late life.

Much longer follow-up information on hospital samples is provided by Angst (1981) and by Ciompi (1969). In both cases however the samples are of subjects whose illnesses began prior to the age of 65 but who have been followed up into old age. Angst (1981) reports that 37%

of unipolar depressives and 15% of those with bipolar illnesses had no relapses during a follow-up period that averaged more than 20 years. Unipolar subjects with early onset of illness and bipolar subjects had a relapse rate of about 25% after the age of 65 whereas late onset unipolars had a relapse rate of over 40% until the age of 74 which then fell to 25%. Angst emphasizes that none of his subjects received lithium prophylaxis but the use of other drugs or ECT is not specified and no information is given about other prognostic features or mortality rate.

Ciompi's (1969) study from Lausanne consisted of a follow-up of all patients admitted to the University Psychiatric Hospital aged less than 65 and followed up in 1963 when aged between 66 and 90. A total of 555 subjects had been admitted with depressive illnesses and 97% were retraced. The average duration of follow-up was 20.5 years. It was concluded that depressive symptomatology became gradually less severe in the majority of patients, one-third of whom had no relapse after the age of 65 and another third had less frequent and less severe attacks in old age than previously. One third however exhibited chronic depressive symptoms in old age. Even of those subjects with relatively good outcomes, many developed minor neurotic symptoms and loss of interest and social contact. Only 11% were 'really well adjusted and completely free from all kinds of mental disorders' at the time of follow-up. Good outcome was associated with good physical health and continuing work. Life expectancy was significantly reduced in the depressed sample (5.1% reduction in men and 7.6% in women). This was accounted for almost completely by a 7–8 times higher suicide rate in depressives than in the general population.

3.4.2 Community studies

Studies of the prognosis of depression in old age in community samples are still thinner on the ground. Gianturco and Busse (1978) followed up a sample of 'normal elderly volunteers' for a total of 20 years. Of those subjects depressed when first seen, 87% had had at least one other depressive episode and by the end of the 20-year period nearly three-quarters had had at least one episode of depression. Surprisingly, episodes of depression were related to financial status in women and physical health in men but age, sex and marital status did not seem related to likelihood of becoming depressed. MacDonald (1986b) in a nine month follow-up of patients attending their GPs found that of those depressed when first seen, one-third had improved and two-thirds remained depressed; during the nine month period 12% of those initially well had become depressed.

3.5 CONCLUSION

This chapter has reviewed available data on the age-related prevalence of depression with particular reference to the problems of diagnosis; the epidemiology of suicide and attempted suicide in old age; and the prognosis of, including the impact of treatment on, depression in the elderly.

Estimates of the prevalence of depression in the elderly vary widely largely due to difficulty in the selection of subjects, the problem of defining 'caseness' and the clinical challenge of detecting depressive illness in elderly subjects who frequently have co-existent physical illnesses and cognitive impairment. Studies using rating scales are particularly prone to result in over-estimates; for this reason many recent studies have favoured structured clinical interviews linked to operational diagnostic systems. The clearest conclusions to emerge are that depression, especially if relatively mild, is commoner in elderly women than in elderly men and that physical ill-health is the variable most consistently associated with the presence of depression.

Suicide is increasingly common with increasing age. Rates for elderly men are approximately twice those for women and although less than 15% of the population of most Western countries is aged 65 and over, up to 30% of suicides occur in this age group. Almost all successful suicide in old age is associated with depressive illness. Insomnia, weight loss, and hypochondriasis are frequent symptoms preceding successful suicide in old age and GP consultation for physical illness in the weeks prior to suicide is very common. Parasuicide in old age is much more frequently followed by successful suicide than in younger subjects. Clinical awareness of these pointers to a high suicide risk may be lifesaving.

A number of follow-up studies of depressed subjects indicate that only a minority recover fully and do not relapse, and up to a quarter become chronically depressed. Severity of illness, physical ill-health and long duration of illness prior to hospitalization are predictors of poor prognosis; there is however increasing evidence that an energetic approach to treatment improves the long-term outlook.

It is clear that depression in old age is common and disabling. Suicide is a particularly important risk in old age depression. A better understanding of the social and biological factors involved in the aetiology and prognosis of depression in the elderly, and an optimistic approach to its assessment and treatment may well improve its currently disappointing prognosis.

REFERENCES

American Psychiatric Association (1980) *Diagnostic and Statistical Manual of Mental Disorders (DSM-III)* (3rd edn.), American Psychiatric Association, Washington D.C.

Angst, J. (1981) Clinical indications for a prophylactic treatment of depression. *Adv. Biol. Psychiat.*, **7**, 218.

Baldwin, R.C. and Jolley, D.J. (1986) Prognosis of depression in old age. *Brit. J. Psychiat.*, **151**, 129.

Barraclough, B.M. (1971) Suicide in the elderly. In: *Recent Developments in Psychogeriatrics* (eds. D.W.K. Kay and A. Walk), Headley Brothers, Ashford, pp. 87–97.

Blazer, D. and Williams, C.D. (1980) Epidemiology of dysphoria and depression in an elderly population. *Am. J. Psychiat.*, **137**, 439.

Blessed, G. and Wilson, I.D. (1982) The contemporary natural history of depression in old age. *Brit. J. Psychiat.*, **141**, 59.

Bulbena, A. and Berrios, G.E. (1986) Pseudodementia: facts and figures. *Brit. J. Psychiat.*, **148**, 87.

Christie, A.B. (1982) Changing patterns in mental illness in the elderly. *Brit. J. Psychiat.*, **140**, 154.

Ciompi, L. (1969) Follow-up studies on the evolution of former neurotic and depressive states in old age. *J. Geriat. Psychiat.*, **3**, 90.

Copeland, J.R.M., Dewey, M.E. and Griffiths-Jones, H.M. (1986) A computerised psychiatric diagnostic system and case nomenclature for elderly subjects: GMS and AGECAT. *Psychol. Med.*, **16**, 89.

Copeland, J.R.M., Gurland, B.J., Dewey, M.E. *et al.* (1987a) Is there more dementia, depression and neurosis in New York? *Brit. J. Psychiat.*, **151**, 466.

Copeland, J.R.M., Dewey, M.E., Wood, N. *et al.* (1987b) Range of mental illness amongst the elderly in the community: prevalence in Liverpool using AGECAT. *Brit. J. Psychiat.*, **150**, 815.

Durkheim, E. (1951) *Suicide: A Study in Sociology* (Trans. J. Spaulding and G. Simpson), Free Press of Glencoe, New York.

Gianturco, D.T. and Busse, E.W. (1978) Psychiatric problems encountered during a long-term study of normal ageing volunteers. In: *Studies in Geriatric Psychiatry* (eds. A.D. Isaacs and F. Post), John Wiley, New York, pp. 1–16.

Jacoby, R.J., Levy, R. and Bird, J.M. (1981) Computed tomography and the outcome of affective disorder: a follow-up study of elderly patients. *Brit. J. Psychiat.*, **139**, 288.

Katona, C.L.E. and Aldridge, C.R. (1985) The dexamethasone supression test and depressive signs in dementia. *J. Aff. Dis.*, **8**, 83.

Kay, D.W.K., Beamish, P. and Roth, M. (1964) Old age mental disorders in Newcastle-upon Tyne. *Brit. J. Psychiat.*, **110**, 146.

Kay, D.W.K. and Bergmann, K. (1980) Epidemiology of mental disorders among the aged in the community. In: *Handbook of Mental Health and Ageing* (eds. J.E. Birren and R.B. Slone), Prentice-Hall, Englewood Cliffs, pp. 34–56.

Kay, D.W.K., Henderson, A.S., Scott, R. *et al.* (1985) Dementia and depression

41

among the elderly living in the Hobart community: the effect of the diagnostic criteria on the prevalence rates. *Psychol. Med.*, **15**, 771.

Kral, V.A. (1983) The relationship between senile dementia (Alzheimer type) and depression. *Can. J. Psychiat.*, **28**, 304.

Kreitman, N. (1976) Age and parasuicide ('attempted suicide'). *Psychol. Med.*, **6**, 113.

MacDonald, A.J.D. (1986a) Do General Practitioners 'miss' depression in elderly patients? *Br. Med. J.*, **292**, 1365.

MacDonald, A.J.D. (1986b) *The prevalence and recognition of depression in elderly patients attending their General Practitioners.* M.D. Thesis, University of Glasgow.

MacDonald, A.J.D and Dunn, G. (1982) Death and the expressed wish to die in the elderly: an outcome study. *Age Ageing*, **11**, 189.

McClure, G.M.G. (1984) Trends in suicide rate for England and Wales 1975–80. *Brit. J. Psychiat.*, **144**, 119.

Mann, A.H., Graham, R. and Ashby, D. (1984) Psychiatric illness in residential homes for the elderly: a survey in one London borough. *Age Ageing*, **13**, 257.

Murphy, E. (1983) The prognosis of depression in old age. *Brit. J. Psychiat.*, **142**, 111.

Murphy, E., Lindesay, J. and Grundy, E. (1986) 60 years of suicide in England and Wales. *Arch. Gen. Psychiat.*, **43**, 969.

Murphy, G.E. and Wetzel, R.D. (1980) Suicide risk by birth cohort in the United States: 1949–1974. *Arch. Gen. Psychiat.*, **37**, 519.

Myers, J.K., Weissman, M.M., Tischler, G.L. *et al.* (1984) Six-month prevalence of psychiatric disorders in three communities. *Arch. Gen. Psychiat.*, **41**, 959.

Parkin, D. and Stengel, E. (1965) Incidence of suicidal attempts in an urban community. *Br. Med. J.*, **2**, 133.

Post, F. (1972) The management and nature of depressive illnesses in late life: a follow-through study. *Br. J. Psychiat.*, **121**, 393.

Post, F. and Shulman, K. (1985) New views on old age affective disorders. In: *Recent Developments in Psychogeriatrics No. 1* (ed. T. Arie), Churchill Living-stone, London.

Raymond, E.F., Michals, T.J. and Steer, R.A. (1980) Prevalence and correlates of depression in elderly persons. *Psychol. Rep.*, **47**, 1055.

Roth, M. (1955) The natural history of mental disorder in old age. *J. Ment. Sci.*, **101**, 281.

Sainsbury, P. (1955) *Suicide in London*, Chapman and Hall, London.

Sainsbury, P. (1973) Suicide: opinions and facts. *Proc. Royal Soc. Med.*, **66**, 579.

Shulman, K. (1978) Suicide and parasuicide in old age: a review. *Age Ageing*, **7**, 201.

Stenback, A. (1980) Depression and suicidal behaviour in old age. In: *Handbook of Mental Health and Ageing* (eds. J.E. Birren and R.B. Slone), Prentice-Hall, Englewood Cliffs, pp. 616–52.

Whitlock, F.A. (1973) Suicide in England and Wales 1959–63, Part 1: the county boroughs. *Psychol. Med.*, **3**, 350.

Chapter Four

Neuroendocrine abnormalities in depression and the influence of drugs

IAN McKEITH

CONTENTS

4.1 INTRODUCTION

The original observations bridging the disciplines of psychiatry and endocrinology were those in which abnormal psychopathology was described in association with disordered endocrine states. These descriptive reports of abnormal mental function were subsequently included in the recognized symptomatology of endocrine disease, ranging from the insidious cognitive decline of hypothyroidism to the less common but more florid paranoid psychosis of 'myxoedema madness', and from the anxiety state associated with hyperthryoidism to the profound depressive states seen in Cushing's disease.

Psychological disturbances of this type were thought to reflect the effects of altered or fluctuating levels of peripheral endocrine hormones on the central nervous system, and treatment correcting such imbalance was often found to reverse the psychiatric abnormality. This was not inevitably the case however, endocrine disorder sometimes appearing to act as a trigger for mental disorder, management of which then required orthodox psychiatric treatment in addition to correction of hormonal abnormalities.

In the late 1960s researchers were able for the first time to measure circulating hormone levels using the new highly specific, accurate and sensitive methods of radioimmunoassay (RIA). The brain was quickly recognized to be not only a target for the influence of peripheral hormone secretions but also the most prolific endocrine organ in the body, itself producing a large number of peptide hormones. The distribution and localization of these within the central nervous system have been gradually identified and the associated neuroendocrine regulatory mechanisms described in some detail.

Using new information and techniques the developing field of psychoneuroendocrinology began to pursue the measurement of alterations in neuroendocrine function in response to external influences, both pharmacological – e.g. the suppression of cortisol secretion in response to exogenous corticosteroids, and psychological – e.g. following hospitalization. Having characterized the reactivity of neuroendocrine systems to external influences in this manner psychoneuroendocrinology moved its attention to observation of the relationships between neuroendocrine hormones and classical neurotransmitter activities. This strategy, applicable both in the normal brain and in abnormal psychological states, has been likened to looking through a 'window into the brain', using peripheral measures of endocrine activity to visualize complex neuroendocrine/neurotransmitter interactions. Arising from Edward Sachar's insight that biogenic amines particularly serotonin (5–HT), noradrenaline (NA), dopamine (DA) and acetylcholine (ACH) are of central importance to both neuroendocrine hormone regulation and possibly also to mood disorders, a large proportion of neuroendocrine investigation in psychiatry has involved such observation through the neuroendocrine window.

High hopes were held that such investigations would reveal important information about the underlying biochemical disturbances in psychiatric illness, might assist in refining diagnostic categories on the basis of particular neuroendocrine profiles and would aid in the prediction of response to treatment and/or long-term prognosis.

The enthusiastic introduction of the modified dexamethasone suppression test into clinical psychiatry by Dr Bernard Carroll (Carroll *et al.*, 1981) greatly heightened the awareness of clinicians to the powerful potential of these developments. The inclusion of a brief chapter on the topic in this book about antidepressant treatments reflects this interest, but it must be said that clinical psychoneuroendocrinology remains in its infancy and its applications remain predominantly in the arena of clinical research.

Bearing this in mind the following review is largely occupied with the most extensively studied neuroendocrine system in depression, namely the hypothalamic–pituitary–adrenal axis (HPA axis). The majority of work has been in younger patients although a number of studies have examined elderly depressives and these will be highlighted. HPA axis function associated with the ageing process and with psychiatric disorders of the elderly other than depression (particularly degenerative dementia) are also considered. Reference is made to the growing knowledge about mechanisms involving growth hormone (GH), thyroid hormones including thyroid releasing hormone (TRH) and melatonin.

4.2 THE HPA AXIS IN 'STRESS' AND DEPRESSION

It has been known for over quarter of a century that some depressed patients hypersecrete cortisol as demonstrated by; 1) increased 24 h urinary free cortisol; 2) increased plasma cortisol concentrations; 3) disturbances in the diurnal rhythm of cortisol secretion; 4) increased CSF cortisol concentrations; and 5) a failure to suppress serum cortisol levels adequately after a low dose of dexamethasone (Carroll and Mendels, 1976; Carroll *et al.*, 1981). Originally these findings were interpreted as part of a non-specific stress response and it is necessary to digress slightly to consider the early investigations into endocrine function in stress as opposed to depression (if such a distinction can be drawn!).

4.2.1 Neuroendocrine response to stress

The original concept, embodied in Cannon's description of changes in adrenal medullary hormones and the sympathetic nervous system, was of a stress response which had a positive survival value. This concept was later extended to include the function of the HPA axis and 'more recently' changes in growth hormone, gonadal steroids, prolactin and other endocrine products have been associated with exposure to stressful stimuli (reviewed in Reichlin, 1987). Munck has proposed that an additional function of the endocrine response to stress is to protect not only against the stress itself but also against the normal defence reactions that are activated by stress. This physiological function of stress-induced increased glucocorticoid levels might be achieved by turning off some of the body's defence reactions thus preventing them from overshooting and themselves threatening homeostasis. The defence reactions referred to include a range of inflammatory mediators such as prostaglandins, leukotrienes, endogenous pyrogen and other compounds with potential tissue-damaging effects (Reichlin, 1987); a stress response of this type is recognizable as beneficial in dealing with viral or bacterial challenge. The potential provocation of a similar response by 'psychological stress' in man may prove to be the basis for alterations not only in endocrine (and hence probably neurotransmitter) function with the potential to induce behavioural and psychological abnormality, but may also mediate changes in immunological competence, increasing vulnerability to autoimmune, infective and neoplastic disease. The fields of psychoneuroendocrinology and neuroimmunology may be seen to overlap in work such as that of (Lowy, A. *et al.*, 1984) who found that depressed patients who showed persistently raised cortisol following dexamethasone also showed a non-suppression of lymphocyte function despite the high cortisol levels which would normally produce immune suppression.

The HPA axis is one of the most responsive systems in the body to stressful stimuli with rapid adaptive change in response to novel situtations. This is seen for example in the relatively short-lived elevation of cortisol levels with a return to normal within three or four days following hospitalization, compared with the much more persistent reduction in testosterone secretion in the same circumstances. The HPA axis was extensively studied in stress partly because of this reactivity, and researchers then became interested in determining whether the observations of HPA axis dysfunction made in depressed patients were part of a stress response or more specific to the depressed state.

Normally cortisol secretion is maximal at 08.00 h and almost ceases between midnight and 02.00 h. In a stress response the peak levels of cortisol output might be expected to occur by day and diminish at night when subjects are sleeping and this does appear to be the case. In depression the opposite is seen with the most signficant elevation in cortisol levels compared with controls occurring between 02.00 h and 06.00 h. Using multiple point time sampling, Sachar concluded that the abnormality in depression was not simply a transient general increase in cortisol output but a more persistent dysregulation of the control of the HPA axis with a loss of the normal diurnal rhythm. He speculated that such a disturbance might reflect 'apparent limbic system dysfunction consistent with disturbances in mood, affect, appetite, sleep, aggressive and sexual drives and autonomic nervous system dysfunction seen in certain depressive illnesses' (Sachar *et al.*, 1973).

It is important to recognize that a stress response may be occurring in depression in addition to any depression-specific HPA axis abnormality. For example there are now a number of reports that dexamethasone non-suppression occurs following admission to hospital and this effect is seen not only in medical and surgical in-patients (Connolly *et al.*, 1968) but also in psychiatric patients. In one study (Coccaro *et al.*, 1984) 71% of a group of depressives were dexamethasone non-suppressors on day two of their admission whereas only 33% of a similar group were non-suppressors when tested between days three and six. These findings are similar to those of increased levels of urinary corticosteroids and urinary catecholamines in normal volunteers following hospital admission and the implications are clear – HPA axis testing is extremely reactive to external influence and for clinical application should not be performed for at least three or four days after hospitalization or if the patient is under conditions of 'novel' stress.

Intensity of depressed mood has been proposed as a continuing stress in depression which may be responsible for persistent HPA axis dysfunction. The balance of evidence so far does suggest a relationship between severity of depressed mood and cortisol levels when measured over time in individual patients, removing the variance due to differences between individuals or because of diagnostic considerations (Braddock, 1986). Whether this should be interpreted as evidence for an additive effect of stress, or alternatively as a correlation indicating the depression-specific nature of the cortisol dysregulation is not yet resolved.

4.2.2 Neuroendocrine function in depression

Before moving on to review the information which has resulted from attempts to look through the neuroendocrine window in depression, reference will be made to the growing body of knowledge about control systems within the HPA axis, which is shedding new light on the possible site of cortisol dysregulation in depression and attempting to explain abnormal responses to dexamethasone challenge.

Secretion of cortisol is of course modulated by adrenocorticotrophic hormone (ACTH) secretion and it is possible that alterations in cortisol levels and abnormal responses to dexamethasone challenge are secondary to an underlying ACTH abnormality. ACTH is secreted synchronously with beta endorphin, one of the principal endogenous opioid peptides, both being contained within a common precursor molecule proopiomelanocortin (POMC) which is cleaved in response to the release of corticotrophin releasing factor (CRF) produced not only in the hypothalamus (where a negative feedback occurs mediated by circulating cortisol) but also widely distributed throughout the limbic system and cortex and in close association with the autonomic nervous system and the locus ceruleus.

ACTH is technically difficult to assay using standard radioimmunoassay (RIA) techniques due to poor specificity, insensitivity and the need to sample large volumes of plasma. Ferrier *et al.* (1988) using a more sensitive two-site recognition immunoradiometricassay (IRMA) which uses antibodies directed at both ends of the ACTH molecule, found a tendency for elderly (mean age 76 years) depressed patients to have raised ACTH levels at three time points compared with controls. Although cortisol levels were also raised in the patient group, ACTH levels and cortisol levels did not appear to be correlated. This lack of correlation between cortisol and ACTH has been reported previously and may be due in part to the varying sensitivity of the adrenal cortex to ACTH stimulation throughout the 24-hour cycle. Following dexamethasone, depressives exhibited significantly higher levels of ACTH than controls. The interpretation of this hypersecretion of ACTH may be that steroid feedback at the pituitary level is less effective in depression, perhaps resulting from down-regulation of glucocorticoid receptors at the pituitary or hypothalamus.

Corticotropin releasing factor (CRF) has been synthesized and when the ovine form, which is cleared less rapidly from plasma than human CRF, is given to depressed patients blunted ACTH responses have been recorded (Good *et al.*, 1984) suggesting that pituitary ACTH-releasing cells may have been made less sensitive to CRF stimulation by increased circulating cortisol levels. The finding of a significant negative correlation between basal cortisol levels and the ACTH response to CRF in depression further supports this hypothesis. Nemeroff *et al.* (1984) have shown an increase in cerebrospinal fluid CRF-like immunoreactivity in 11 of 23 DSM-III major depressives. This has raised the possibility that CRF hypersecretion is the basis of the disordered cortisol regulation and Nemeroff *et al.* (1988) further reported a reduction (23% compared to controls) in CRF binding in the frontal cortex of 26 suicide victims thought to reflect down-regulation secondary to chronic hypersecretion. In contrast, Ferrier and McKeith (in preparation) did not find reductions in CRF binding in the frontal cortex of patients known to have been depressed and dying of natural causes.

One analysis of the CRF hypersecretion hypothesis is that in depressed patients the ACTH-producing pituicytes are in a balance between high CRF drive to produce ACTH (perhaps with adaptive blunting of this response) and the inhibitory influence of high circulating cortisol levels. The net effect on ACTH levels is at most a modest increase but this is sufficient to maintain excessive cortisol secretion by hyperplastic adrenals. A primary hypersecretion of CRF would predict a transient increase in ACTH early in the depression, but alterations in HPA axis activity may occur throughout the course of the illness as adaptive mechanisms come into play.

4.3 CLINICAL APPLICATION OF THE DST IN DEPRESSED ELDERLY PATIENTS

Discussion of the utility of the dexamethasone suppression test (DST) in clinical practice with elderly depressed patients is complicated by the fact that both age and dementia have been suggested to substantially alter dexamethasone resistance. Both of these proposals will be discussed in some detail (see 4.6).

The most instructive way of approaching this uncertain area is to consider the conclusions drawn to date in the wider arena of investigation of the use of the DST in younger depressives and then to return to the special case of elderly patients. Interpretation of findings is heavily influenced by variation in the details of test procedure which are considered (see 4.4).

4.4 TECHNICAL ASPECTS OF THE DST.

The non-suppression rate following administration of dexamethasone is highly dependent on the dose given. A dose of 1 mg of dexamethasone is known to suppress cortisol levels strongly for at least 24 h in normal subjects. One study of depressed patients found relative sensitivities for a 1 mg and a 2 mg (dose of dexamethasone) DST to be 43.5% and 30.7% respectively (Arana and Baldessarini, 1987) with little difference in specificity, suggesting that the 1 mg dose is sufficient for this purpose. (Sensitivity refers to the proportion of depressed patients in whom abnormal DST results are found, and specificity refers to the proportion of normal controls in whom normal results are found.)

Studies based on comparisons of depressed versus normal subjects suggest that both sensitivity and specificity rates are relatively stable at sampling times between nine and 24 h after a midnight dose of dexamethasone for an individual subject. Therefore the form of test in which a 1 mg oral dose of dexamethasone at 23.00 h is followed by a single point sample at 16.00 h the following day appears adequate for routine clinical use. Carroll recommended a cut-off value of 5.0 μg/dl as achieving the highest sensitivity without a significant loss of specificity in his laboratory, and slavish adherence to this value may explain a large part of the variation in sensitivity and specificity rates reported by numerous other workers testing apparently similar patients and normal controls. This was well illustrated by a WHO collaborative study using Research Diagnostic Criteria (RDC) to standardize diagnosis of major depressive disorder and a standard, kit-form RIA cortisol assay. In 12 different countries mean post-dexamethasone cortisol levels varied from 22.5 µg/dl in Moscow to 116.5 µg/dl in Copenhagen (Coppen, 1987). Sex distribution, age and severity of illness were examined but did not account for these differences. Using a fixed cut-off point of 5.0 µg/dl the sensitivity rates (i.e. of non-suppressors) would have been 71% and 15% respectively. A similarly large variation in non-suppression rates was also seen in non-depressed controls. The importance of standardizing the test in a local laboratory by a normative study using local controls and adopting an appropriate cut-off value to define non-suppression is apparent. The further suggestion is made that such controls are age-matched, particularly for subjects over the age of 65.

4.4.1 Dexamethasone levels

Individual or illness-related variations in absorption or metabolism of dexamethasone influence the DST, and variance in dexamethasone availability may contribute to the limited sensitivity of the DST in major depression. Several studies have found a tendency for lower dexamethasone levels in subjects categorized as non-suppressors (Morris *et al.*, 1983; Johnson *et al.*, 1984). In Ferrier's study of elderly DSM-III major depressives and controls there was a signficant negative correlation between plasma cortisol and dexamethasone levels but plasma dexamethasone levels did not vary significantly between patients and controls. Age-related changes in dexamethasone metabolism are not well established (Greden *et al.*, 1986) and require further investigation if the DST is to be applied to groups of elderly patients.

As a final practical point, measurement of dexamethasone levels can be a useful way of checking compliance with medication, sometimes questioned when the test is given as an out-patient to an elderly depressed individual.

4.4.2 Exclusion factors

The list of factors which may influence the DST and produce an abnormal result is slowly expanding and is summarized in Table 4.1. Normal doses of psychotropics including tricyclic antidepressants, neuroleptics and lithium do not appear to influence the DST, whereas

Table 4.1 External factors influencing DST response

Increased post-dexamethasone cortisol (i.e. false positive results may be enhanced by:

Significant medical illness
  hepatic
  adrenal
  hypothalamic
  diabetes mellitus, even under adequate control
  severe acute medical illness

Unusually severe or rapid weight loss

Other psychiatric disorders
  particularly dementia or psychosis

'Stress'
  e.g. within four days of hospitalization

Drug administration or withdrawal
  particularly hepatic microsomal enzyme inducers including alcohol,
  barbiturates, anticonvulsants and carbamazepine
  (ordinary doses of tricyclics, neuroleptics and lithium do not appear to
  influence the DST)

Non-compliance or increased metabolism of dexamethasone

Decreased post-dexamethasone cortisol (i.e. false negative results) may be related to:

High dose benzodiazepines
Decreased dexamethasone metabolism

---

carbamazepine which is being increasingly used in recurrent affective disorder may produce false positive results by enhancing dexamethasone metabolism. The effects of monoamine oxidase inhibitors are not known with certainty.

Electroconvulsive treatment (ECT) may cause normalization of DST non-suppression without corresponding change in clinical presentation (Greden *et al.*, 1983).

4.5 CLINICAL ASPECTS

As indicated already, the majority of studies have been in young or middle-aged patients, but the findings may be regarded as relevant to elderly populations, subject to several qualifications. Age-specific considerations will be discussed later.

4.5.1 Diagnosis

Direct comparison between different studies of younger patients is made difficult, not only because of the technical variations discussed above, but also by differences in the diagnostic procedures used in order to define a 'case' of depression. Carroll's original suggestion (Carroll *et al.*, 1981) was that the DST enabled identification of 'melancholic' patients with a sensitivity of 67% and a specificity of 96% with cortisol levels at 16.00 h and 23.00 h and with a reduced sensitivity of 50% in a 16.00 h sample only.

Melancholia appears in DSM-III as a clinical syndrome based on symptoms of the current illness and is similar to the endogenous subtype of RDC major depressive disorder. Such depressions are characterized by anhedonia (loss of the ability to experience any pleasure), loss of reactivity of mood, positive diurnal variation and vegetative disturbance with sleep, appetite and psychomotor change. These concepts are similar to those embodied in the Newcastle Scale (Carney, Roth and Garside, 1965) which uses not only information about the current episode such as guilt, nihilistic delusions, weight loss and depressive psychomotor activity, but also draws upon the assessment of an adequate premorbid personality and occurrence of previous episodes. Negative weight is given to anxiety symptoms, a tendency to blame others, and the presence of an adequate psychological stress to explain symptoms.

Most studies have found the Newcastle Scale to correlate better with DST status than either DSM-III or Research Diagnostic Criteria. Arana has reviewed this field extensively (Arana, 1987) and concludes that the DST achieves 49% sensitivity for patients with major depression using either DSM-III or RDC, but this sensitivity is increased to 78% for patients with mixed mania and depression and to 68% for those with major depression and psychosis. Family history of depression, increased severity of symptoms (as measured for example on a Hamilton Depression Rating Scale), and age over 60 years, appeared to contribute to non-suppression less markedly than the presence of severe, acute and psychotic illness.

4.5.2 Relationship of the DST to clinical course and treatment

DST non-suppression has been considered as a state marker in depression with a return to normal on clinical recovery. It has no apparent use as a marker of trait vulnerability. Early studies suggested that it could therefore be used either to predict treatment response and/or prognosis (Carroll *et al.*, 1981). Non-suppressors were thought to respond better to physical treatments (Brown, Johnston and Mayfield, 1979; Brown, Haier and Qualls, 1980) and a failure of normalization of DST status with recovery to carry a poor prognosis (Greden *et al.*, 1980). These proposals have received some support from more recent investigations although Greden *et al.* (1986) have shown a tendency for non-suppression to revert to normal within a few weeks of treatment regardless of change in clinical status. This may occur particularly during electroconvulsive treatment. Arana has estimated the contribution of a positive test result towards predicting good treatment response in major depression, particularly with melancholia, at about 10%, increasing response rates to adequate doses of antidepressants from 64–74% in normally suppressing major depressives to 76–82% in non-suppressors. Brown, Haier and Qualls (1980) had proposed that non-suppressors responded better to noradrenergic antidepressants such as imipramine and desmethylimipramine and that suppressors improved more with serotinergic drugs such as amitryptiline or clomipramine. Larger studies have so far not been able to replicate these findings.

An increased suicide rate of patients who remain non-suppressors at completion of treatment (about four-fold) is supported by several case reports but there is a possibility of a selection bias. The further suggestion that surveillance of patients with recurrent depression by the DST may enable relapse to be predicted (by observing a switch into non-suppression before clinical relapse) is interesting (Greden *et al.*, 1983) but so far is only applicable to a very small number of selected cases and requires replication. The available evidence suggests that serial change in the DST during a course of treatment is not in itself a sufficient guide to response, but failure to revert to normality may be associated with higher subsequent morbidity.

4.6 CLINICAL USE OF THE DST IN PSYCHOGERIATRIC PRACTICE

The effect of age on the DST has been extensively investigated although few studies have included many patients over the age of 65. Earlier findings in the age range 20–60 years showed little change in dexamethasone resistance with age (Carroll *et al.*, 1981). When older patients are included a positive correlation is repeatedly shown between age and post-dexamethasone cortisol levels (Alexopoulous *et al.*, 1984; Davis *et al.*, 1984; Georgotas *et al.*, 1986; Oxenkrug *et al.*, 1983) although one study did not find this difference between young and elderly healthy volunteers (Tourigny-Rivard, Raskind and Rivard, 1981). Georgotas *et al.* were able to explain this finding by greater severity of depression in the elderly patients, but this was not so for the other studies cited.

This tendency to higher post-dexamethasone cortisol has been interpreted as reflecting either a higher rate of non-suppression in elderly melancholics or alternatively a higher proportion of melancholic depression in old age. Neither conclusion can be drawn from the evidence available. If dexamethasone resistance is an age-related phenomenon affecting healthy individuals as well as depressives, the cut-off point for discriminating non-suppression will be shifted. Suitably age-matched control studies are therefore necessary for testing these hypotheses.

Technical aspects of the procedure are unchanged for the elderly as are the exclusion criteria. Studies in cognitively intact elderly depressives (McKeith, 1984; Davis *et al.*, 1984; Alexopoulous *et al.*, 1984; Georgotas *et al.*, 1986; Fogel, Satel and Levy, 1985; Greden *et al.*, 1986; Magni *et al.*, 1986) have reported essentially similar correlations with clinical data to those summarized for the much larger body of evidence in younger patients. McKeith (1984) showed non-suppression in elderly patients to be restricted to those with endogenous symptoms as measured by the Newcastle Scale in whom the test sensitivity was 70%.

Such patients however represent only a minority of elderly patients complaining of depressive symptoms. Epidemiological data suggests that whereas the prevalence of major depression in the over-65s is around 5% there are at least twice as many individuals with complaints of depressive symptoms insufficiently severe to be classed as major depression but nevertheless significant. These cases, which represent the bulk of elderly depressives, are not easily accommodated in current diagnostic schemes and have been described by Blazer and Williams (1980) as 'senile dysphorics', a group with personal health problems and loss events similar to major depressives and with poorly coping personality types but no previous affective illness. It has been suggested that brain ageing may contribute to this high rate of minor affective disturbance and if this were so, abnormalities of HPA axis functioning might be expected. No studies of DST response in this group of elderly depressives have yet been published.

4.6.1 Depressive pseudodementia

When the DST was first introduced into clinical practice it was soon advocated (McAllister *et al.*, 1982; Rudorfer and Clayton, 1982) as an aid in the differential diagnosis of depressive pseudodementia from true organic dementia. Pseudodementia may occur in the course of a melancholic depression and Table 4.2 based on Wells' (1979) checklist summarizes the usual clinical distinguishing features.

The proposed use of the DST to aid in this distinction was based on the assumption that non-suppression occurs significantly less often in

Table 4.2 Clinical features aiding in the distinction of depressive 'pseudodementia' from organic dementia

Self reports of memory failure
Clear onset and rapid progression
Variable performance on memory testing on different occasions
'Equal' short and long term memory deficits
'Don't know' answers rather than confabulation
Other depressive symptoms
Past history of psychiatric disorder

dementia than depression but, as discussed in the following paragraph, this is not the case.

Dexamethasone resistance has been shown in a wide range of psychiatric disorders in the elderly. McKeith (1984) found high non-suppression rates (Fig. 4.1) in patients with both acute and chronic brain syndromes in the absence of any significant depressive symptomatology. It may be difficult to recognize depression in demented individuals either because of the pathoplastic effect of the organic brain disease on the depressive syndrome or alternatively because of difficulties for patients in communicating their feelings. Greenwald *et al.* (1986) also found no correlation between DST result and depressive symptoms in demented patients, although using a specially constructed scale for detecting depressive signs in severely demented patients, Katona and Aldridge (1985) were able to do so. Unfortunately both they and McAllister and Hays (1987) found neither clinical improvement nor DST normalization with tricyclic antidepressants. The earlier suggestion (Coppen *et al.*, 1983) that an abnormal DST response in a patient with dementia is sufficient indication for a trial of antidepressant medication does not appear justified, particularly since patients with dementia are more likely to experience adverse side effects.

Abnormal HPA axis function in dementia may well be related to the diffuse disturbances in central neurotransmission which are known to occur and as such may be unrelated to the depressive syndrome (McKeith, 1984).

4.7 GROWTH HORMONE IN DEPRESSION

The secretion of growth hormone (GH) from the anterior pituitary is probably under the control of alpha–adrenergic, dopaminergic and possibly serotinergic excitatory stimulation and by beta–adrenergic and GABA–ergic inhibition. Since these neurotransmitters have been implicated in depressive illness, interest has focused on GH responses to a

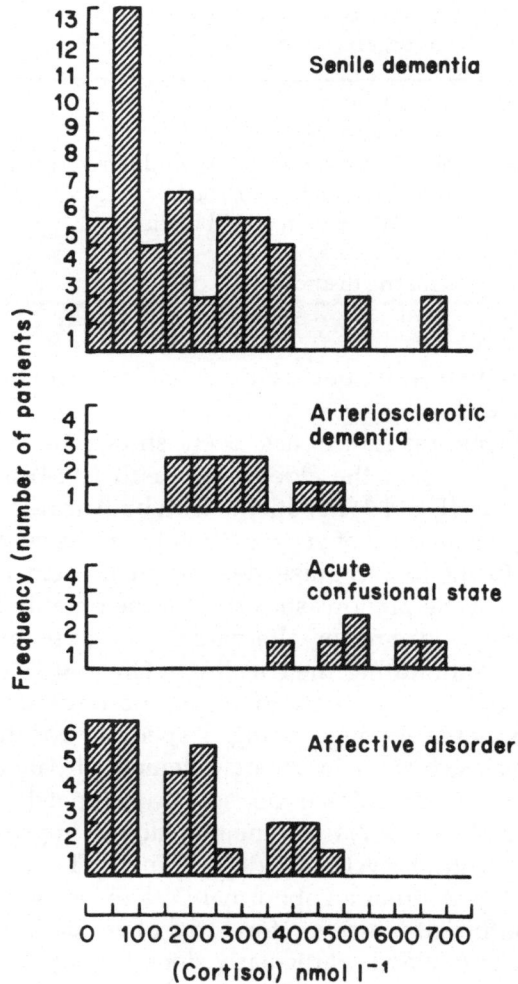

Fig. 4.1 Distribution of cortisol levels (expressed in nmol/l) at 16.00 h following 1 mg dexamethasone in 100 psychogeriatric clinic attenders. Using a cut-off point of 140 nmol/l (approximately 5 µg/dl) non-suppression rates were: senile dementia (Alzheimer type) 58%; arteriosclerotic dementia 100%; acute confusional state 100%; affective disorder (endogenous) 70%, (reactive) 0%. Diagnosis with Newcastle Scale (McKeith, 1984).

variety of pharmacological challenges. No consistent findings have emerged in measurement of basal GH secretion levels between depressives and controls (Ansseau *et al.*, 1988) and the majority of studies have found no differences in GH response to the dopamine agonist apomorphine.

The alpha–adrenergic agonist clonidine stimulates GH release and since this response is not blocked by pretreatment with presynaptic monoamine depleters (e.g. reserpine), but is abolished by alpha–2 antagonists such as yohimbine, the response is thought to be post-synaptic. Matussek *et al.* (1980) found that this GH response to intravenous clonidine was impaired in patients with endogenous depression compared with neurotic depressives and normal controls, and this finding has been replicated several times (Checkley *et al.*, 1984). Most studies have included age-matched controls, important in that GH secretion falls markedly with age and the stimulation response also becomes attenuated.

The impaired GH response in endogenous depression has been interpreted as an indicator of a defect in post-synaptic alpha–adrenergic neurotransmission and since the hypotensive response to clonidine (known to be mediated by stimulation of hind brain alpha–2 receptors) remains intact in these patients, the receptor abnormality in depression is postulated to be in the forebrain adrenergic system.

Serial testing in patients receiving antidepressant treatments ranging from desimipramine (Glass *et al.*, 1982) and electroconvulsive treatment (Slade and Checkley, 1980) to stereotactic subcaudate tractotomy (Corn *et al.*, 1984) have shown no alteration in GH responses correlated either with treatment or clinical improvement. Mitchell *et al.* (1988) retested ten patients with endogenous depression on average 2.1 years following recovery. Growth hormone responses were abnormal on both occasions in all but one patient, suggesting a persistent abnormality in alpha–adrenergic function. The interpretation of these findings must be made cautiously because of the relatively small numbers of patients tested, but an impaired GH reponse to clonidine may become recognized as a biological trait marker in a subtype of depressed individuals. In this it is distinct from the state-dependent abnormality detected using the DST.

4.7.1 Technical aspects

The standard form of the clonidine test, described by Checkley, Slade and Shur (1981) involves the patient fasting overnight and having an intravenous cannula inserted at 09.30 h. After one hour without observations baseline recordings of pulse, blood pressure and observer-rated sedation are made. Clonidine (1.3 or 2.0 µg/kg body weight) diluted in 10 ml of normal saline is slowly infused over 10 min, and 5 ml blood samples taken for GH estimation every 15 min. GH estimations can be made by double antibody radioimmunoassay. The GH response is defined by the area under the time-plotted curve.

Test results in normal volunteers may be enhanced by antidepressant drugs within the first week of treatment, followed by an attenuation after three weeks (Corn, Thompson and Checkley, 1984); Glass *et al.,* 1982 saw similar changes in depressed patients following desipramine.

If confirmed in larger patient samples, the clonidine test may prove valuable as an indicator of vulnerability to endogenous depressive illness and would also hold theoretical implications both for the aetiology and treatment of depression. It is of interest that this blunted neuro-endocrine response, seen in depression, is similar to that seen in normal elderly individuals. Brain ageing as a contributory factor in the aetiology of depression in the elderly has long been proposed – however the fact that blunted GH responses to clonidine are not specific to depression but are also seen in obsessional disorder and panic disorder, neither of which diagnoses appear increased in old age, does not support a simple link between age-related change in adrenergic systems, abnormal GH control and depressive illness.

4.8 THYROID HORMONES AND DEPRESSION

Historically the connections between thyroid disease and mental symptoms have been well recognized. The irritability, anxiety and emotional lability of hyperthyroidism are contrasted with the apathy, depression, memory loss and generalized slowing of hypothyroidism. Much of the published information is in the form of case reports and therefore subject to selection bias. Review of unselected thyroid patients (Loosen, 1987) suggests that depression is associated with both thyroid hypo and hyperactivity but is more common in deficiency states.

Turning to patients with primary psychiatric diagnoses in whom thyroid function has been assessed, and recognizing that L–triodo-thyronine (T3), L–thyroxine (T4) and free thyroxine index (FTI) are all elevated during the first few days of hospitalization as part of a stress response, most depressed patients are euthyroid. In Whybrow *et al.'s* 1972 study a small number were found to have elevated thyroid hormone levels and this was correlated with a prompt clinical response to imipramine. Following Whybrow's observations, four studies have shown that the antidepressant effect of imipramine or amitryptiline is accelerated by concurrent administration of as little as 20 μg of T3 daily. This effect is more marked in women. Similarly, T3 has been shown in seven studies to 'convert' tricyclic non-responders to responders in about 60% of cases and this effect does not appear to be dependent on elevation of inadequate tricyclic levels into the usual therapeutic range by displacement. An enhancement of noradrenergic neurotransmission is thought to underlie these clinical observations and it remains unclear whether or not the response is restricted to patients with faulty hypothalamo–pituitary–thyroid (HPT) axis function.

4.8.1 The TRH test

Thyrotrophin releasing hormone (TRH), when given in an intravenous dose of 500 μg, stimulates release of TSH which is measured at 15-minute intervals over the next hour in a standard TRH test. Blunted responses are found in about 25% of depressed patients. Loosen (1987) has proposed an increase of less than 5.0 μ units/ml as significantly blunted. The TRH test is influenced by a wide range of drugs including neuroleptics and lithium which increase TSH response and by carbamazepine which attenuates it. The test is not specific for depression, with up to 50% of alcoholics and patients with personality disorders showing abnormalities. Abnormalities in TRH test and DST in depressed patients do not show any clear association and although persistent blunting of the TSH response has been associated with early clinical relapse, it cannot be advocated as a predictor of treatment outcome.

Of some theoretical interest is the blunting of TSH response seen in normal elderly people (Snyder and Utiger, 1972) and the increased incidence of hypothyroidism in old age. The effect of T3 enhancement of tricyclic antidepressants in elderly depressives has not yet been systematically reported.

4.9 MELATONIN AND THE PINEAL GLAND IN DEPRESSION

Melatonin (5–methoxy–N–acetyltryptamine) is secreted at night by the pineal gland in response to beta–adrenergic stimulation deriving from the suprachiasmatic nucleus which is the primary internal pacemaker influencing circadian rhythms.

Melatonin secretion has been reported to be decreased in depression (Wetterburg *et al.*, 1979), accompanied by a rise in cortisol secretion and DST non-suppression. It is suggested that melatonin or another pineal factor could act as an inhibitor for CRF and that in depression, with release of CRF from inhibitory feedback by reduced melatonin, the melatonin/cortisol ratio might be used as a state-dependent marker.

Nair, Hariharasubramanian and Pilapil (1984) found the melatonin peak to be not only reduced but also phase advanced in depression. Early morning awakening and diurnal variation in mood – worsening in the morning – have been associated with the endogenous type of depression (corresponding approximately to melancholic major depression) and these characteristics may be related to phase shifts in central biological mechanisms.

One possible explanation for the seasonal variation in incidence of depressive illness with spring and autumn peaks may be changes in melatonin secretion in response to alterations in daylight intensity and duration.

Thompson *et al.* (1988) did not find reductions in overnight melatonin secretion in nine Newcastle Scale endogenous depressives nor phase shift when compared with closely age and sex-matched controls. Reviewing earlier studies they noted these had not allowed adequately for the effects of psychotropic drugs (particularly tricyclic antidepressants), age, sex or season of testing, all of which may be influential.

4.10 CONCLUSION

Neuroendocrine investigations in psychiatric patients and healthy controls have attempted:

1. To correlate abnormal neuroendocrine function, either in baseline secretion or in response to pharmacological challenge, with clinical syndromes.
2. To study central nervous system neurotransmitter responses to external stimuli by observation 'through the neuroendocrine window', measuring peripheral endocrine hormone changes.

Both approaches have been described in this Chapter in relation to depressive illness. Neuroendocrine abnormalities have been particularly identified to date in the secretion of cortisol and growth hormone which, although not specific for depression, do appear to be related to a particular clinical syndrome (endogenous depression/melancholia) and which are not adequately explained as general reactions to stress.

Further refinement of such methods may provide trait markers of vulnerability to depression (e.g. GH responses to adrenergic stimulation) and state markers useful in monitoring treatment and/or relapse (e.g. dexamethasone resistance).

Increased information about neurotransmitter system dysfunction obtained from neuroendocrine testing may aid in the prescription of existing antidepressant treatments and direct the development of new ones.

Although any such developments in young depressives are likely to have implications for elderly patients, the influence of age and degenerative brain disease on neuroendocrine function will need to be taken into account.

REFERENCES

Alexopoulous, G.S., Young, R.C., Kocsis, J.H. *et al.* (1984) Dexamethasone suppression test in geriatric psychiatry., *Biol. Psychiat.*, **19**, 1567–71.

Ansseau, M., Von Frenckell, R., Cerfontaine, J.L. *et al.* (1988) Blunted response of growth hormone to clonidine and apomorphine in endogenous depression. *Brit. J. Psychiat.*, **153**, 65–71.

Arana, G.W. and Baldessarini, R.J. (1987) Development and clinical application of the dexamethasone suppression test in psychiatry. In: *Hormones and Depression* (ed. U. Halbreich), Raven Press, New York.

Blazer, D.G. and Williams, C.D. (1980) Epidemiology of dysphoria and depression in an elderly population. *Am. J. Psychiat.*, **137**, 439–44.

Braddock, L. (1986) The dexamethasone suppression test – fact and artefact. *Brit. J. Psychiat.*, **148**, 363–74.

Brown, W.A., Johnston, R. and Mayfield, D. (1979) The 24 hour dexamethasone suppression test in a clinical setting: relationship to diagnosis, symptoms and response to treatment. *Am. J. Psychiat.*, **136**, 543–7.

Brown, W.A., Haier, R.J. and Qualls, C.B. (1980) Dexamethasone suppression test identifies subtypes of depression which respond to different antidepressants. *Lancet*, **i**, 928–9.

Carney, M.W.P., Roth, M. and Garside, R.F. (1965) The diagnosis of depressive syndromes and the prediction of ECT response. *Brit. J. Psychiat.*, **111**, 659–74.

Carroll, B.J. and Mendels, J. (1976) Neuroendocrine regulation in affective disorders. In: *Hormones, Behaviour and Psychopathology* (ed. E.J. Sachar), Raven Press, New York.

Carroll, B.J., Feinberg, M., Greden, J.F. *et al.* (1981) A specific laboratory test for the diagnosis of melancholia. *Arch. Gen. Psychiat.*, **38**, 15–22.

Checkley, S.A., Slade, A.P. and Shur, E. (1981) Growth hormone and other responses to clonidine in patients with endogenous depression. *Brit. J. Psychiat.*, **138**, 51–5.

Checkley, S.A., Glass, I.B., Thompson, C. *et al.* (1984) The growth hormone response to clonidine in endogenous as compared to reactive depression. *Psychol. Med.*, **14**, 773–7.

Coccaro, E.F., Prudic, J. Rothpearl, A. and Nurnberg, H.G. (1984) Effect of hospital admission on DST results. *Am. J. Psychiat.*, **141**, 982–5.

Connolly, C.K., Gore, M.B.R., Stanley, N. and Wills, M.R. (1968) Single dose dexamethasone suppression in normal subjects and hospital patients. *B.M.J.* (i): 665–7.

Coppen, A. (1987) The dexamethasone suppression test in depression – a World Health Organization collaborative study. *Brit. J. Psychiat.*, **150**, 459–62.

Coppen, A. Abou-Saleh, M. Millin, P., *et al.* (1983) Dexamethasone suppression in depression and other psychiatric illnesses. *Brit. J. Psychiat.*, **142**, 498–504.

Corn, T., Thompson, C. and Checkley, S.A. (1984) Effects of desipramine treatment upon central adrenoreceptor function in normal subjects. *Brit. J. Psychiat.*, **145**, 139–45.

Corn, T., Hoenig, A., Thomson, C. *et al.* (1984) A neuroendocrine study of stereotactic subcaudate tractotomy. *Brit. J. Psychiat.*, **144**, 417–20.

Davis, K.L., Davis, B.M., Mathe, A.A. *et al.* (1984) Age and the dexamethasone suppression test. *Am. J. Psychiat.*, **141**, 872–4.

Ferrier, I.N., Pascual, J., Charlton, B.G. *et al.* (1988) Cortisol, ACTH and dexamethasone concentrations in a psychogeriatric population. *Biol. Psychiat.*, **23**, 252–60.

Fogel, B.S., Satel, S.L. and Levy, S. (1985) Occurrence of high concentrations of post-dexamethasone cortisol in elderly psychiatric in-patients. *Psychiat. Res.*, **15**, 85–90.

Georgotas, A., McCue, R.E., Kim, M.O. *et al.* (1986) Dexamethasone suppression in dementia, depression and normal ageing. *Am. J. Psychiat.*, **143**, 452–6.

Glass, I.B., Checkley, S.A., Shur, E. and Dawling, S. (1982) The effect of desipramine upon central adrenergic functions in depressed patients. *Brit. J. Psychiat.*, **141**, 372–6.

Good, P.W., Chrousos, G., Kellner, C. *et al.* (1984) Psychiatric implications of basic and clinical studies with corticotrophin releasing factor. *Am. J. Psychiat.*, **141**, 619–27.

Greden, J.F., Abala, A.A., Haskett, R.F. *et al.* (1980) Normalization of dexamethasone suppression test: a laboratory index of recovery from endogenous depression. *Biol. Psychiat.*, **15**, 449–58.

Greden, J.F., Gardner, R., King, D. *et al.* (1983) Dexamethasone suppression tests in antidepressant treatment of melancholia. *Arch. Gen. Psychiat.*, **40**, 493–500.

Greden, J.F., Flegel, P., Haskett, R. *et al.* (1986) Age effects in serial hypothalmic – pituitary – adrenal monitoring. *Psychoneuroendocrinology.*, **11**(2), 195–204.

Greenwald, B.S., Mathe, A.A., Mohs, R.C. *et al.* (1986) Cortisol and Alzheimer's disease II: dexamethasone suppression, dementia, severity of symptoms and affective symptoms. *Am. J. Psychiat.*, **143**, 442–6.

Johnson, G., Hunt, G., Kerr, K. and Caterson, I. (1984) Dexamethasone suppression test and plasma dexamethasone levels in depressed patients. *Psychiat. Res.*, **13**, 305–13.

Katona, C.L.E. and Aldridge, C.R. (1985) The dexamethasone suppression test and depressive signs in dementia. *J. Affect. Disorders.* **8**, 83–9.

Loosen, P.T. (1987) Thyroid hormones and affective state. In: *Hormones and Depression* (ed. U. Halbreich), Raven Press, New York.

Lowy, M.T., Reder, A.T., Antel, J.P. *et al.* (1984) The D.S.T. and lymphocyte sensitivity to dexamethasone. *Am. J. Psychiat.*, **141**, 1365–8.

McAllister, T.W., Ferrell, R.B., Price, T.R.P. and Neville, M.B. (1982) The dexamethasone suppression test in two patients with severe depressive pseudodementia. *Am. J. Psychiat.*, **139**, 479–81.

McAllister, T.W. and Hays, L.R. (1987) TRH test, DST and response to desipramine in primary degenerative dementia. *Biol. Psychiat.*, **22**, 189–93.

McKeith, I.G. (1984) Clinical use of the DST in a psychogeriatric population. *Brit. J. Psychiat.*, **145**, 389–93.

Magni, G., Schifano, F., de Leo, D. *et al.* (1986) The dexamethasone suppression test in depressed and non-depressed geriatric medical patients. *Acta Psychiat. Scand.*, **73**, 511–14.

Matussek, N., Achenheil, M., Hippius, H. *et al.* (1980) Effect of clonidine on growth hormone release in psychiatric patients and controls. *Psychiat. Res.*, **2**, 25–36.

Mitchell, P.B., Bearn, J.A., Corn, T. and Checkley, S.A. (1988) Growth hormone response to clonidine after recovery in patients with endogenous depression. *Brit. J. Psychiat.*, **152**, 34–8.

Morris, M., Carr, V., Gilliland, J. and Hooper, M. (1983) Dexamethasone concentrations and the dexamethasone suppression test in psychiatric disorders. *Brit. J. Psychiat.*, **148**, 66–9.

Nair, N.P.V., Hariharasubramanian, N. and Pilapil, C. (1984) Circadian rhythms of plasma melatonin in endogenous depression. *Progress in Neuropsychopharmacology and Biological Psychiatry*, **8**, 715–18.

Nemeroff, C.B., Widerlov, E., Bissette, G. *et al.* (1984) Elevated concentrations of CSF corticotropin releasing factor-Like immunoreactivity in depressed patients. *Science*, **226**, 1342–4.

Nemeroff, C.B., Owens, M.J., Bissette, G. *et al.* (1988) Reduced corticotrophin releasing factor binding sites in the frontal cortex of suicide victims. *Archives of General Psychiatry*, **45**, 577–81.

Oxenkrug, G.F., Pomara, N., McIntyre, I.M. *et al.* (1983) Ageing and cortisol resistance to dexamethasone suppression. *Psychiatry Research*, **10**, 125–30.

Reichlin, S. (1987) Basic research of hypothalamic–pituitary–adrenal neuroendocrinology: an overview. The physiological function of the stress response. In: *Hormones and Depression* (ed. U. Halbreich), Raven Press, New York.

Rudorfer, M.V. and Clayton, P.J. (1982) Pseudodementia – use of the DST in diagnosis and treatment monitoring. *Psychosomatics*, **23**, 429–31.

Sachar, E.J., Hellman, L. Roffwarg, H.P. *et al.* (1973) Disrupted 24 hour patterns of cortisol secretion in psychotic depression. *Archives of General Psychiatry*, **28**, 19–21.

Slade, A.P. and Checkley, S.A. (1980) A neuroendocrine study of the mechanism of action of ECT. *British Journal of Psychiatry*, **137**, 217–21.

Snyder, P.J. and Utiger, R.D. (1972) Response to thyrotrophin releasing hormone (TRH) in normal man. *Journal of Clinical Endocrinology and Metabolism*, **34**, 380–5.

Thompson, C., Franey, C., Arendt, J. and Checkley, S.A. (1988). A comparison of melatonin secretion in depressed patients and normal subjects. *British Journal of Psychiatry*, **152**, 260–6.

Tourigny-Rivard, M.F., Raskind, M. and Rivard, D. (1981) The dexamethasone suppression test in an elderly population. *Biological Psychiatry*, **16**, 1177–84.

Wells, C.E. (1979) Pseudodementia. *American Journal of Psychiatry*, **136**, 895–900.

Wetterberg, L., Beck-Friis, J., Aperia, B. and Petterson, U. (1979) Melatonin/cortisol ratio depression. *Lancet*, **ii**, 1361.

Whybrow, P.C., Coppen, A., Prange, A.J. *et al.* (1972) Thyroid function and the response of L–liothyronine in depression. *Archives of General Psychiatry*, **26**, 242–5.

TWO

Lithium Salts

Chapter Five

Metabolic and endocrine effects of lithium

JOHN H. LAZARUS

CONTENTS

5.1 INTRODUCTION

The use of lithium in psychiatric patients has increased remarkably since the recognition of its anti-manic effect by Cade (1949). It is estimated that about two in a thousand of the population are taking the drug in the United Kingdom. The main psychiatric indications for the use of lithium carbonate are the treatment of mania and the prophylaxis of recurrent affective disorders of the manic-depressive (bipolar) type. It has been claimed to be effective in the treatment of acute unipolar depression and in the prophylaxis of recurrent episodes of this affective disorder.

Adverse effects of lithium may be observed soon after starting the drug. These include gastrointestinal symptoms, such as anorexia, nausea, vomiting, and diarrhoea; together with disorders of the central nervous system, including tremor, weakness, and dizziness (Ghose, 1977). Exaggeration of these symptoms is seen in gross overdosage with lithium and coma may follow.

The mechanism of action of lithium is unclear; over the past 20 years interest has been focused on its long-term endocrine and metabolic effects both because they are important in patients taking lithium and because they may shed some light on the cellular action of the cation. Recently there has been much interest in the concept that lithium may act by interfering with phosphoinositol metabolism in cell membranes, particularly the brain. This Chapter attempts to highlight the main endocrine and metabolic effects of the drug. These have been discussed in greater detail elsewhere (Lazarus, 1982; Lazarus, 1986).

5.2 LITHIUM AND CELLULAR FUNCTION

Lithium is actively transported across cell membranes but the subsequent removal of the ion is much slower than that of sodium. There are four transport mechanisms in red cells (Duhm and Becker, 1978): a sodium dependent lithium counter-transport system, a purely passive pathway stimulated by bicarbonate, a sodium–potassium pump, and a 'leak' pathway. The clinical relevance of lithium transport mechanisms has been extensively investigated in manic depressive patients (Pandey, Dorus and Davis, 1979). It was hoped that the lithium ratio, namely the intracellular lithium divided by extracellular lithium concentration to give a steady-state distribution ratio, would be useful in predicting response to therapy. This has not been found to be the case. The sodium–lithium counter-transport mechanism has also been widely studied in essential hypertension but there is no consensus about the prevalence and importance of transport abnormalities in the red cells of hypertensive patients. Lithium transport has also been studied in frog's skin, intestine and toad bladder where it is dependent on other ion concentrations, particularly sodium and potassium. In the heart, lithium produces changes in potassium permeability and a reduction in calcium uptake. Lithium transport in different tissues has yielded interesting physiological data but these have not been of much clinical importance.

In an attempt to explain the action of lithium on the cell, attention has been paid to the various well known enzyme systems and signalling transduction systems. For example, studies in erythrocyte membranes have shown increases in sodium potassium adenosine triphosphatase (ATPase) in lithium-treated depressed patients (Dick, Naylor and Dick, 1978) but other studies have shown no changes in this enzyme (Hesketh *et al.*, 1978). Magnesium ATPase has also been found to be altered by lithium. More attention has been paid to the well known second messenger, cyclic adenosine monophosphate (cAMP) which is formed from ATP within the cell following hormonal stimulation of a hormone receptor in the cell membrane. Lithium inhibits the formation or action of the adenylate cyclase cAMP system in many tissues but the precise mode of action is unclear (Belmaker, 1981). Many studies have shown that lithium has these actions only at very high concentrations, much higher than used in therapeutic studies. However, the immunological modulatory effects of lithium are thought to be mediated by its inhibitory action on lymphocyte cAMP. Data on plasma cAMP and plasma GMP in humans taking lithium are difficult to interpret because the studies have been small and measurement of these compounds only reflects a net result of many cellular events.

A transduction signalling system in the cell which has been intensively studied recently is the inositol phospholipid system (Downes, 1983). Following stimulation of a membrane receptor, phosphatidyl inositol, (PI) a complex membrane lipid, is broken down to inositol phosphate and diacyl glycerol. The inositol phosphates are further broken down to myoinositol phosphate. The enzymatic action of myoinositol–1–phosphatase, which converts myoinositol phosphate to inositol, is inhibited by lithium. The hydrolysis of PI plays an important part in the function of receptors that use calcium. As lithium interacts with calcium in many sites it is tempting to speculate that its action on the PI pathway may provide the unifying concept for the action of lithium in many tissues including the brain. There is no doubt that lithium is capable of having quite profound effects on brain phosphoinositol metabolism. The consequence of this effect on cell function and its relationship to the therapeutic effect of the ion is not known. It is not clear which receptors in the brain operate through inositol phospholipid breakdown. Nevertheless, this recent work on inositol phospholipid metabolism has opened up new routes for lithium research to follow and like so many new discoveries in clinical science it poses more questions than it has answered.

Lithium interacts with many cellular enzymes both *in vitro* and *in vivo* (Birch, 1978). Unfortunately many of the studies have not used lithium in therapeutic concentrations. Lithium has been shown to inhibit several magnesium-dependent enzymes relating to the glycolysis pathway. Lithium also affects cell growth by influencing the function of DNA and RNA in the cell and has been shown to inhibit hormonal stimulation of DNA synthesis and protein formation. In some experimental tumour models lithium could actually increase and stimulate tumour growth. However, this is not thought to occur in man.

The effects of lithium on many cellular functions have been investigated. While there has been agreement on transport mechanisms of lithium in and out of cells, the relevance of these mechanisms to clinical disease is still questionable. The importance of other effects of lithium on cellular metabolism is also disputed. However, recent data on the phosphoinositol pathway has opened up a new area of enquiry. This is important not only because it may provide a clue as to the mechanism of action of lithium, but the use of lithium in this system is also helping to elucidate the detailed biochemistry of many hormonal signalling mechanisms within the cell.

5.3 MINERAL METABOLISM

Electrolyte abnormalities have been described in patients with affective disorders (Coppen, 1965). There is a substantial sodium accumulation in depresssive states and intracellular sodium may increase dramatically during mania. Sodium transport may also be altered in depression and lithium resembles sodium in some of its physical and biological properties. There is a sodium diuresis during the first few days of lithium administration with subsequent sodium retention. Consequently, a positive sodium balance is produced due to a decrease in the urinary excretion of sodium accompanied by increased excretion of aldosterone. Long-term balance studies have indicated a continuing retention of sodium with reduced sodium excretion.

There is an initial water diuresis with the increased sodium excretion. However, total body water increases during the first week of therapy.

There are relatively few data on potassium changes and no significant clinical effects of lithium are observed. There are significant increases in serum magnesium levels in patients given lithium, and urinary magnesium also increases. It is not known whether these effects have any long-term consequences.

Many groups have described hypercalcaemia, and high serum immunoreactive parathyroid hormone (PTH) values in patients on lithium, though not all studies agree with this (Mallette and Eichhorn, 1986). Clinical hyperparathyroidism responsive to surgical treatment has also been reported but in the cases not operated on, the metabolic abnormalities have reverted to normal on cessation of lithium. The published prevalence of hyperparathyroidism in the normal population makes it difficult to be sure that this is a definite lithium-associated condition. In practice, the biochemical changes in patients on lithium are usually mild and not associated with any clinical manifestation. It appears that the lithium ion *in vitro* renders the parathyroid cell less sensitive to calcium which may be thought of as a reset of the 'calciostat'. The clinical implications of mild hyperparathyroidism in the lithium-treated patient are unknown. Further evaluation of lithium-associated hyperparathyroidism is necessary, in particular to note the onset of the hypercalcaemia in relation to lithium therapy and to monitor any long-term adverse effects.

Lithium accumulates in bones to a higher concentration than in any other organ except the thyroid and parts of the kidney. The ion causes a reduction of bone mineralization in growing female rats possibly due to suppression of osteoid formation. In humans a difference in the rate of bone loss has been found in lithium-treated female patients and controls. Long-term controlled studied to further assess the potential effect of lithium on bone mineral content have not been performed.

There is a reduction in urinary calcium excretion in manic depressive patients after starting lithium. Lithium interferes with the phosphaturic response of PTH and cAMP in animals but not in man. Infusion of PTH into normal healthy people results in a significant rise in renal tubular reabsorption of calcium and an increase in nephrogenous cAMP. PTH infusion into the same subject receiving short term lithium therapy did not alter these parameters, suggesting that the hypercalcaemic effect of lithium could be due to an inhibitory effect of the ion calcium transport, independent of a parathyroid mechanism (Lazarus *et al.*, 1987).

5.4 LITHIUM AND RENAL FUNCTION

Lithium is excreted mainly by the kidneys and impairment of renal function will contribute to lithium toxicity. Lithium has effects on renal morphology, glomerular filtration rate and tubular function. Extensive light and electron microscopy studies in animals have shown morphological damage to cortical collecting tubules and distal convoluted tubules (McAuliffe and Olesen, 1983). Increase in DNA synthesis and mitochondrial oxidative enzymes with increased glycogen deposition has also been noted. The changes may be species-specific and they may be difficult to separate histologically from natural biological variability especially, for example, in rat kidney. In humans there have been isolated reports of renal failure associated with lithium intoxication. Renal biopsy specimens in patients on lithium have shown lithium-associated distal tubular lesions characterized by ballooning of cells, vacuolation of cytoplasm and the presence of PAS-positive material (glycogen) present in clumps, granules or strands. In addition a focal interstitial nephropathy characterized by cortical interstitial fibrosis, tubular atrophy, and tubular PAS-positive casts, has been documented. There is debate on the interpretation of renal biopsy findings in patients on lithium compared with patients on other psychotropic drugs (Walker *et al.*, 1982). Nevertheless, there are specific studies which do document varying degrees of damage to the distal convoluted tubule in patients on the drug.

The renal lithium clearance ranges from 10–30 ml/min and the fractional excretion of lithium is around 0.2–0.3 (compared to inulin) indicating that 70–80% of the filtered load is reabsorbed. The renal lithium clearance is unaffected by water loading and is thus independent of urine flow. This implies active tubular lithium reabsorption. Lithium clearance is significantly affected by sodium excretion but the ion is not handled identically to sodium. A significant reduction of lithium clearance is seen after thiazide treatment, and drugs that exert a natriuretic effect in the distal nephron will lower the lithium clearance. Thus the renal handling of lithium is complex and extreme care should be taken in the clinical management of patients on lithium who are receiving other drugs known to affect renal function.

Lithium has little or no effect on glomerular function in those patients who are well controlled on the drug although a small reduction in GFR (glomerular filtration rate) has been seen in a few patients. Urinary albumin is not significantly affected. Nephrotic syndrome associated with lithium therapy has been reported but renal biopsy data are sparse. The condition has remitted when lithium was stopped and recurred in one patient when rechallenged with the drug. Nephrotic syndrome is not a toxic phenomenon but appears to be a rare idiosyncratic response to lithium (Depner, 1982).

The development of diabetes insipidus characterized by polydipsia and polyuria associated with lithium therapy occurs in at least 40% of patients often after a few days of treatment (Forrest *et al.* 1974). It usually ceases after a week or so but may present for the first time months or years after lithium has been started. Central mechanisms may play a minor role. Lithium has been found to stimulate thirst in rats and can increase plasma renin concentrations in animals and man. There is circumstantial evidence that lithium may stimulate thirst mechanisms independent of antidiuretic hormone (ADH) and the ion is capable of inhibiting angiotensin-induced stimulation of cAMP accumulation in isolated rats neurohypophyses. Lithium may inhibit ADH release from the posterior pituitary. However, the fully developed syndrome is usually consistent with a nephrogenic type of diabetes insipidus with high plasma arginine vasopressin (AVP) levels (Padfield *et al.*, 1977). There is a markedly impaired concentrating ability after dehydration that resists exogenous vasopressin in patients on long-term lithium therapy. Infusion of AVP does not significantly change urine volume or osmolarity, suggesting a lack of renal response to this hormone, a similar finding being seen in rats. The mechanism of lithium-induced impairment of AVP action involves the effect of lithium on cAMP generation. Lithium appears to inhibit the action of AVP at the level of the regulating protein or the catalytic unit of the membrane adenylate cyclase. The result of the diminished activity of adenylate cyclase is a decreased ability of the medullary collecting tubules and the collecting ducts to generate and accumulate cAMP. Other mechanisms involved in the production of diabetes insipidus include interference with microtubular assembly in the renal medulla, direct renal damage and alteration of intrarenal electrolyte concentrations (Christensen *et al.*, 1985).

Lithium also causes renal tubular acidosis resulting in impairment of urinary acidification. However, this condition in clinical practice is mild and causes few if any clinical problems.

The clinical aspects of the nephrotoxic effects of lithium have received great attention during the past decade. Clearly, any drug that is given for many years must be very carefully assessed in relation to any potential long-term side effect. It has been suggested that kidney function should be assessed in psychiatric patients prior to starting lithium treatment (Waller and Edwards, 1985). A reasonable procedure is to estimate serum creatinine and predict creatinine clearance. If the GFR is less than 60 ml/min the patient should be referred to a physician and the use of lithium reconsidered. If the GFR is less than 30 ml/min lithium treatment should be avoided. It may also be useful to measure the osmolality of an early morning specimen as a baseline for assessment during the treatment period. If it is low then a measurement in response to desmopressin (DDAVP), a synthetic analogue of AVP, should be done. During therapy with lithium, serum creatinine should be monitored, probably six-monthly and clearance measurements should be done if a rise in serum creatinine occurs. The osmolality of early morning urine specimens should also be monitored if there is a progressive impairment of the response to DDAVP, and it may be necessary to stop the lithium. In practice, however, most patients remain on lithium and although mild degrees of impairment of renal function may occur they are not significant in the vast majority of patients.

An important clinical aspect of lithium handling by the kidney is in lithium toxicity (Hansen and Amdisen, 1978). Fifty percent of intoxication cases occur during routine maintenance treatment and up to 75% of patients may have some degree of pre-exisiting renal impairment. Very often patients are on diurectics – usually thiazides. These drugs by virtue of their action on the distal nephron decrease the renal clearance of lithium with a consequent increase in serum lithium.

Patients on lithium who have developed polydipsia and polyuria must be adequately hydrated before surgery. It is important to note that there are many other agents that may also raise plasma lithium levels, for example non-steroidal anti-inflammatory drugs. The aim of treatment of gross intoxication must be to eliminate lithium from the body as rapidly as possible. Haemodialysis has been suggested as the best method. Peritoneal dialysis is slower but still effective.

Much of the data on renal effects of lithium in humans were obtained when the optimal therapeutic lithium concentration was thought to be best above 1 mmol/l. The recent reduction in recommended therapeutic levels to between 0.6 and 1 mmol/l has meant that long-term renal effects are of less importance although they should still be sought (Lokkegaard *et al.*, 1985). In addition to reducing the average therapeutic levels avoidance of peak serum lithium levels is important in preventing long-term renal effects.

Therapeutic doses of lithium are associated with a tubulointerstitial nephropathy in 20–30% of patients, and other renal histological changes may also occur. Although it is important to establish the pathogenesis of these complications, their effect on routine lithium therapy must not be overestimated. In general the renal complications of lithium therapy do not give rise to serious renal functional impairment.

5.5 CARBOHYDRATE METABOLISM

An early report described an increase in body weight, and improved glucose tolerance, together with decreased urinary glucose and ketone bodies in diabetic patients given lithium. Following the introduction of lithium into psychotherapeutics, it has been appreciated that the drug has definite effects on carbohydrate metabolism. Lithium causes an increase in weight in patients receiving the drug (Peselow *et al.*, 1980). In one study it was reported that 63% of lithium-treated patients gained 5% of their total body weight compared with only 15% of a controlled group over 12 months. The mechanisms for weight increase may involve effects on lipid metabolism or increased cortisol production. There does not seem to be any relation between the weight gain and therapeutic response and most of the weight gain occurs in the first few months of treatment. Reports of the effect of lithium on carbohydrate metabolism are conflicting (Vendsborg, 1978). *In vivo* studies of humans have described impaired, unchanged, or improved glucose tolerance during lithium treatment. Studies are often difficult to interpret because of differences in experimental technique. An increase in glucose disposal rate has been found following intravenous glucose in lithium-treated patients and in normal volunteers. In animals lithium may have an insulin-like effect and thus be antidiabetic. On the other hand, lithium has been shown to inhibit the acute insulin release in response to tolbutamide in both animals and man.

The occurrence of diabetes mellitus in patients taking lithium does not necessarily imply cause and effect although deterioration of the diabetic state has been described in one insulin-dependent diabetic taking lithium. Administration of lithium in therapeutic doses to maturity onset diabetics for one week caused no deterioration in glucose and insulin response to a standard carbohydrate meal. The relatively high prevalence of diabetes mellitus makes it impossible to state whether lithium therapy is associated with the condition. The metabolic responses to glucose have been repeatedly studied in lithium-treated patients with variable results. During a glucose tolerance test (GTT) symptomatic reactive hypoglycaemia occurs in lithium-treated patients but not in controls. Chronic lithium treatment may be associated with a rise in serum cortisol during a GTT (unlike controls) and by a lack of appropriate rise in plasma glucagon concentrations (Shah *et al.*, 1986).

The biochemical explanation of these clinical findings remains to be clarified. Lithium for example can promote glucose uptake into some tissues and in animal experiments there is a variable effect of lithium on liver glycogen concentrations, the data being confounded by different experimental methods. Lithium appears to increase glycogen synthesis in cultured rat liver hepatocytes at pharmacologically appropriate concentrations. The ion affects the activity of many enzymes related to glycogen synthesis presumably altering the specific ionic milieu for their correct functioning. Thus, lithium activates hexokinase and inhibits pyruvate kinase and protein kinase. Lithium has many effects upon the cellular aspects of carbohydrate metabolism when studied in whole tissue or isolated subcellular systems. In high concentrations it inhibits glucose and amino acid-induced insulin release from isolated rat islets of Langerhans.

From the clinical point of view, the main effect of lithium is weight gain. No significant deterioration or impairment of glucose metabolism occurs during long-term therapy in humans on the drug. The recent report of symptomatic hypoglycaemia following oral GTT may however point to the fact that there are abnormalities of glucose-regulating hormones in lithium-treated patients which have as yet not been elucidated.

5.6 BRAIN METABOLISM (Collard, 1986)

It is clearly important to understand how lithium acts on the brain in view of its therapeutic efficacy. Studies using *in vitro* preparations, whole animals and cultured brain cells have provided data on lithium transport into the brain and its effect on central neurotransmitters. It has been appreciated that there are regional variations in the effects of lithium in the brain. Specific brain areas have been examined, and in some cases the influence of other drugs on the lithium effect has been demonstrated. *In vitro* investigations of specific brain areas with lithium have also been performed (Wood and Goodwin, 1987).

The effects of lithium on inositol phospholipid metabolism have already been discussed. Suffice it to say that these effects are easily seen in brain tissue. It is possible that the continued presence of lithium may gradually deplete the membrane content of phosphatidyl inositol in the brain. This would decrease the sensitivity of those receptors in which inositol phospholipids are important components of the transducing mechanism. The identity of these receptors is at present not known but it seems that this is an important pathway by which lithium could modulate brain activity.

There have been many studies on the effects of lithium on brain neurotransmitters. Of the transmitter amino acids, most work has been conducted on gamma amino butyric acid (GABA). The most common effect of lithium treatment is an increase in the overall activity of the brain GABA system in experimental animals and an increase in the level of GABA in the CSF and plasma of patients. It is not clear whether these increases in GABA have any significance for the therapeutic effect of the ion. GABA activity may be reduced in depression and the reversal of this effect would be consistent with the antidepressant effects of lithium.

The complex relationships that exist between choline transport, acetylcholine, choline synthesis and acetylcholine release in brain tissue make any interpretation of acetylcholine metabolism effects difficult. Many experiments have shown an increased level of acetylcholine in the brain following lithium although other studies have observed that there was no change in total brain acetylcholine suggesting that regional differences may exist.

As the biochemical basis of affective disorders has been thought to involve a disorder of noradrenaline metabolism, the effects of lithium on this amine have been intensively studied. However, although some definitive data are available, there is difficulty in extrapolating from animal results to man, especially with regard to the concentrations of lithium used in some animal experiments. In general, there is no change in noradrenaline concentrations in the brain following lithium. Synthesis of the amine may be increased shortly after lithium administration but subsequently there is no change. Noradrenaline turnover has been reported to be both decreased or increased in the hypothalamus. Neuronal uptake of noradrenaline is generally increased following lithium though there are regional differences. Thus, in general, lithium increases the turnover of noradrenaline and its catabolism. Of interest are several studies relating to the effect of lithium on new properties of noradrenergic receptors in brain tissue although the data are difficult to interpret. Some experiments have shown a decreased beta–receptor activity, others have shown no effect on antidepressant-induced down regulation of beta–receptors. It appears that lithium can attenuate beta–receptor supersensitivity.

Available data does not offer an easy explanation for lithium's anti-manic action, though it has been suggested that overactivity in central dopaminergic pathways may be important in the aetiology of manic states. Several workers have examined the effects of lithium on dopamine metabolism both in brain slices and subcellular systems. Data suggests that striatal dopamine synthesis is decreased or increased by chronic lithium. The overall effect of lithium seems to be to decrease synaptic dopamine activity due merely to a decrease in the amount of dopamine released from nerve terminals. There is a decrease in dopaminergic activity at the dopamine receptor, and a decrease in dopamine receptor binding produced by lithium; the ion also attenuates the behavioural and endocrinological effects of haloperidol-induced dopamine receptor supersensitivity. In a similar fashion to noradrenaline available data does not make it easy to provide a unifying hypothesis of the action of lithium on brain metabolism.

Investigations have been performed to evaluate the effect of lithium on the transport of precursors, synthesis, concentration, storage and release of 5–hydroxytryptamine (5–HT) from synaptic vesicles. The synthesis of 5–HT is increased by short-term lithium treatment but returned to normal over longer treatment periods. During lithium treatment 5–HT storage is reduced but metabolism is increased. There is conflicting data on the release and uptake of 5–HT depending to some extent on the experimental methods used. There seems to be agreement that lithium induces a decrease in the density of 5–HT receptors in the hippocampus but not in the cortex.

Taken overall, the effects of lithium on brain metabolism are complex. It is important to note that there are clear regional differences in the effects of lithium on a number of neurotransmitters. It may be speculated that the effect of lithium will involve multiple interactions between several neurotransmitters with varying degrees of involvement among the different brain regions. This should encourage further research on a regional basis; detailed studies of the interaction of neurotransmitters in the regulation of both synthesis and release in specific brain regions would prove very useful as an experimental framework against which the effects of lithium could be studied.

5.7 LITHIUM AND THE THYROID

Goitre was first reported as a side-effect of lithium in 1968 (Schou *et al.*, 1968). Since then the effect of lithium on thyroid physiology has been examined in animals, normal humans, psychiatric patients, and patients with thyroid disease (Wolff, 1978). Lithium is concentrated in rat thyroid and the ion reduces radioactive iodine uptake into the gland. In animals there is evidence of an intrathyroidal blocking effect of lithium but the main physiological action is its inhibition of thyroid hormone secretion from the thyroid. The detailed biochemistry of this action is not fully understood but may relate to action of lithium on tubulin polymerization.

Thyroid function tests may be altered in patients on lithium. Assessment of the hypothalamic pituitary thyroid axis by monitoring the response of thyroid stimulating hormone (TSH) to the intravenous administration of thyrotrophin releasing hormone (TRH) has shown exaggerated TSH responses in up to 50% of patients. However, only about 10% of patients have elevated basal TSH levels. Lithium probably affects both hypothalamic function and neurotransmitter modulation of TSH release. In patients on long-term lithium therapy, serum thyroid hormone concentrations are indistinguishable from control subjects. However, short-term prospective studies have shown slight rises of TSH during the first three months of lithium therapy. This may be due to the transient inhibition of secretion of thyroid hormones which will affect feedback at the pituitary level.

The result of these thyroidal effects of lithium is that goitre is found in patients on lithium therapy (Mannisto, 1980). The prevalence varies but may well be around 30% when more sensitive techniques such as ultrasound are used to assess thyroid size. A significant increase in thyroid volume can be demonstrated in normal volunteers after four weeks of lithium, the goitre being produced as a result of the increased TSH levels already referred to. The goitre is usually smooth and non-tender although nodular enlargement may occur when there is pre-existing thyroid disease and, as mentioned, may be a transient phenomenon and spontaneously resolve. Treatment with L–thyroxine in normal dosage will speed its resolution. There is no evidence that lithium causes thyroid cancer although one patient has been reported who developed papillary adenocarcinoma of thyroid while on lithium therapy. It should be remembered that lithium crosses the placenta and therefore may cause foetal goitre during pregnancy.

Lithium-associated hypothyroidism has been widely studied, occurring in about 5% of patients. It is an important side-effect which may influence the underlying psychiatric condition but is readily treated. Several factors are involved in the pathogenesis of lithium-associated hypothyroidism. The prevalence of thyroid autoantibodies in patients on long-term lithium has been noted to be about 25%, and many patients on lithium who develop hypothyroidism are found to have Hashimoto's autoimmune thyroiditis. Lithium appears to be able to act as an immunomodulatory agent as shown by *in vitro* experiments with cultured lymphocytes (Hassman *et al.*, 1985). In addition, prospective studies have shown that lithium can increase the titres of antibodies to thyroglobulin and microsomes in lithium-treated patients who possess them at the start of treatment (Lazarus *et al.*, 1986). There is also some evidence that lithium may be able to induce antibody formation in appropriately susceptible patients. Lithium, then, has immunological effects as demonstrated by animal studies on T–cells, and may also affect clonal balance. If lithium is an immunomodulatory agent, the question may be asked as to whether it has any effect on Graves' hyperthyroidism.

There are many reports of the occurrence of hyperthyroidism in patients on lithium. Most patients who have developed hyperthyroidism on lithium have been taking the drug for extended periods but the association between lithium therapy and thyrotoxicosis has not been adequately explained. There is little data examining the effect of the concurrent iodine status in such patients although it is known that iodine and lithium can act synergistically to produce hypothyroidism. It is possible that, considering the large number of patients on lithium, the reported incidence of thyrotoxicosis may represent nothing more than the expected incidence of that disease. However, in view of the immunological actions of lithium, no definitive conclusion can be reached and the subject merits further investigation. Lithium is such an effective antithyroid agent that it can be used to treat thyrotoxicosis, especially in patients who are sensitive to standard antithyroid drugs. It may also be used as an adjunct to conventional antithyroid drug therapy in the initial treatment of severe hyperthyroidism. More recently, attempts have been made to exploit the iodine-retaining properties of lithium in patients with thyroid cancer. Radioiodine administration to patients with thyroid cancer can be rendered more effective by the concurrent administration of lithium (Robbins, 1981).

5.8 OTHER ENDOCRINE EFFECTS

5.8.1 Pituitary gland

Lithium is thought to be concentrated in the hypothalamus and may be expected to have effects on the hypothalamic anterior pituitary axis. The effects on TRH testing and the response to TSH have already been discussed. Although basal serum prolactin concentrations do not change after lithium administration, an increased prolactin response to TRH has been noted. The effect of lithium on dopaminergic mechanisms of prolactin release is variable and may be partly dependent on alterations produced by the psychiatric disease as well as the lithium. Lithium can enhance the sensitivity of 5–HT receptors in the neuroendocrine axis and this may be an indirect method of influencing prolactin levels. Similarly, abnormal positive growth hormone responses to TRH may occur in manic patients during lithium treatment. Lithium does not appear to affect apomorphine or insulin-induced increase in GH but can inhibit GH release produced by clonidine (a beta–2 adrenergic agonist) in healthy male volunteers.

5.8.2 Gonadal function

The data on luteinizing hormone (LH) and testosterone levels in lithium-treated patients are controversial (Banerji, Parkening and Collins, 1982). Lithium can be found in the ejaculate and in the genital organs of rats following administration. There appear to be differences in distribution between acute and chronic administration in animal experiments. Lithium appears to inhibit testosterone production from the testis in the rat at early times, giving rise to a high LH level. While reproductive capacity may be impaired in the mouse there is no data in humans although lithium is known to be teratogenic.

5.8.3 Adrenal function (Berens and Wolff, 1975)

There are pronounced changes in plasma corticosteroid concentrations in patients with manic depressive psychosis thus making interpretation of any lithium-associated change rather difficult. Small changes in plasma cortisol levels have been noted without loss of diurnal rhythm. Cortisol production rates and excretion of cortisol metabolites are unaffected by lithium. Measurements of urinary aldosterone have shown variable results although there may be an initial increase during the first few days after starting lithium.

From animal and *in vitro* studies it appears that lithium can alter the sensitivity of the glucocorticoid receptor *in vitro*. The ion may have an inhibitory effect on steroid synthesis in cultured adrenal tumour cells. From the clinical point of view the effects of lithium on cortisol metabolism are unimportant.

There is evidence from animal experiments that lithium can induce suppression of pineal activity. In view of the pineal gland's important role in modulating circadian rhythmicity, it is clear that further work on the interaction between lithium and pineal function should be encouraged.

REFERENCES

Banerji, T.K., Parkening, T.A. and Collins, T.J. (1982) Lithium: short-term and chronic effects on plasma testosterone and luteinizing hormone concentrations in mice. *Life Sci.*, **30**, 1045–50.

Belmaker, R.H. (1981) Receptors, adenylate cyclase, depression, and lithium. *Biol. Psychiat.*, **16**, 333–50.

Berens, S.C. and Wolff, J. (1975) The endocrine effects of lithium. In: *Lithium Research and Therapy* (ed. F.N. Johnson), Academic Press, New York, pp. 443–72.

Birch, N.J. (1978) Metabolic effects of lithium. In: *Lithium in Medical Practice* (eds. F.N. Johnson and S. Johnson), MRP Press, Lancaster, pp. 89–114.

Cade, J.F.J. (1949) Lithium salts in the treatment of psychotic excitement. *Med. J. Aust.*, **36**, 349–52.

Christensen, S., Kusano, E., Yusufi, A.N.K. *et al.* (1985) Pathogenesis of nephrogenic diabetes insipidus due to chronic administration of lithium in rats. *J. Clin. Invest.*, **75**, 1869–879.

Collard, K.J. (1986) Effects of lithium on brain metabolism. In: *Endocrine and Metabolic Effects of Lithium* (ed. J.H. Lazarus), Plenum Press, New York, pp. 55–97.

Coppen, A. (1965) Mineral metabolism in affective disorders. *Br. J. Psychiat.*, **111**, 1133–42.

Depner, T.A. (1982) Nephrotic syndrome secondary to lithium therapy. *Nephron*, **30**, 286–9.

Dick, D.A.T., Naylor, G.J. and Dick, E.G. (1978) Effects of lithium on sodium transport across membranes. In: *Lithium in Medical Practice* (eds: F.N. Johnson and S. Johnson), MTP Press, Lancaster, pp. 183–92.

Downes, C.P. (1983) Inositol phospholipids and neurotransmitter receptor signalling mechanisms. *Trends Neurol. Sci.*, **6**, 313–16.

Duhm, D. and Becker, B.F. (1978) Mechanisms of Li^+ transport across the human erythrocyte membrane. In: *The Red Cell* (ed. G. Brewer), Alan R. Liss, New York, pp. 551–70.

Forrest, J.N. Jr., Cohen, A.D., Torretti, J. *et al.* (1974) On the mechanism of lithium-induced diabetes insipidus in man and the rat. *J. Clin. Invest.*, **53**, 1115–123.

Ghose, K. (1977) Lithium salts: therapeutic and unwanted effects. *Br. J. Hosp. Med.*, **3**, 710–13.

Hansen, H.E. and Amdisen, A. (1978) Lithium intoxication. (Report of 23 cases and review of 100 cases from the literature.) *Q. J. Med.*, **47**, 123–44.

Hassman, R.A., Lazarus, J.H., Dieguez, C. *et al.* (1985) The influence of lithium chloride on experimental autoimmune thyroid disease. *Clin. Exp. Immunol.*, **61**, 49–57.

Hesketh, J.E., Loudon, J.B., Reading, H.W. and Glen, A.I.M. (1978) The effect of lithium treatment on erythrocyte membrane ATPase activities and erythrocyte ion content. *Br. J. Clin. Pharmacol.*, **5**, 323–9.

Lazarus, J.H. (1982) Endocrine and metabolic effects of lithium. *Adv. Drug. React. Ac. Pois. Rev.*, **1**, 181–200.

Lazarus, J.H. (1986) *Endocrine and Metabolic Effects of Lithium*. Plenum Press, New York, pp. 1–208.

Lazarus, J.H., Davis, C.J., Woodhead, J.S. *et al.*(1987) Effect of lithium on the metabolic response to parathyroid hormone. *Min. Electrolyte. Metab.*, **13**, 63–6.

Lazarus, J.H., McGregor, A.M., Ludgate, M. *et al.* (1986) Effect of lithium carbonate therapy on thyroid immune status in manic depressive patients: a prospective study. *J. Affect. Dis.*, **11**, 155–60.

Lokkegaard, H., Andersen, N.F., Henriksen, E. *et al.* (1985) Renal function in 153 manic-depressive patients treated with lithium for more than five years. *Acta. Psychiat. Scand.*, **71**, 347–55.

Mallette, L.E. and Eichhorn, E. (1986) Effects of lithium carbonate on human calcium metabolism. *Arch. Intern. Med.*, **146**, 770–6.

Mannisto, P.T. (1980) Endocrine side-effects of lithium. In: *Handbook of Lithium Therapy* (ed. F.N. Johnson), MTP Press, Lancaster, pp. 310–22.

McAuliffe, W.G. and Olesen, O.V. (1983) Effects of lithium on the structure of the rat kidney. *Nephron*, **34**, 114–24.

Padfield, P.L., Park, S.J., Morton, J.J. *et al.* (1977) Plasma levels of antidiuretic hormone in patients receiving prolonged lithium therapy. *Br. J. Psychiat.*, **130**, 144–7.

Pandey, G.N., Dorus, E. and Davis, J.M. (1979) Lithium transport in human red cells: genetic and clinical aspects. In: *Lithium Controversies and Unresolved Issues* (eds. T.B. Cooper, S. Gershon, N.S. Kline, and M. Shou), Excerpta Medica, Amsterdam, pp. 736–57.

Peselow, E.D., Dunner, D.L., Fieve, R.R. and Lautin, A. (1980) Lithium carbonate and weight gain. *J. Affect. Dis.*, **2**, 303–10.

Robbins, J. (1981) The role of TRH and lithium in the management of thyroid cancer. In: *Advances in Thyroid Neoplasia* (eds. M. Andreoli, F. Monaco and J. Robbins), SPC-Casino, Rome, pp. 233–44.

Schou, M., Amdisen, A., Jensen, S.E. and Olsen, T. (1968) Occurrence of goitre during lithium treatment. *Br. Med. J.*, **3**, 710–13.

Shah, J.H., DeLeon-Jones, F.A., Schickler, R. *et al.* (1986) Symptomatic reactive hypoglycemia during glucose tolerance test in lithium-treated patients. *Metabolism*, **35**, 634–9.

Vendsborg, P.B. (1978) Lithium and glucose tolerance. In: *Lithium in Medical Practice* (eds. F.N. Johnson and S. Johnson), MTP Press, Lancaster, pp. 153–8.

Walker, R.G., Bennet, W.M., Davies, B.M. and Kincaid-Smith, P. (1982) Structural and functional effects of long-term lithium therapy. *Kidney Int.*, **21**, (suppl. 11), S13–S19.

Waller, D.G. and Edwards, J.G. (1985) Investigating renal function during lithium treatment. *Psychol. Med.*, **15**, 369–75.

Wolff, J. (1978) Lithium interactions with the thyroid gland. In: *Lithium Contro-*

versies and Unresolved Issues (eds. T.B. Cooper, S. Gershon, N.S. Kline and M. Shou), Excerpta Medica, Amsterdam, pp. 552–64.

Wood, A.J. and Goodwin, G.M. (1987) A review of the biochemical and neuropharmacological actions of lithium. *Psychol. Med.*, **17**, 579–600.

Chapter Six

Clinical pharmacology of lithium salts

KARABI GHOSE

CONTENTS

6.1 HISTORICAL BACKGROUND

Ever since its discovery in the early nineteenth century, the possible medicinal properties of lithium have been considered by many. It was first used in the treatment of urinary bladder calculi without any effect. Similar disappointment was experienced in patients with gout (Garrod, 1873). Neither the local application of lithium solution nor the administration of oral salts was effective in dissolving uric acid crystals. In the late nineteenth century, lithium was also considered in the treatment of various neuropsychiatric disorders, including depression and epilepsy, but no obvious benefit was found.

In the thirties, lithium chloride was recommended to replace sodium salts for patients with hypertension and patients requiring sodium restricted diet, with inevitable disastrous consequences. The modern era of lithium therapy started following the discovery of its antimanic property by an Australian Psychiatrist (Cade, 1949). However, in view of the previously observed adverse effects in hypertensive patients, lithium was understandably labelled as a very toxic drug, and there was a lack of enthusiasm to verify Cade's report. Lithium became a popular therapeutic agent only after Professor Schou's extensive work demonstrating its efficacy and safe use by monitoring plasma lithium levels in the late sixties (Baastrup and Schou, 1967). It is now widely accepted as an established prophylactic agent in affective disorders.

6.2 CHEMISTRY

Lithium is a monovalent cation and is the lightest of all the alkali metals. In the biological system it competes with sodium, potassium, magnesium and calcium for enzyme sites and displaces them according to its affinity (Li<Na<K<Mg<Ca). It therefore influences almost all systems producing many biochemical, metabolic and neuroendocrinal changes. These are discussed in Chapter 5.

6.3 THERAPEUTIC INDICATIONS AND POTENTIAL

As mentioned above, lithium produces many biochemical and nueroendocrinal changes and therefore probably has much wider therapeutic potential than is at present appreciated. Its role in the management of acute episodes of mania and in the prophylaxis of recurrent affective disorders is beyond doubt. Lithium has also been shown to be effective during an acute attack of depression (Worrall *et al.*, 1979); in the prophylaxis of chronic alcoholism and in schizoaffective disorders. The combination of lithium and an antidepressant drug is considered to be superior to an antidepressant drug alone in some patients with 'resistant' depression (Cowen, 1988).

Lithium is also beneficial in many non-psychiatric conditions. It has been shown to reduce both frequency and severity of attacks of cluster headaches (Kudrow, 1976). In the treatment of thyrotoxicosis it can be used successfully alone or in combination with radio-iodine therapy.

Lithium is known to produce leucocytosis and may be helpful in patients with drug-induced neutropenia.

This drug has been tried in many other psychiatric and non-psychiatric disorders. Its clinical application is likely to widen with further expansion of our knowledge about its mode of action in affective disorders and with improvements in methodology to minimize its side-effects.

6.4 PREPARATIONS OF LITHIUM SALTS

Lithium carbonate and lithium citrate are the two salts available for clinical use in the UK. Lithium citrate has only one conventional formulation but both conventional and slow-release formulations of lithium carbonates are used in clinical practice. Several formulations of slow-release lithium carbonates are available. They vary widely in bioavailability and special care should be taken if a change in preparation is required. These preparations are summarized in Table 6.1.

Table 6.1 Preparations of lithium available for prescription in the UK.

Chemical nature	*Formulations*			
	Slow-release		*Conventional*	
	Trade name	*Li+(mmol)*	*Trade name*	*Li+(mmol)*
Lithium carbonate	Camcolit	10.8	Camcolit	6.8
	Liskonum	12.2	Liskonum	12.2
	Phasal	8.1		
	Priadel	5.4		
		10.8		
Lithium citrate	Litarex	6.0		

6.5 PHARMACOKINETICS

Clinical pharmacokinetics of lithium preparations have been studied extensively both in healthy subjects and in patients with affective disorders. As mentioned above, bioavailability of different preparations of lithium salts varies enormously. There appears to be some disagreement regarding their relative pharmacokinetic characteristics. This apparent lack of agreement is probably, at least partly, related to methodological differences. For example, using comparable doses, Shelley and Silverstone (1986) observed no significant differences in 12 and 24 h plasma lithium levels following single oral doses of four

Table 6.2 Some recent studies on the pharmacokinetics of lithium in young subjects

Investigators	Subjects	Parameter studied	Proprietary name			
			Priadel	Camcolit	Liskonum	Litarex
Shelley and	Healthy,	Dose (mmol)	27.0	27.0	30.5	27.0
Silverstone	after single	*Tmax (h)	2.5	2.5	5.0	3.25
(1986)	dose	†Cmax (mmol/l)	0.60	0.63	0.55	0.41
		‡C12 (mmol/l)	0.30	0.30	0.34	0.27
		§C24 (mmol/l)	0.24	0.24	0.24	0.21
Phillips and	Patients,	Dose (mg)	400	400		
Birch (1987)	after 3	*Tmax (h)	1.94	2.11		
	weeks'	Cmax (mmol/l)	0.44	0.43		
	medication	‡C12 (mmol/l)	0.30	0.29		

* Time of maximum concentration
† Maximum concentration
‡ Concentration at 12 h.
§ Concentration at 24 h.

slow-release formulations. These are summarized in Table 6.2. The pharmacokinetic parameters of Priadel and Camcolit were almost identical. Similar comparable plasma lithium levels following three weeks' medication with Priadel and Camecolit (Table 6.2), were reported by Phillips and Birch (1987).

Greil and co-workers (Greil *et al.*, 1985) studied the pharmacokinetics of lithium salts in young adults and patients aged 65 years or over. Although there was no difference in plasma levels, the elderly required significantly lower doses. A 36% decline in the ratio of weight-related lithium dose to plasma level was reported, the authors also indicating that at the age of 50, the dosage requirement decreases abruptly.

Hardy *et al.* (1987) studied the pharmacokinetics of slow-release lithium carbonate in nine female patients aged between 67 and 80 years.

Lithium clearance and volume of distribution were significantly reduced in the elderly as compared with a younger adult cohort (Neilsen-Kudsk and Amidsen, 1979). Based on these pharmacokinetic differences (as summarized in Table 6.3), elderly patients probably require 0.3 to 0.5 times less lithium than younger adults. Hardy *et al.* (1987) concluded that lithium is almost entirely excreted by the kidneys. The age-related reduction in glomerular filtration rate and renal blood flow are considered to be responsible for the altered pharmacokinetics of lithium in the elderly.

Table 6.3 Pharmacokinetics of slow-release lithium carbonate during steady state in elderly and young patients (mean (SD) values are shown)

Investigators	Patients' age (yr)	Dose (mmol/kg)	Distribution half life (hr)	Elimination half life (hr)	*Volume of D (l/kg)	Clearance (ml/min)
Hardy et al. (1987) n = 9	Elderly 73 (5.0)	0.21 (0.06)	‡2.7 (1.2)	26.9 (5.5)	‡0.64 (0.16)	‡15.6 (4.0)
Nielsen–Kudsk and Amidsen (1979) n = 7	Young 35 (10)	0.39 (0.08)	1.1 (0.5)	21.5 (6.8)	0.83 (0.18)	27.8 (5.3)

*Volume of distribution.
‡Significantly different than the young patients.

6.6 CHOICE OF A LITHIUM PREPARATION

Slow-release formulations of lithium carbonate for a once-daily dosage regime are most commonly used. In the past, nephrotoxicity of lithium was considered to be associated with a high peak serum lithium level following a single large oral dose. Many psychiatrists previously preferred to prescribe a multiple daily dosage regime of a conventional lithium preparation. Divided daily dosage regime used to be specifically recommended for elderly patients (Roose, *et al.*, 1979). However, further research in this field indicates that a slow-release lithium formulation is relatively safer than a multiple dosage regime. Perry and colleagues (Perry *et al.*, 1981) not only observed that once-daily lithium therapy significantly decreased the 24 h urine volume, but also claimed that this regime reversed some of the lithium-induced changes in renal functions. A similar advantage of once-daily medication was also suggested by a Danish group (Plenge *et al.*, 1982). Nephrotoxicity of lithium, therefore, if not less following a single daily dose, is unlikely to be higher than in a divided daily dosage regime.

There are several advantages of once-daily medication. Prophylactic lithium is usually prescribed for long-term therapy. The patients are required to continue with this maintenance therapy even at times when they are apparently keeping well. In order to encourage compliance, therefore, a slow release preparation of lithium salts for a once-daily regime is preferable.

6.7 BIOCHEMICAL EFFECTS

Lithium inhibits adenylcyclase activity and influences many enzyme systems. It may interfere with hormonal and metabolic functions (discussed in detail in Chapter 5). As mentioned in Section 6.2, lithium displaces other alkali metals according to its affinity. In animal studies, chronic lithium administration had been shown to reduce sodium concentration in various parts of the brain (Edelfers, 1975).

Lithium does not appear to have any significant effect on potassium distribution. Long-term lithium administration was reported to be associated with an increase in organic phosphate in muscle and liver, and a decrease in bone. The concentration of magnesium in muscle and serum were increased but uptake of magnesium and calcium into bone was decreased following long-term lithium administration in rats. An increase in circulating parathormone has also been reported (Christiansen, Baastrup and Transbol, 1976).

The effect of lithium on biogenic amines, especially on 5–hydroxytryptamine (5–HT) has been extensively studied in view of its efficacy in affective disorders. However, despite a great deal of research work, its mode of action in affective disorders is still inconclusive. A large amount of literature exists on its varied effects on the biogenic amines. Briefly, an increase of 5–hydroxytryptamine (5–HT) synthesis and noradrenaline turnover in rats was reported by several investigators. In animals, short-term lithium administration is associated with an increase in cerebral 5–HT uptake. Lithium increases both the uptake of neuronal tryptophan (a precursor of 5–HT) and the release of 5–HT from nerve endings. Long-term effects of lithium in the brain are more complex. The activity of tryptophan hydroxylase (an enzyme necessary for the conversion of tryptophan to 5–HT) is reduced and down regulation of post-synaptic 5–HT receptors occurs in some regions of the brain. Both short and long-term lithium administration has been reported to increase 5–HT-mediated behaviour (Harrison-Read, 1981).

In man, lithium is considered to prevent the release of 5–HT from platelets and to increase platelet 5–HT uptake. These effects may be responsible for its anti-migrainous activity. Recently, lithium has been reported to enhance prolactin response in man (Glue *et al.*, 1986). The enhancement of some aspects of cerebral 5–HT function during lithium therapy may be important in its mode of action in affective disorders (Glue *et al.*, 1986). Lithium is known to produce several morphological and functional changes in the kidneys which are discussed in Chapter 5.

6.8 SIDE-EFFECTS

Side-effects can be defined as the other effects of a drug which are therapeutically undesirable and which usually occur within the 'therapeutic' range of drug level. They should be distinguished from the toxic effects of a drug. Hypersensitivity or allergic reaction to lithium is rare: when it occurs, it is usually due to the presence of dyes in the drug preparation (Clark and Jefferson, 1987).

Lithium therapy is known to be associated with a number of side-effects, both subjective and biochemical (Vestergaard, Amdisen and Schou, 1980). However, with continued therapy, most patients are able to tolerate these effects but in some further dosage reduction may be necessary. Even so a small number of patients may continue to suffer from severe symptoms and may not be able to tolerate this medication.

Side-effects of lithium therapy usually fall into two categories, some which appear at the early stage of therapy and some which develop during continuing medication. Common side-effects and their clinical significance are summarized in Table 6.4.

Table 6.4 Common side-effects of lithium therapy

Symptoms	Early stage	Long-term therapy	Impending toxicity	Comments
Nausea	+			Supportive drug
Loose motions				therapy may be required.
Vomiting and severe diarrhoea			+	Stop lithium.
Fine finger tremor	+	+		Beta-blockers may be helpful, but should be avoided in the old.
Coarse tremor			+	Check lithium level.
Polydipsia and polyuria	+	+		Usually no treatment required
Weight gain	+	+		
Hypothyroidism	+	+		Replacement therapy.
Muscle weakness and lethargy		+		Need reassurance.
Oedema		+		Thiazides should not be prescribed.
Dysarthia		+	+	Stop lithium.
Vertigo			+	Check level.
Unsteadiness				Observe.
Sluggishness				Facilitate Li excretion.
Drowsiness				?Dialysis.

6.8.1 Early stage

The most common symptom at the early stage is nausea. It is usually experienced by the majority of patients. It may be associated with loose bowel motions. These symptoms are considered to be harmless and usually are not severe enough for therapy to be discontinued. It may sometimes be necessary to prescribe an anti-emetic drug during the first four weeks, but the symptoms usually disappear after 2–6 weeks' medication.

The other common socially disabling symptom is fine tremor of the fingers which is an exacerbation of physiological tremor and is common in the elderly. This is dose related and may improve with slight dosage reduction. Betablockers may be helpful in alleviating this symptom, but they are not devoid of hazards in the elderly. Symptoms of diabetes insipidus (polyuria and polydipsia) may also commence as early as 1–2 weeks after starting therapy. These symptoms, like tremor, tend to persist throughout the lithium therapy.

6.8.2 Long-term effects

Long-term treatment with lithium is usually defined as treatment lasting six months or more. Side-effects of lithium can be divided into two groups, subjective effects and functional abnormalities.

(a) Subjective effects
The symptoms of diabetes insipidus and finger tremor, which develop in the early stage, usually persist. They may also occur during long-term medication. Polyuria and polydipsia usually occur in 50% of patients (Vestergaard, 1983). Finger and hand tremor also develop in a similar proportion of patients.

The incidence of weight gain was observed in 60% of patients (Vendsborg, Bech and Rafaelsen, 1976). The frequency of diarrhoea and oedema was reported to be 10–20% and 10–15% respectively of patients of all age groups (Vestergraad, 1983). Lithium-induced tremor occurs more frequently in patients above 60 years of age (Bech *et al.*, 1979). Other symptoms of which patients receiving long-term lithium therapy frequently complain are poor memory and concentration, palpitations, blurred vision, vertigo, dry mouth and goitre (Ghose, 1977). Acne, exacerbation of psoriasis and loss of libido were reported in young patients.

(b) Functional abnormalities
Biochemical changes associated with lithium therapy have been discussed above. Lithium, by altering mineral metabolism, influences the electrical activity of the heart and brain. Disturbances of cardiac conduction and conductivity may be observed in electrocardiographic studies (Albrecut and Muller-Oerlinghausen, 1980).

The electroencephalograph may demonstrate changes in brain contractility, and cognitive disturbances (Tyrer and Shopsin, 1980). However, these are usually mild clinical changes.

Altered carbohydrate metabolism may precipitate overt diabetes mellitus. Its effect on thyroid is discussed in Chapter 5. Lithium is well known to produce clinical hypothyroidism in 5–15% of patients receiving long-term therapy.

During recent years considerable work has been carried out to study the effect of long-term lithium therapy on kidneys. In all studies 85–90% of patients showed normal glomerular function when the age-related changes were taken into consideration. Renal tubular function, however, has been shown to be impaired. Lithium has been shown to interfere with the action of antidiuretic hormone in the renal distal tubules and may produce a syndrome of nephrogenic diabetes insipidus. Its effect on renal concentrating ability is unclear. No change was reported by Coppen *et al.* (1980), but was considered to be reduced in 20–40% of patients by Vestergaard (1983). Similar controversy exists regarding lithium-induced morphological changes in the kidneys (Vestergaard, 1983).

6.9 INTERACTIONS WITH OTHER DRUGS

Broadly speaking, all drug–drug interactions fall into two categories: pharmacokinetic and pharmacodynamic.

6.9.1 Pharmacokinetic interactions

Lithium is mainly excreted by the kidneys and is also dependent on sodium metabolism. Therefore, any drug which influences renal functions and sodium metabolism by reducing lithium clearance, increases plasma lithium levels and vice versa. Diuretics, especially thiazides (Petersen *et al.*, 1974) potentiates the effect of lithium by decreasing its clearance. However, loop diuretics, such as frusemide, are considered to be relatively safer (Saffer and Coppen, 1983). Other drugs which are known to reduce lithium levels are acetazolamide and theophylline.

Conversely, drugs containing sodium bicarbonates such as antacids, increase lithium excretion. Both diuretics and gastric antacids are frequently prescribed for elderly patients and obviously require special caution when used concomitantly with lithium.

Nonsteroidal anti-inflammatory drugs are widely prescribed in the elderly. These drugs cause water and sodium retention and also have some deteriorating effects on renal blood flow and glomerular filtration rate. In general, they tend to increase lithium levels (Reiman and Frolich, 1981; Ragheb and Powell, 1986). Enalepril, an angitensin-converting enzyme inhibitor drug, also increases the lithium level, probably via its effect on the kidneys.

6.9.2 Pharmacodynamic interactions

Neurotoxicity due to interaction between lithium and neuroleptic drugs is well established. Sixty percent of elderly bipolar patients who previously were stabilized on lithium and maintained therapeutic plasma levels, were observed to develop neurotoxicity when a neuroleptic was added (Miller, Menhinger and Whitcup, 1986). Neurotoxicity occurred despite the use of neuroleptic dosages that were considered safe when administered alone. In addition to the increase in extrapyramidal side-effects of neuroleptics, the patients may also have other central nervous system effects, such as ataxia, dysarthia and altered levels of consciousness. These interactions may occur without any change in serum lithium levels (Smith and Helms, 1982). It is advisable either to avoid such drugs during lithium therapy or to use a lower dosage regime. Neurotoxicity may also occur in patients maintained on long-term therapy receiving anticonvulsants (carbamazepine, phenytoin) (Ghose, 1980) and calcium antagonists (dildaizem and verapamil) concomitantly.

In general, concomitant therapy with monoamine oxidase inhibitor antidepressants, tryptophan, tricyclic and related antidepressants are usually tolerated by patients receiving lithium therapy. Addition of another antidepressant drug is usually found to be beneficial in some patients with resistant depression. However, drugs with significant anticholinergic effects may produce some neurotoxic side-effects, such as mental confusion and tremor. Patients maintained on long-term lithium therapy usually tolerate benzodiazepines, but drugs with central depressant effects should be used with caution.

6.10 TOXICITY

6.10.1 Presentations

Symptoms of impending toxicity of lithium therapy are diarrhoea, vomiting, coarse tremor, ataxia, dysarthia, sluggishiness and drowsiness. These symptoms are usually associated with plasma lithium levels between 1.2 mmol/l and 2.6 mmol/l, but toxic symptoms may appear even at lower dosage levels. At higher levels (usually over 2 mmol/l) signs of neurotoxicity are common and patients may even present with coma. However, the severity of toxicity may not always correlate with plasma lithium levels. Some neurological symptoms may become apparent even 2–3 days after the discontinuation of lithium following the diagnosis of a biochemical toxicity.

Lithium toxicity produces a wide spectrum of signs and symptoms related to the central and peripheral nervous system. Neurotoxicity such as cerebellar signs, paresis and extrapyramidal signs are well documented (Sansone and Ziegler, 1985). Most of these toxic effects are reversible and usually improve with a reduction of the lithium dosage or with the discontinuation of therapy. However, permanent cerebellar degeneration and cerebral atrophy (diagnosed by computed tomography) in a 32-year-old man was considered to be related to previous lithium toxicity (Bejar, 1985). Although this clearly requires further confirmation, the elderly are obviously at greater risk in view of age-related changes in the brain, and the need for close supervision in this age group cannot be over-emphasized.

Table 6.5 Some common causes of lithium toxicity and intolerance in the elderly

Mechanisms	Causes	Remarks
Salt/water depletion	Low-salt diet Fluid restrictions Dehydration/sweating Diarrhoea/vomiting Polyuria	Lithium should be avoided or stopped immediately.
Renal disorders	Renal failure Infection Drug-induced	Close monitioring is required. In severe case, stop lithium.
Acute physical illnesses	Pyrexia Infection Heart failure etc.	Stop or if mild, monitor closely, encourage drinking of water and sodium-containing fluids.
Drugs	Diuretics	Thiazides contraindicated. Frusemide may be tolerated. Stop lithium if large dose required.
	Neuroleptics	Higher doses of these drugs should be avoided; or stop lithium.
	MAO inhibitors	Not contraindicated.
	Tricyclic and second generation anti-depressants	Usually synergistic effect. Lithium level should be reassessed.
	Carbamazepine Phyenytoin	Increased incidence of side-effects. Doseage readjustment.
	Antihypertensives	Beta-blockers can be used. Ca-antagonists with care ACE-inhibitors should be avoided.
	Nonsteroidal anti-inflammatory drugs Anticholinergics	Lithium level may alter. Readjust dose or stop. Preferably to be avoided.

6.10.2 Precipitating factors

Lithium is excreted almost exclusively by the kidneys. During the steady state, the amount of urinary excretion of lithium is usually equal to the daily lithium dosage. Therefore any factor which influences this close relative relationship between daily dose, plasma level and urinary excretion of lithium is likely to alter the lithium status of the body. A decrease in lithium excretion will increase plasma level and may precipitate toxicity. There are several precipitating factors and some common causes are discussed below.

Salt deficiency is the commonest cause of lithium toxicity. Lithium competes with sodium in the biological system and its excretion diminishes in presence of sodium deficiency. Any condition which produces a negative sodium balance is likely to increase lithium concentration. Severity of clinical toxicity depends on the degree of sodium deficiency and on the lithium levels.

Water deficiency also increases lithium levels by reducing renal excretion of lithium. Common conditions such as a low-salt diet, fluid restriction or excessive fluid and salt loss (diarrhoea, vomiting, sweating and polyuria), are known to precipitate lithium toxicity. Patients with pyrexia and/or infection are also at risk.

Other underlying physical illnesses, for example heart failure, may be responsible for an attack of lithium toxicity. Drugs which influence the sodium and water metabolism, such as diuretics or nonsteroidal anti-inflammatory drugs, may be responsible for toxicity. A number of other drugs are known to interact with lithium and alter the lithium status of the body, as discussed in section 6.9. Some common causes of lithium toxicity are shown in Table 6.5.

6.10.3 Management

All patients suspected of having lithium toxicity should be hospitalized and lithium should be discontinued immediately. Plasma lithium level, renal functions and other relevant investigations to evaluate any underlying precipitating factor, such as infection or interaction with another drug, should be performed. The patient should be treated either in a general medical ward or admitted to an intensive care unit, depending on the clinical severity of toxicity.

Although, as mentioned above, plasma lithium level may not reflect the severity of symptoms, treatment is usually designed according to the plasma lithium level. Renal clearance of lithium, any precipitating factor and general condition of the patient should be assessed. If plasma lithium level is less than 2 mmol/l and the patient is ambulating and not very drowsy, no corrective treatment is required, especially if the renal function is adequate. Supportive therapy such as electrolyte containing fluid (milk or intravenous saline), may be required for some patients. Treatment should be directed towards the cause of toxicity.

In patients with higher plasma lithium concentration (for example, 4 mmol/l or above) and/or if the patient is drowsy or comatose, it is advisable to treat such a patient in an intensive care unit and the plasma lithium level should be monitored at 1–3 hourly intervals, depending on the severity of toxicity. If the plasma lithium comes down rapidly within six hours and the level is not too high and the severity of neurotoxicity is mild, dialysis is usually not required. In patients with slow neurological progress and poor renal clearance of lithium, haemodialysis should be considered. There is very little place for ion-exchange resins, as lithium is lighter than other alkali metals, but it should be tried if immediate facilities for dialysis are not available.

6.11 PRESCRIBING IN THE ELDERLY

6.11.1 Special problems

In addition to the usual problems and side-effects of lithium therapy, there are two major predisposing risks of this medication in the elderly. Firstly, lithium is almost entirely excreted by the kidneys and age-related deterioration in renal functions occurs in the elderly. Routine renal function tests may not show any deterioration as the synthesis of urea and creatinine may also be reduced in this population. Secondly, old people tend to suffer from multiple pathology and as a result receive polypharmacy, which increases the risks of drug–drug interactions. For example, heart failure and osteoarthritis are common in old people and they may require concomitant diuretics and nonsteroidal anti-inflammatory drugs, both of which influence sodium balance. The elderly, therefore, are particularly vulnerable to lithium toxicity.

6.11.2 Selection of patients

The widely accepted indication for long-term lithium therapy in affective disorders is that it is prescribed in patients with three or more episodes (usually within a period of five years or less) of depression, or mania, or both. In elderly patients, it is less commonly used for other indications such as manic attacks or for an acute episode of depression, unless the patient is resistant to other conventional therapy.

Prior to the initiation of therapy, each patient's physical state should be assessed and routine laboratory investigations, particularly renal and thyroid functions, should be evaluated. There is no absolute contra-indication, but appropriate precautions and dosage adjustments may be required in some conditions, as shown in Table 6.5. Lithium should be avoided in patients who are noncompliers, have significant renal impairment and/or evidence of early dementia.

6.11.3 Dosage guidance

It is advisable to start with a small dose even if the renal functions are apprently 'normal'. The usual starting dose is 200 mg of a slow-release preparation of lithium carbonate in a once-daily dosage regime. The dose should be slowly raised to achieve the therapeutic plasma lithium concentration in 2–4 weeks' time. A lithium clearance test may provide guidance regarding the daily dosage requirement. The aim is to achieve a steady state therapeutic plasma concentration between 0.5 and 0.8 mmol/l usually 12 hours after the last dose of a slow-release preparation. Average dosage requirement for slow-release lithium carbonate in this age group also varies enormously and is usually between 200 and 800 mg daily.

6.11.4 Assessment

It is initially necessary to measure plasma lithium concentration on alternate days or at least at weekly intervals but once the steady state has been achieved, this can be monitored at 4–8 weekly intervals. In addition, routine biochemical tests (such as renal and thyroid functions), mental state and side-effects are also evaluated at regular 8–12 weekly intervals. Patients with associated physical illness, especially renal insufficiency, should be mointored more frequently.

6.11.5 Lithium clinic

The role of the lithium clinic in the management of patients receiving long-term therapy is discussed in Chapter 7.

6.11.6 Instructions to patients/carers

In addition to the patients, their carers should ideally be interviewed. Compliance is usually better if information is provided regarding the purpose of long-term therapy, the importance of maintaining lithium therapy even during remission, the need for regular plasma drug level monitoring and what to do if they become ill or require any additional medication. Carers should have some idea about the side-effects, particuarly the symptoms of impending toxicity. Consideration should be given to the patient carrying a card indicating the name of lithium preparation and current dose, and the name of the supervising hospital/ clinic.

6.11.7 Communications with other health care staff

The importance of liaison with the patient's General Practitioner and other staff involved in the care of an elderly patient cannot be over-emphasized. Frequent home visits by a community nurse or a health visitor, particularly for patients who live alone, are desirable. Patients who fail to keep an out-patients appointment should be visited by staff as soon as possible. Lithium should preferably be avoided without facilities of adequate supervision in this age group.

REFERENCES

Albrecut, J.W. and Muller-Oerlinghausen, B. (1980) Cardiovascular side-effects of lithium. In: *Handbook of Lithium Therapy* (ed. F.N. Johnson), MTP Press, Lancaster, pp. 323–33.

Baastrup, P.C. and Schou, M. (1967) Lithium as a prophylactic agent. Its effect against recurrent depressions and manic-depressive psychosis. *Arch. Gen. Psychiat.*, **16**, 162–72.

Bech, P., Thomsen, J., Prytz, S. *et al.* (1979) The profile and severity of lithium-induced side-effects in mentally healthy subjects. *Neuropsychobiology*, **5**, 160–6.

Bejar, J.S. (1985) Cerebellar degeneration due to acute lithium toxicity. *Clin. Neuropharmac.*, **8**, 379–81.

Cade, F.J.J. (1949) Lithium salts in the treatment of psychiatric excitement. *Med. J. Aust.*, **2**, 349–52.

Christiansen, C., Baastrup, P.C. and Transbol, I. (1976) Lithium hypercalcaemia, hypermagnesaemia and hyperparathyroidism. *Lancet*, **ii**, 969.

Clark, K.J. and Jefferson, J.W. (1987) Lithium allergy. *J. Clin. Psychopharmac.*, **7**, 287–9.

Coppen, A., Bishop, M., Bailey, J. *et al.* (1980) Renal function in lithium and non-lithium-treated patients with affective disorders. *Acta. Psychiat. Scand.*, **62**, 343–55.

Cowen, P.J. (1988) Depression resistant to tricyclic antidepressants. *Brit. Med. J.*, **297**, 435.

Edelfers, S. (1975) Distribution of sodium, potassium and lithium in the brain of lithium-treated rats. *Acta. Pharmacol. Toxicol.*, **37** (5), 387–8.

Garrod, A.B. (1873) Renal calculus, gravel and gouty deposits and the value of lithium salts in their treatment. *Med. Times and Gazette*, **83–4**, 216–17, 299–300.

Ghose, K. (1977) Lithium salts: therapeutic and unwanted effects. Br. J. Hosp. Med., **18**, 578–83.

Ghose, K. (1980) Interactions between lithium and carbamazepine. *Brit. Med. J.*, **1**, 1122.

Glue, P.J., Cowen, P.J., Nutt, T. *et al.* (1986) The effect of lithium on 5–HT-mediated neuroendocrine responses and platelet 5–HT receptors. *Psychopharmacol.*, **90**, 398–402.

Greil, W., Stoltzenburg, M.C., Mairhofer, M.L. and Haag, M. (1985) Lithium dosage in the elderly. A study with matched age groups. *J. Affect. Disorder*, **9**, 1–4.

Hardy, B.G., Shulman, K.I., Mackenzie, S.E. *et al.* (1987) Pharmacokinetics of lithium in the elderly. *J. Clin. Psychopharmac.*, **7**, 153–8.

Harrison-Read, P.E. (1981) Behavioural studies with lithium in rats: implications for animal models of mania and depression. In: *Neuroendocrine Regulation and Altered Behaviour* (eds. P.U. Hrdina and R.L. Singhal), Croom Helm, London.

Kudrow, L. (1976) Prophylactic lithium in the treatment of chronic cluster headaches. Presentation at the *18th Annual Meeting of the American Association for the Study of Headaches*, Dallas, Texas.

Miller, F., Menninger, J. and Whitcup, S.M. (1986) Lithium-neuroleptic neurotoxicity in the elderly bipolar patient. *J. Clin. Psychopharmacol.*, **6**, 176–8.

Neilsen-Kudsk, F. and Amidsen, A. (1979) Analysis of the pharmacokinetics of lithium in man. *Eur. J. Clin. Pharmacol.*, **16**, 271–7.

Perry, P.J., Denner, F.J., Hann, R.L. *et al.* (1981) Lithium kinetics in single daily dosage. *Acta. Psychiat. Scand.*, **64**, 281–94.

Petersen, V., Hvidt, S., Thomsen, K. and Schou, M. (1974) Effect of prolonged thiazide treatment on renal lithium clearance. *Br. Med. J.*, **3**, 143–5.

Phillips, J.D. and Birch, N.J. (1987) The effect of lithium formulations on peak serum concentrations. *Med. Sci. Res.*, **15**, 943–4.

Plenge, P., Mellerup, E.T., Bolwig, T.G. *et al.* (1982) Lithium treatment – does the kidney prefer one daily dose instead of two? *Acta. Psychiat. Scand.*, **66**, 121–8.

Ragheb, M. and Powell, R.L. (1986) Lithium interaction with sulindac and naproxen. *J. Clin. Psychopharmacol.*, **6**, 150–4.

Reiman, I.W. and Frolich, J.C. (1981) Effects of diclofenac on lithium kinetics. *Clin. Pharmacol. Ther.*, **30**, 348–52.

Roose, S.P., Bone, S., Haidorfer, C. *et al.* (1979) Lithium treatment in older patients. *Am. J. Ther.*, **136**, 843–4.

Saffer, D. and Coppen, A. (1983) Fusemide: a safe diuretic during lithium therapy. *J. Affect. Disord.*, **5**, 289–92.

Sansone, M.E. and Ziegler, D.K. (1985) Lithium toxicity: a review of neurologic complications. *Clin. Neuropharmac*, **8**, 242–8.

Shelley, R.K. and Silverstone, T. (1986) Single dose pharmacokinetics of 5 formulations of lithium: a controlled comparison in healthy subjects. *Int. Clin. Psychopharm.*, **1**, 324–31.

Smith, R.E. and Helms, P.M. (1982) Adverse effects of lithium therapy in acutely ill patients. *J. Clin. Psychiat.*, **43**, 94–9.

Tyrer, S. and Shopsin, B. (1980) Neural and neuromuscular side effects of lithium. In: *Handbook of Lithium Therapy* (ed. F.N. Johnson), MTP Press, Lancaster, pp. 289–309.

Vendsborg, P.B., Bech, P. and Rafaelsen, O.J. (1976) Lithium treatment and weight gain. *Acta. Pyschiat. Scand.*, **53**, 139–47.

Vestergaard, P. (1983) Clinically important side effects of long-term lithium treatment: a review. *Acta. Psychiat. Scand.*, **67**, 10–33.

Vestergaard, P., Amdisen, A. and Schou, M. (1980) Clinically significant side effects of lithium treatments. A survey of 237 patients in long-term treatment. *Acta. Psychiat. Scand.*, **62**, 193–200.

Worrall, E.P., Moody, J.P., Peet, M. *et al.* (1979) Controlled studies of the acute antidepressant effects of lithium. *Brit. J. Psychiat.*, **135**, 255–62.

Chapter Seven

Lithium in the prophylaxis of depressive illness in late life

KARABI GHOSE and ALEC COPPEN

CONTENTS

7.1 INTRODUCTION

Depression is one of the most common symptoms presented by the elderly (Kantor and Glassman, 1980). Depressive illness is a recurrent condition in 60% of cases and usually presents for the first time in the 40s. Depression in the older age group consists of patients whose illness arose earlier in life and persists until the older ages, and patients in whom depression presents for the first time in late life after 70.

Prognosis of depressive illness in late life is poor (Murphy, 1983), yet prophylactic drug therapy is not always considered for elderly patients suffering from recurrent episodes of depression. There are two main reasons for this. Firstly, until recently, elderly patients were systematically excluded from most drug trials. As a consequence, only a limited number of published reports are available on the role of prophylactic drug therapy in elderly patients suffering from recurrent episodes of depression. It is even more difficult to obtain published data on the tolerance and efficacy of lithium salts in the elderly. Secondly, the elderly tend to suffer from serious adverse effects more frequently and are known to be less tolerant to most psychotropic drugs (Thompson, Moran and Nies, 1983). Lithium therapy is associated with a number of metabolic and neuroendocrine abnormalities and is responsible for many side-effects (Ghose, 1977). Lithium is mainly excreted by the kidneys and it was thought to have a narrow therapeutic range. In view of age-related deterioration in renal functions, the risk of toxicity is likely to be greater in the elderly. However, the decision for any therapeutic intervention, particularly in this age group, is usually based on the balance of benefits against risks of a particular therapy. Lithium is an established prophylactic agent and has also been shown to reduce morbidity in elderly patients suffering from affective disorders. The incidence and severity of side-effects of lithium in the elderly are comparable to patients below the 60 years age group (Coppen, *et al.*, 1983). Old people therefore should not be denied an effective thera-peutic agent in anticipation of toxicity or serious side-effects, but close monitioring of such therapy in a hospital clinic should be provided and other appropriate precautions should be taken.

7.2 PROPHYLACTIC EFFECT OF LITHIUM IN UNIPOLAR DEPRESSION

7.2.1 Long-term prophylaxis

Baastrup and Schou (1967) first reported the prophylactic activity of lithium salts in patients with affective disorders. They studied 88 patients of whom 22 were suffering from uniploar depressive illness. In an open study, during one year's lithium therapy, the average number of depressive episodes was observed to be significantly less than the preceding year. Using this method ('before and after design'), both Hullin, McDonald and Allsopp (1972) and Angst, Weis and Grof (1973) observed similar beneficial results. These studies were later criticized as evaluations were not carried out in a double-blind situation.

Further evidence to support the prophylactic effect of lithium in recurrent episodes of depression came from Baastrup, Poulsen and Schou (1970). Thirty-four patients with unipolar depression received open lithium for at least one year. The patients were then randomly selected to receive either lithium or matched placebo for one year. In this 'double-blind discontinuation study', nine patients who received placebo relapsed within five months, but all lithium-treated patients remained well.

In 1971, Coppen *et al.* published the first prospective double-blind trial in which there was an 80% reduction in morbidity in patients given prophylactic lithium compared with patients treated with conventional *ad hoc* antidepressant or neuroleptic treatment. Fieve, Dunner and Kumbarachi (1975) followed up to 29 patients with unipolar depression for four years in a placebo controlled double-blind study. The mean number of depressions in the placebo group was 1.60, whereas this was only 0.59 in patients treated with lithium. Severity of depression was significantly less in the lithium-treated patients than in the placebo group.

7.2.2 Continuation therapy

In view of the high incidence of relapse, prophylactic drug therapy is usually considered after recovery from an acute episode in patients who have had at least two previous attacks. There is ample evidence that the incidence of relapse is high in this vulnerable group. Relapse sometimes occurred within a month after recovery from an acute attack in patients who were not prescribed an antidepressant drug as continuation therapy (Mindham, Howland and Shepherd, 1973; Coppen *et al.*, 1978a). Continuation therapy, usually for 6–12 months, is also indicated in patients recovering from an acute episode of depression (Coppen *et al.*, 1978a). In a retrospective study, lithium and tricyclic antidepressants were found to be equally effective in reducing subsequent relapse rates (Perry and Tsuang, 1979). Coppen and co-workers (Coppen *et al.*, 1981) made a double-blind parallel comparison on the effect of lithium as continuation therapy with matched placebo tablets. Thirty-eight patients who responded to electroconvulsive therapy (ECT) were randomly selected to receive one of these two treatments for one year. The lithium-treated group spent significantly less time with a relapse (1.7 weeks per year) than the placebo group (over 7.8 weeks). This difference was greater during the second six months of the study. Mean duration of relapses in the lithium group was only 0.2 weeks, whereas this was 5.6 weeks in the placebo group. Lithium is clearly an effective continuation therapy after recovery from the acute episode.

7.2.3 Lithium versus antidepressants

Long-term prophylactic effect of lithium has been shown to be either superior or equal to any antidepressant drug in a number of studies. Prien, Klett and Caffey (1973) found both lithium and imipramine superior to placebo in a double-blind study involving 78 unipolar patients with depression who received medication for two years. They observed no difference between lithium and imipramine. Quitkin,

Table 7.1 Prophylactic effect of lithium in unipolar depression

Study design	Investigators	Duration	Number	Outcome
'Before and after' design	Baastrup and Schou, (1967)	1 year	22	Relapse rate: 0.40 after lithium 1.56 before lithium
'Double-blind discontinuation'	Baastrup et al. (1970)	5 months	34	No relapse – lithium 9 relapse – placebo
Double-blind (prospective) study	Coppen et al. (1971)	2.25 years	27	Time spent with depression: 4.3% – lithium 30% – placebo
	Fieve et al. (1975)	4 years	29	Number with depression: 0.59 – lithium 1.60 – placebo
Comparison with a tri-cyclic antidepressant	Prien et al. (1973)	1 year	78	Lithium and imipramine better than placebo
	Quitkin et al. (1978)	1 year	27	Lithium, but not imipramine superior to placebo
	Coppen et al. (1976)	1 year	30	Lithium superior to maprotiline
	Coppen et al. (1978b)	1 year	32	Lithium superior to mianserin
	Glen (1981)	1 year		Lithium and amitriptyline superior to placebo

Rifkin and Kane (1978) studied 27 patients in an identical protocol. Contrary to Prien *et al.*'s study, they observed lithium, but not imipramine, better than placebo. In two further separate studies, prophylactic effects of lithium were observed to be superior to maprotiline and mianserin by Coppen's team (Coppen *et al.*, 1976; Coppen *et al.*, 1978b). Glen (1981) compared the effect of lithium with amitriptyline and placebo in a prospective study. His observations were similar to Prien *et al.*, that is, both lithium and amitriptyline-treated patients responded better than the placebo group. No difference between lithium and amitriptyline groups was observed.

Lithium, therefore, undoubtedly is a prophylactic agent and should be considered for patients with recurrent episodes of depression.

Table 7.1 summarizes the results of these various studies.

7.2.4 Therapeutic plasma level

Therapeutic plasma concentrations were previously considered to be between 0.8 and 1.2 mmol/l usually 12 h after a single slow-release or twice-daily oral preparation (Coppen *et al.*, 1971). However, in a prospective double-blind study, Coppen and colleagues (Coppen *et al.*, 1983) found that a 12 h plasma concentration of 0.5–0.7 mmol/l was more effective than the high doses. Benefits and side-effects profiles in patients over 60 years of age were similar to the younger patients. It is, therefore, suggested that lithium should be considered in the prophylactic therapy for recurrent episodes of depression in old age.

7.2.5 Side-effects

Lithium is known to produce many biochemical changes and is associated with many subjective side-effects. Symptoms such as thirst, tremor, dryness of mouth, weight gain and polyuria have been specifically related to lithium therapy. These are discussed in detail in Chapters 5 and 6.

7.3 PROPHYLACTIC LITHIUM IN THE ELDERLY

7.3.1 Efficacy during long-term therapy

At present there is no published report of any investigation designed to study the efficacy and tolerance of lithium in the elderly suffering from affective disorders. Prophylactic lithium therapy, however, once started, is usually indicated for an indefinite period, probably life-long unless the patient develops any specific problem. This therapy, in a stabilized patient aged 60 years or over, is usually continued by most clinicians. Once faces the dilemma of whether to initiate lithium therapy only when a patient presents with recurrent episodes of depression in late life.

In a lithium clinic at the Medical Research Council Neuropsychiatric Laboratories, Epsom, 49 male and 104 female patients with affective disorders were followed up for a period between 1 and 14.5 years (mean 4.9 years). They all received a slow-release tablet (lithium carbonate) at bedtime. Plasma lithium concentrations were maintained between 0.8 and 1.2 mmol/l 12 h after dosing. Prophylactic lithium therapy was started in 47 of these patients after 60 years of age. There was no significant difference in the affective morbidity index between the younger patients and these elderly subjects as shown in Table 7.2 (Abou-Saleh and Coppen, 1983a). Thus, elderly patients showed a very good response to lithium therapy that was at least as good as that observed in younger patients. Side-effects in the older group were similar to the younger patients.

Table 7.2 Affective morbidity index during lithium therapy in young and elderly patients (after Coppen and Abou-Saleh, 1983)

Age when lithium started (year)	Polarity unipolar (n)	bipolar (n)	*Episodes before lithium (year)	*Years on lithium	*Affective morbidity index
Less than 40	17	5	4.4	5.3	0.14
40–59.9	58	21	4.2	5.5	0.17
60 and above	42	5	4.9	3.8	0.18

* Mean values are shown.

7.3.2 Lower dosage regime started in late life

In a further study, 22 elderly patients (over 60 years of age) who started lithium in late life received a 25–50% reduction in lithium dosage in a double-blind situation (Coppen *et al.*, 1983). A significant reduction in side-effects without any deterioration in affective morbidity index in these patients was observed. Response to lithium therapy over one year showed a relationship with the Newcastle scores. The patients classified on this scale as endogenous had the best response to lithium. Endogenous depressive illness is an illness of middle and old age (Abou-Saleh and Coppen, 1983b). Lithium therapy is clearly indicated in these patients.

7.3.3 Special problems

Lithium carbonate is a water-soluble compound which is excreted mainly by the kidneys and it produces a negative sodium balance. In view of age-related deterioration in renal functions (Greenblatt *et al.,* 1982), the elderly are likely to be more sensitive to lithium therapy. That is, they will require, in theory, lower dosage than the younger patients and are under greater risk of developing toxicity. The incidence of thyroid disorders is also higher in old people. It is therefore advised to assess renal and thyroid functions prior to initiation of therapy. Patients should be closely monitored in a clinic even when their conditions are apparently stable. The dose of lithium may require further adjustment (reduction) in patients who were previously stabilized, particularly during an attack of infection. Elderly patients are known sufferers of a number of neurological conditions, including cerebrovascular episodes and Parkinsonism. They may also require concurrently other drugs acting on the central nervous system or a thiazide diuretic. Consequently, these patients are vulnerable to lithium toxicity. It is possible to detect signs of side-effects or toxicity in an elderly patient at an early stage and the importance of regular supervision in a clinic cannot be overemphasized.

The need for additional supportive therapy in some patients with thyroid or renal disorders should also be closely monitored.

7.4 GUIDANCE FOR LITHIUM THERAPY IN DEPRESSIVE ILLNESS

7.4.1 Indications for lithium therapy

As discussed above, patients with recurrent episodes (three or more) of depression are likely to benefit from lithium therapy. This was extensively discussed by Angst (1981). He examined numerous criteria to identify those patients at risk. He concluded that if a patient, in addition to the present attack, had had one episode or more in the previous five years, it is likely that he will suffer from two further attacks in the following five years. According to his observations at least 40% of unipolar patients would require prophylactic therapy. More than one episode of depression in the previous year is clearly a strong indication for prophylactic lithium therapy.

7.4.2 Dosage regimes

Lithium should be administered once daily (usually in the evening) as a slow-release preparation. There is no standard dose. The required dose is that which achieves a steady state 12 h plasma concentration of about 0.5 mmol/l. This is usually 200–600 mg in the older age group. This drug therefore has a very narrow therapeutic window.

Previously, therapeutic plasma levels were considered to be between 0.8 and 1.2 mmol/l which was associated with a high incidence of side-effects (Ghose, 1977). In addition to Coppen *et al.*'s (1983) study, as mentioned above, a number of other investigations now also suggest that the prophylactic effect of lithium can be achieved at lower dosage levels (Jerram and McDonald, 1978; Sashidhoran, McGuire and Glen, 1982). In a double-blind study where the affective morbidity index and side-effects of 72 patients were studied, the patients were randomly selected to continue either with their usual dose of lithium or to receive a 25% or 50% reduction in lithium dosage (Coppen, Abou-Saleh, Milln *et al.*, 1983). The patients who underwent dosage reduction had lower plasma lithium levels (0.5–0.8 mmol/l). No change in affective morbidity index was observed in patients with lower plasma levels, but the incidence of side-effects was less in these patients as shown in Table 7.3.

Table 7.3 Affective morbidity and side-effects of patients during lithium therapy (mean values are shown)

Age (year)	n	Affective morbidity Index	Beck	Side-effects
Less than 60	61	0.16	6.3	8.8
60–69.9	51	0.14	5.8	8.7
70 and above	16	0.06	6.9	7.6

7.4.3 Response to therapy

The relationship between response to therapy and various factors such as sex, age at start of lithium therapy, age at onset of affective disorders, duration of lithium therapy, number of previous episodes, family history and red blood cell (intracellular) lithium concentrations was extensively studied by a number of investigators. None of these factors appear to influence the outcome of therapy (Coppen, Metcalfe and Bailey, 1979). Poor response correlated with neuroticism, as measured by the Eysenck Personality Inventory (Eysenck and Eysenck, 1964). The patients with neurotic depression had a worse prognosis than those suffering from endogenous depression on the Newcastle Scale (Carney, Roth and Garside, 1965).

More recently, addition of folic acid (200 μg per day) has been shown to enhance lithium prophylaxis (Coppen, Chaudhury and Swade, 1986). The patients with highest plasma folate concentrations showed a significant reduction in their affective morbidity and patients who had their plasma folate increased to 13 ng/ml or above had a 40% reduction in their affective morbidity. Coppen *et al.*, therefore, suggested folic acid supplementation to patients receiving long-term lithium therapy. This is probably more applicable to elderly patients as many of them tend to have folate deficiency (probably related to poor diet).

7.4.4 Duration of therapy

As discussed above, prophylactic lithium therapy is indicated in patients with recurrent (three or more) episodes of depression. Although no published data is available regarding duration of therapy in elderly patients, prophylactic therapy is in general required for this vulnerable group who respond to lithium for an indefinite period. In the case of elderly patients who have developed several neurological disorders or other multiple problems, it is advisable to stop lithium therapy. Such a decision should ideally be made on the basis of a patient's general condition, other associated illnesses and concomitant medication, rather than by his chronological age.

7.4.5 The lithium clinic

The lithium clinic plays an important role in the prophylaxis of affective disorders. Obviously, the main functions of the clinic are to monitor plasma lithium levels, assess mental state, evaluate side-effects and identify early signs of toxicity. At the Medical Research Council Neuropsychiatry Laboratory, a standardized chart is used to record plasma lithium levels and mental state, as assessed by a four-point scale. From this chart, yearly affective morbidity index (AMI) can be calculated by the area above the baseline (0 morbidity). Side-effects are usually monitored by administering a self-administered standardized check-list containing 37 questions (Ghose, 1977).

It should be emphasized that these patients are suffering from a chronic recurrent illness characterized by spontaneous remissions and relapses. It is therefore necessary to motivate and educate them to continue their prophylactic medication regularly even during the periods when they are keeping apparently well. This can best be achieved with the help of trained staff in a regular clinic.

The patients should be instructed to take their medication at a particular time of day, preferably at night, thus building up this habit as a part of daily routine. They should be provided with an information booklet on lithium and asked to carry a card and remind all attending doctors regarding this medication. The clinic environment should be such that patients will be encouraged to come back to the clinic or telephone (during working hours) for advice if they encounter any problem or develop early symptoms of toxicity. The clinic also serves the purpose of group therapy.

Facilities for lithium estimates in the clinic can provide instant feedback to the patients of their lithium status, which encourages compliance. The clinician has the opportunity to follow up these high-risk patients and to detect early signs of lithium toxicity or the recurrence of illness at an early stage.

7.4.6 Community support

In addition to the lithium clinic, regular community support is required for elderly patients. The patients in this age group are likely to suffer from many other physical illnesses which may require them to take other medication. Lithium is known to interact with a number of drugs. They are also likely to develop toxicity following a slight change in their renal functions and electrolyte status by other concomitant medication or infection. They are also likely to be more forgetful than the younger generation. Physically, many of them may be too frail to attend a clinic regularly.

The elderly patients on long-term lithium therapy, therefore, should be closely supervised in the community. This can be provided, depending on a patient's situation and mental state, by regular visits (daily to fortnightly) from a district nurse or a health visitor. Lithium should never be prescribed first time for an elderly patient who lives alone, without facilities of supervision.

7.5 CONCLUSION

There is now good evidence that prophylactic lithium is effective in unipolar and in bipolar patients over 70 years old. The effective dosage of slow-release lithium carbonate given once a day is that which will produce a plasma concentration of 0.5 mmol/l 12 h after the dose. The dose usually varies between 200 and 600 mg daily. With such a dosage regime subjective side-effects and thyroid interaction are very low. However, as with all long-term medication in older people regular clinical assessments should be made and the patient's plasma lithium concentration should be checked, both to avoid overdosage and to encourage compliance.

REFERENCES

Abou-Saleh, M.T. and Coppen, A. (1983). Subjective side-effects of amitriptyline and lithium in affective disorders. *Br. J. Psychiat.*, **142**, 527–8.

Abou-Saleh, M.T. and Coppen, A. (1983b) Classification of depression and response to antidepressive therapies. *Br. J. Psychiat.*, **143**, 601–3.

Angst, J., Weis, P. and Grof, P. (1970) Lithium prophylaxis in recurrent affective disorders. *Br. J. Psychiat.*, **116**, 604–14.

Angst, J. (1981) Clinical indications for a prophylactic treatment of depression. *Adv. Biol. Psychiat.*, **7**, 218–29.

Baastrup, P. and Schou, M. (1967) Lithium as a prophylactic agent: its effect against recurrent depressions and manic-depressive psychosis. *Arch. Gen. Psychiat.*, **16**, 162–72.

Baastrup, P., Poulsen, J.C. and Schou, M. (1970) Prophylactic lithium. Double-blind discontinuation in manic depressive and recurrent depressive disorders. *Lancet*, **ii**, 326–30.

Carney, M.H.P., Roth, M. and Garside, R.F. (1965) The diagnosis of depressive syndromes and the prediction of ECT response. *Br. J. Psychiat.*, **111**, 659–74.

Coppen, A. and Abou-Saleh, M.T. (1983) Lithium in the prophylaxis of unipolar depression. *J. Roy. Soc. Med.*, **76**, 297–301.

Coppen, A., Abou-Saleh, M.T., Milln, P. *et al.* (1981) Lithium continuation therapy following ECT. *Br. J. Psychiat.*, **139**, 284–7.

Coppen, A., Abou-Saleh, M.T., Milln, P. *et al.* (1983) Decreasing lithium dosage reduces morbidity and side-effects during prophylaxis. *J. Affect. Disord.*, **5**, 353–62.

Coppen, A., Chaudhury, S. and Swade, C. (1986) Folic acid enhances lithium prophylaxis. *J. Affect. Disord.*, **10**, 9–13.

Coppen, A., Ghose, K., Montgomery, S. *et al.* (1978a) Continuation therapy with amitriptyline in depression. *Brit. J. Psychiat.*, **133**, 28–33.

Coppen, A., Ghose, K., Rao, V.A.R. *et al.* (1978b) Mianserin and lithium in the prophylaxis of depression. *Br. J. Psychiat.*, **133**, 206–10.

Coppen, A., Metcalfe, M. and Bailey, J. (1979) Lithium prophylactic therapy in unipolar depression and some possible prognostigators of response. In: *Lithium Controversies and Unresolved Issues* (eds. T.B. Cooper, S. Gershon, N.S. Kline and M. Scholl), Excerpta Medica, Amsterdam, pp. 401–12.

Coppen, A., Montgomery, S.A., Gupta, R.K. and Bailey, J. (1976) A double-blind comparison of lithium carbonate and maprotiline in the prophylaxis of affective disorders. *Br. J. Psychiat.*, **128**, 479–85.

Coppen, A., Noguera, R., Bailey, J. *et al.* (1971) Prophylactic lithium in affective disorders – controlled trial. Lancet, **ii**, 275–9.

Eysenck, H.J. and Eysenck, S.B.G. (1964) *Manual of Eysenck Personality Inventory*, University of London Press, London.

Fieve, R.R., Dunner, D.L. and Kumbarachi, T. (1975) Lithium carbonate in affective disorders. *Arch. Gen. Psychiat.*, **32**, 1541–4.

Ghose, K. (1977) Lithium salts: therapeutic and unwanted effects. *Br. J. Hosp. Med.*, **18**, 578–83.

Glen, A. (1981) Lithium and antidepressants in the prophylaxis of depression. *Adv. Biol. Pyschiat.*, **7**, 208–17.

Greenblatt, D.J., Divoli, M., Abernethy, D.R. and Shader, R.I. (1982) Physiologic change in old age: relation to altered drug disposition. *J. Am. Geriat. Soc.*, **30**, (Suppl.) S6–S10.

Hullin, R.P., McDonald, R. and Allsopp, M.N.E. (1972) Prophylactic lithium in recurrent affective disorders. *Lancet*, **i**, 1044–6.

Jerram, T.C. and McDonald, R. (1978) Plasma lithium control with particular reference to minimum effective levels. In: *Lithium in Medical Practice* (eds. F.N. Johnson and S. Johnson), MTP Press, Lancaster, pp. 407–13.

Kantor, S.J. and Glassman, A.H. (1980) In: *Psychopharmacology of Ageing* (eds. C. Eisdorfer and W.E. Fann), MTP Press, Lancaster, pp. 99–117.

Mindham, R.H.S., Howland, C. and Shepherd, M. (1973) An evaluation of continuation therapy with tricyclic antidepressants in depressive illness. *Psychological Medicine*, **3**, 5–17.

Murphy, E. (1983) The prognosis of depression in old age. *Br. J. Psychiat.*, **142**, 111–13.

Perry, P.J. and Tsuang, M.T. (1979) Treatment of unipolar depression following electroconvulsive therapy: relapse rate comparisons between lithium and tricyclic therapies following ECT. *J. Affect. Disord.*, **1**, 123–9.

Prien, R.F., Klett, C.J. and Caffey, E.M. (1973) Lithium carbonate and imipramine prevention of affective psychoses. *Arch. Gen. Psychiat.*, **29**, 303–13.

Quitkin, F., Rifkin, A. and Kane, J. (1978) Prophylactic effect of lithium and imipramine in unipolar and bipolar II patients: a preliminary report. *Am. J. Psychiat.*, **133**, 570–2.

Sashidhoran, B., McGuire, R.J. and Glen, A.I.M. (1982) Plasma lithium levels and therapeutic outcome in the prophylaxis of affective disorders: a retrospective study. *Br. J. Psychiat.*, **140**, 619–22.

Thompson, T.L., Moran, M.G. and Nies, A.S. (1983) Psychotropic drug use in the elderly (parts 1 and 2). *N. Eng. J. Med.*, **308**, 134–8; 194–9.

THREE

Tricyclic and Related Antidepressants

Chapter Eight

Pharmacokinetics of tricyclic and related antidepressants

PETER CROME and SHEILA DAWLING

CONTENTS

8.1 INTRODUCTION

The last decade has seen growing concern over the use of medication in the elderly. Many drugs, including some antidepressants (nomifensine and zimeldine), have been introduced only to be withdrawn shortly afterwards because of side-effects. Although in the case of these antidepressants aged-related changes in pharmacokinetics were not the reason for their withdrawal, it has become clear that with increasing years the body's ability to handle drugs declines and this has important implications both for therapeutic efficacy and for side-effects.

8.2 PHARMACOKINETICS: GENERAL CONSIDERATIONS

The term pharmacokinetics is used, as the name suggests, to describe the way in which drugs are handled by the body. A number of

Table 8.1 Physiological changes with ageing which affect pharmacokinetics

Pharmacokinetic process	*Physiological change*
Absorption	Reduction in gastric acid production
	Reduction in gastrointestinal motility
	Reduction in gastrointestinal blood flow
	Reduction in absorptive surface
Distribution	Increase in proportion of body fat
	Decrease in proportion of body water
	Decrease in plasma albumin
	Increase in alpha 1–acid glycoprotein
Metabolism	Reduction in liver size
	Reduction in liver blood flow
	Reduction in hepatic metabolic capacity
Excretion	Reduction in glomerular filtration
	Reduction in renal tubular function

physiological changes take place with age which in turn may influence the various factors – absorption, distribution, metabolism and excretion (Table 8.1) which determine a drug's pharmacokinetic profile. Additionally, a number of disease states, common in old age and often associated with depression, may affect the various processes described below.

8.2.1 Absorption

The most important route of administration for drugs is by mouth. Age-related changes taking place in the gastrointestinal tract include elevation of gastric pH and reduction of gastrointestinal motility, gut blood flow and absorptive surface. These changes might be expected to result in reduced absorption of drugs but in practice this is rarely so and most drugs are absorbed to the same extent and at the same rate in the elderly as in younger subjects. Where changes have been reported they are usually considered to be of little clinical significance. This is also true of the antidepressants. Although peak blood concentrations in elderly people may be higher, at steady state this has little overall effect because most of the body load of drug is in the tissues. Co-administration of drugs which alter gut motility can affect absorption (anticholinergics, narcotics, laxatives, etc.). The anticholinergic effects of tricyclic anti-depressants can of course affect absorption of other co-prescribed drugs.

Following absorption of the drug from the gut a proportion may be deactivated during its passage through the liver before it reaches the systemic circulation (first-pass effect) (Rawlins *et al.*, 1987). This first-pass effect may be much reduced in the elderly. Thus Castleden and George (1979) found that propanolol concentrations were two and a half times higher following oral administration of the drug in elderly subjects compared to younger ones.

8.2.2 Distribution

Body mass declines with age, so that as a general rule in the elderly a smaller dose of drug would be expected to give the same tissue concentration. The proportion of adipose tissue increases whilst body water declines. As a consequence, for water-soluble drugs, plasma concentrations will be higher and the effect may be greater. On the other hand, for fat-soluble drugs (including the antidepressants) plasma concentrations will be lower.

Most studies have shown a decline in plasma albumin with age. This can result in an increased free concentration of acidic drugs which are bound to plasma albumin, and an enhanced effect. On the other hand basic drugs including some antidepressants are bound to alpha 1–acid glycoprotein. This protein is raised in a variety of disease states thus increasing plasma concentrations of the drug. A smaller proportion of free drug might be expected to decrease pharmacological effect but on the other hand there is also less drug available for metabolism. The clinical consequences of altered protein binding are not thought to be particularly significant (Curry, 1980).

8.2.3 Metabolism

Drugs which are metabolized in the liver fall into two main categories. Firstly, there are drugs with a high hepatic excretion ratio whose metabolism is largely dependent on liver blood flow. Since this falls with age, and may also be affected by drugs which are commonly given to the elderly (e.g. propranolol), clearance of these highly extracted drugs is reduced. The other main group of drugs are those with low extraction ratios where clearance is more dependent on drug-metabolizing capacity. This group can again be divided into two. For Phase 1 reactions which include oxidation, reduction and hydrolysis there is often but by no means invariably a reduction in metabolic capacity in the elderly. For Phase 2 reactions involving conjugation, often with sulphate or glucuronide, the results have usually shown there to be no age-related changes in pharmacokinetics.

8.2.4 Excretion

Glomerular filtration rate falls by about half in old age. Drugs which are

Table 8.2 Summary of studies of tricyclic antidepressant pharmacokinetics in young and elderly people

Drug	Group half-life (hours) Mean (range)		Group clearance (l/h) Mean (range)		Steady state concentration	References
	Young	Elderly	Young	Elderly		
Amitriptyline	22 (18–30)[12]	37 (21–61)[14]	79 (61–105)[12]	15 (12–21)[14]	Higher[6,8,21]	
	16 (10–27)[23]	22 (17–24)[23]	55 (36–72)[23]	47 (26–65)[23]		
	35 (17–84)[9]		71 (16–155)[9]			
Nortriptyline	26 (14–51)[11]	45 (24–79)[11]	54 (16–115)[11]	20 (8–39)[11]	Higher[6,21]	
	46 (22–88)[5]	37 (23–59)[24]	26 (8–56)[5]	37 (18–67)[24]		
	27 (18–35)[3]		44 (28–69)[3]			
	44 (18–93)[4]		46 (14–100)[4]			
Imipramine	28 (19–34)[22]	26 (21–35)[15]	96 (40–172)[22]	21 (17–28)[15]	Higher[21]	
	19 (not given)[21]	24 (not given)[21]				
	13 (8–16)[13]		63 (42–102)[13]			
Desipramine	34 (not given)[21]	76 (not given)[21]			Higher[21]	
	17 (14–25)[4]		108 (63–177)[4]			

References:

1 Abernethy and Todd, 1986
2 Abernethy et al., 1984
3 Alexanderson, 1972
4 Alexanderson, 1973
5 Braithwaite et al., 1978
6 Carr and Hobson, 1977
7 Crampton et al., 1980
8 Dawling, 1982
9 Dawling et al., 1979
10 Dawling et al., 1980a
11 Dawling et al., 1980b
12 Garland et al., 1978

Drug				
	20 (12–30)[22]	69 (46–95)[22]		
	22 (14–35)[25]	141 (90–169)[25]		
Doxepin	17 (8–25)[28]	340 (127–701)[28]		
	13 (7–23)[1]	264 (72–600)[1]		
Dothiepin	22 (14–40)[19]	96 (62–126)[19]		
	19 (not given)[26]	139 (not given)[26]		
	24 (21–30)[7]	56 (22–90)[7]		
Maprotiline	39 (18–75)[9]	62 (25–130)[9]	32 (21–52)[15]	25 (17–31)[15]	Higher[16]
	30 (29–32)[17]	39 (32–51)[17]		
	46 (20–79)[18]	65 (21–121)[18]		
Clomipramine	36 (22–84)[10]	73 (23–122)[10]		
Protriptyline	78 (54–198)[20]	16 (8–24)[20]		
	74 (54–91)[27]	23 (11–35)[27]		
Trimipramine	24 (16–39)[2]	62 (37–98)[2]		

13 Gram and Christiansen, 1975
14 Henry et al., 1981
15 Hrdina et al., 1980
16 John et al., 1980
17 Jones and Luscombe, 1976
18 Maguire et al., 1980
19 Maguire et al., 1981
20 Moody et al., 1977
21 Nies et al., 1977
22 Potter et al., 1980
23 Schulz et al., 1983
24 Turbott et al., 1980
25 de Vane et al., 1981
26 Yu et al., 1986
27 Ziegler et al., 1978a
28 Ziegler et al., 1978b

detoxified by renal elimination have almost invariably been found to be excreted more slowly in the elderly than in younger individuals. This is perhaps the most consistent change which is found when investigating drugs in the elderly.

For a more extensive review of the pharmacokinetic changes with ageing see Swift and Triggs (1987).

8.3 PHARMACOKINETICS: CONSEQUENCES FOR PRESCRIBING

Of the various pharmacokinetic measurements, knowledge of any age-related changes in half-life and clearance are the two most useful when it comes to prescribing drugs. If the half-life is prolonged then it will take longer to reach steady state and longer for any side-effects to wear off when the drug is withdrawn. As a general rule drugs have to be given for four to five half-lives before steady state is reached. This also applies to any change in dosing so that in elderly patients one might have to wait longer before measuring plasma concentrations to see whether they are in the 'therapeutic' range.

The clearance of the drug is the sole physiological determinant of the steady state plasma concentration, the two being related by the formula:

$$\text{Steady state concentration} = \frac{\text{Dose}}{\text{Dosing Interval}} \times \frac{1}{\text{Clearance}}$$

Thus if clearance is halved, the steady-state concentration will be doubled. Furthermore, clearance itself may be altered by changes in half-life or distribution volume according to the formula:

$$\text{Clearance} = 0.693 \times \text{Distribution volume/Half-life}$$

Thus a drug clearance measurement takes into account all the above processes and is a measure of an individual's 'exposure' to the compound following a given dose.

8.4 TRICYCLIC ANTIDEPRESSANTS

8.4.1 Pharmacokinetics of individual tricyclic antidepressants

There are many different tricyclic antidepressants now on the market throughout the world. Not all of these are available in every country and this review is restricted to those which can be prescribed in the United Kingdom. Of these amitriptyline, imipramine, nortriptyline and desipramine have been investigated most thoroughly, whilst for other drugs information is limited. A comparison of the pharmacokinetics of individual drugs in young and elderly subjects is presented in Table 8.2. The general conclusion from these studies is that half-life is increased, clearance is reduced and steady state concentrations are higher in the elderly. Superimposed on this general reduction in metabolism is a much greater variability amongst individual elderly people.

8.4.2 Pharmacokinetic drug interactions

An underlying problem in the evaluation of pharmacokinetic data with tricyclic antidepressants is that many studies are carried out in healthy, normal subjects. By contrast, these drugs are prescribed in clinical practice to people who are suffering from depression and who may be additionally receiving medication for other disorders. This can have important consequences as a number of drugs have been shown to affect the pharmacokinetics of tricyclic antidepressants.

The metabolism of tricyclic antidepressants takes place almost exclusively in the liver. These drugs have high excretion ratios and their rates of metabolism are thus dependent on hepatic blood flow. Cardiac output, which is generally already lowered in the elderly, can be further reduced by drug administration e.g. betablockers. Thus Tollefson and Lesar (1984) have shown that maprotiline metabolism is inhibited by co-administration of propranolol. Other drugs inhibit cytochrome P450 activity, the enzyme system responsible for tricyclic antidepressant metabolism. Neuroleptics (chlorpromazine, haloperidol and perphenazine) reduce the rate of metabolism of imipramine, desipramine and nortriptyline as shown by rising plasma drug concentrations on addition of one of these compounds (Gram, 1975; Gram and Overø, 1972). The hydroxylation of imipramine, desipramine and nortriptyline can be inhibited by cimetidine, although a similar drug, ranitidine, has no effect (Hessauer and Hollister, 1984; Spina and Koike, 1986; Miller, Sawyer and Duffy, 1983). Desipramine and nortriptyline half-lives are increased and clearances lowered by co-administration of quinidine (Ayesh *et al.*, 1988), while disulfiram has a similar effect on imipramine and desipramine kinetics (Ciraulo, Barnill and Boxenbaum, 1985). This enzyme system may also be induced, for example, co-administration of anticonvulsants and barbiturates has been shown to increase the rate of metabolism of imipramine and nortriptyline, resulting in lower blood drug concentrations (Ballinger, *et al.*, 1974; Braithwaite, Flanagan and Richens, 1975; Perucca and Richens, 1977).

8.4.3 Protein binding

Tricyclic antidepressant drugs bind to a number of different plasma proteins – albumin, lipoproteins and alpha 1–acid glycoprotein (AGP). The relative importance of these binding proteins varies with the specific drug involved. They are, however, all very highly bound (often 95%), and although there is a 2–4 fold variation in free fraction amongst individuals, this is insignificant compared to the variation in steady state concentrations which can be as high as 40–fold (Bertilsson *et al.*, 1979; Bickel, 1975; Breyer-Pfaff *et al.*, 1982; Piafsky and Borgå, 1977).

Unlike albumin and lipoproteins, AGP is an acute phase reactant protein and its concentration can alter markedly over a short space of time: AGP rises in some short-term and long-term inflammatory diseases, malignancy, stress and in various haematological conditions. By contrast, AGP concentrations are low in hepatic disease, nephrotic syndrome and malnutrition. These are not uncommon conditions in elderly people.

Piafsky and Borgå (1977) have shown that the extent of imipramine binding correlates with the plasma AGP concentration. Inflammatory disease and other conditions which result in raised AGP levels give higher circulating concentrations of imipramine, amitriptyline and nortriptyline, as would be predicted from this relationship, bearing in mind that only free drug is available for metabolism (Dawling *et al.*, 1984; Kragh-Sørensen and Larsen, 1980; Piafsky and Borgå, 1977). However, it is only the free drug which is pharmacologically active, and since higher total drug concentrations are accompanied by a higher bound fraction the net effect at receptor level of rising AGP concentrations may not in practice be significant.

In a study of healthy elderly people, Schulz *et al.* (1983) were unable to detect any abnormality in amitriptyline binding. Braithwaite, Heard and Snape (1978) have shown that maprotiline binding, although more variable than in the young, was not grossly altered in elderly hospital patients, but the binding of this drug correlated with the albumin concentration rather than with AGP. Although plasma proteins are known to be abnormal in (chronic) renal failure, Lynn *et al.* (1981) duplicated these findings with maprotiline and Reidenberg (1977) found desipramine binding to be normal in uraemic serum. On the basis of these findings, impaired renal function in the elderly is unlikely to be an important determinant of tricyclic antidepressant binding, although the significance of other effects of renal function on metabolism are discussed later (8.4.4).

8.4.4 Accumulation of active metabolites

A complicating factor in assessing the various age-related changes in pharmacokinetics of tricyclic antidepressants is that many of them produce one or more active metabolites (demethylated and hydroxylated). The majority of studies outlined in Table 8.2 have been confined to examining the kinetics of the parent compound only. However, since the active demethylated metabolites of imipramine and amitriptyline (desipramine and nortriptyline respectively) are also antidepressants they have been studied in their own right and some useful generalizations emerge. An important observation is that the half-lives of the secondary amine compounds usually exceed those of the parent tertiary amine drug. This means that during treatment it will take longer for nortriptyline and desipramine concentrations to attain their steady states on dosage alteration, although it does not necessarily follow that the final concentration of metabolite will be higher in absolute terms. This is a particularly notable feature of clomipramine treatment where plasma concentrations of desmethylclomipramine were reported to be rising in some patients even after four weeks of maintenance dosing (Mellström and Tybring, 1977; Montgomery *et al.*, 1980). The tendency must be for this effect to be more pronounced in the elderly who already have extended tricyclic antidepressant half-lives compared to younger people.

Investigations have consistently shown that elderly people demethylate amitriptyline and imipramine more slowly than those who are younger (Dawling, 1982; Henry *et al.*, 1981; Hrdina *et al.*, 1980; Roy and Dawling, 1987). This means that the steady state ratio of plasma nortriptyline to amitriptyline concentration (known as the demethylation factor – DMF) is lower in the elderly. The significance of this finding for the clinical effects of drug treatment however remains controversial. While Jungkunz and Kus (1980) contend that a lower DMF is detrimental to improvement, Coppen and Rama Rao (1979) indicate a negative trend of DMF with response. Although this conflict may be partly attributed to differences in drug concentrations in the studies, the significance of the DMF in the incidence of drug-induced side-effects remains to be investigated.

In recent years much interest has focussed on the hydroxylated metabolites. They have been found to have antidepressant activity of similar potency (although not necessarily the same specificity of action) to their parent tricyclic compounds (Bertilsson, Mellström and Sjöqvist, 1979; Heikkila, Goldfinger and Orlansky, 1976; Potter *et al.*, 1979).

Investigations show the hydroxylated metabolites to be present at similar concentrations to the tricyclic antidepressants and the available evidence suggests that they also exert toxic effects, particularly cardio-toxicity (Brøsen *et al.*, 1986; Jandhyala *et al.*, 1977; Linnoila *et al.*, 1982; Young *et al.*, 1985).

Plasma concentrations of 10–hydroxynortriptyline were found by Young *et al.* (1984) to be twice as high at steady state in the elderly as in a younger group of patients. The ratio of 2–hydroxydesipramine to desipramine concentration has also been shown to be elevated in elderly people (Kitanaka *et al.*, 1982), while Bertilsson *et al.* (1979) were able to demonstrate a positive correlation between the steady state ratio of 10–hydroxynortriptyline to nortriptyline concentration, and age. The circulating concentration of the hydroxylated metabolites obviously depends on their rate of formation as well as their elimination rate. The first aspect of this has already been discussed in section 8.4.2 under the heading 'Pharmacokinetic drug interactions'. Because of their water-solubility compared to their parent compounds, the hydroxylated metabolites are excreted in the urine, partly in unchanged form, whilst the majority (> 80%) undergoes conjugation prior to excretion. The importance of this pathway in the elderly is that the rate of excretion of these metabolites may be expected to relate to renal function, which is of course impaired with advancing age. Kitanaka *et al.* (1982) have shown that renal clearance of 2–hydroxydesipramine does decrease with age and Young *et al.* (1984) have demonstrated a weak positive correlation of 10–hydroxynortriptyline/nortriptyline concentration at steady state with serum creatinine measurements. Studies in chronic renal failure have shown that at steady state, concentrations of amitriptyline, imipramine and desipramine are not abnormal, concentrations of their hydroxylated metabolites being higher and subject to greater variability than in healthy individuals (Lieberman *et al.*, 1985). Dawling *et al.* (1982) have shown single-dose nortriptyline half-life to be unaffected by chronic renal failure, but the half-life of 10–hydroxynortriptyline to be increased (mean 26 h in healthy volunteers, 47 h in chronic renal failure treated with haemodialysis and 113 h in chronic renal failure managed conservatively). These findings may help to explain the susceptibility of the elderly to the side-effects of tricyclic antidepressants and demonstrate the inadequacy of therapeutic drug monitoring programmes which do not incorporate measurement of all the active metabolites.

8.4.5 Individualization of drug dosage regime

Knowledge of single-dose pharmacokinetics has been used to predict doses necessary to produce target steady state concentrations. The rationale for this is firstly that there is some evidence to show that there is a 'therapeutic range' of plasma tricyclic antidepressant concentrations which give maximal clinical response, and secondly to avoid high plasma concentrations and toxic side-effects (Dawling, 1982).

As described earlier, the single-dose clearance is a measurement of the individual's metabolic capacity which accommodates all the variables discussed above – drug interactions, protein binding, renal function, demethylation and hydroxylation rates, etc. Investigations of single-dose pharmacokinetics followed by multiple dosing regimes in the same subjects demonstrated a strong correlation between the single-dose clearance and the steady state ultimately achieved for a number of tricyclic antidepressants – nortriptyline (Braithwaite, Montgomery and Dawling, 1978; Perry *et al.*, 1984), amitriptyline and maprotiline (Dawling *et al.*, 1979), imipramine and desipramine (Potter *et al.*, 1980). Further inspection showed that a much simpler measurement (a single carefully-timed plasma drug concentration estimation) could produce an equally reliable relationship (Braithwaite, Montgomery and Dawling, 1978; Brunswick *et al.*, 1979; Perry *et al.*, 1984). The practicality of these relationships has been tested prospectively by selecting an individual's dose based on either their single-dose drug clearance or the value of a single timed measurement following a single test-dose of the drug. These studies have been very successful. Based on an amitriptyline plus nortriptyline measurement 18 h after a test dose of amitriptyline, Madaksira and Khazanie (1985) were able to get 90% of their patients within their target range, while Roy and Dawling (1987) using a 24 h measurement, had an 87% success rate. Nelson, Jatlow and Mazure (1987) used a 24 h desipramine estimation following a desipramine test dose to produce a 90% success rate, compared to 23% on a fixed standard dose.

There are a number of equally successful studies in the elderly. Dawling *et al.* (1980) used the single-dose nortriptyline clearance to individualize dosage regimes in elderly hospitalized patients. A mean dose of 43 mg (range 20–90 mg) gave a mean steady state nortriptyline concentration of 106 µg/l with 75% of patients within the 50–150 µg/l target range. The authors calculated that use of a standard 75 mg dose in these patients would have resulted in a mean steady state concentration of 206 µg/l with 25% of patients having toxic blood concentrations above 300 µg/l. Later Dawling *et al.* (1981) used a 24 h nortriptyline concentration, giving a 90% success rate. Once again the mean daily dose required was low, at 50 mg. A 24 h amitriptyline plus nortriptyline measurement was used by Dawling *et al.* (1984) to select individualized doses of amitriptyline in elderly depressed patients. Using a mean daily dose of 60 mg these authors managed to achieve target steady state concentrations in every one of the patients studied.

Such tests obviously have significant practical advantages over previous methods of aiming at 'therapeutic' blood concentrations. However, they do rest on one important assumption – namely that the pharmacokinetics of tricyclic antidepressants are linear within any one individual, i.e. that they do not vary with the dose given. Some evidence is accumulating which challenges the validity of this assumption. All the available data for amitriptyline and nortriptyline uphold the assumption of linear pharmacokinetics, in studies which cover a wide range of observed plasma drug concentrations and include both young and elderly patients (Dawling, 1982; Kragh-Sørensen and Larsen, 1980). Yu *et al.* (1986) have demonstrated linear pharmacokinetics of dothiepin and its metabolites in a study giving increasingly larger single doses (plasma concentration time curve area increased proportionally with dose, and half-life remained constant). Most of the evidence suggesting inhibitory or saturation kinetics arises in studies of desipramine (i.e. metabolism is inhibited at higher doses producing higher than expected plasma drug concentrations). Bjerre *et al.* (1981), who treated six elderly patients with increasing doses of imipramine, noticed steady state desipramine concentrations to be 1.25–2.2 times higher than expected (a similar group treated with nortriptyline had expected-to-observed ratios of 0.91–1.21). In a larger study of younger patients receiving desipramine, Nelson and Jatlow (1987) observed that one-third of patients had linear pharmacokinetics, a further third had some saturation effect and the remaining third had a significant effect such that concentrations were more than 50% higher than expected on dosage increase. The mechanism for this does not appear to be saturation of desipramine hydroxylation, since 2-hydroxydesipramine concentrations did not rise disproportionately to dosage given (Cooke *et al.*, 1984; Nelson and Jatlow, 1987).

There is also some evidence which suggests that tricyclic antidepressants can display autoinduction, i.e. the drug is able to stimulate its own metabolism. Nelson *et al.* (1982) discuss two patients who were unable to maintain a steady state desipramine concentration, and two groups show patients with falling blood concentrations of doxepin despite a constant maintained dose (Joyce and Sharman, 1985; Linnoila *et al.* 1980). These reports are rare compared to those which report saturation kinetics.

8.5 NON-TRICYCLIC ANTIDEPRESSANTS

8.5.1 Fluvoxamine

The pharmacokinetics of fluvoxamine in the elderly have been studied after both single (Duphar, 1984) and multiple (Duphar, 1985a) dosing. Eight elderly subjects (aged 63 to 82 years) received a single 50 mg dose of fluvoxamine and blood samples were taken until 96 h post ingestion. There was no difference in the following pharmacokinetic measurements: area under the plasma concentration time curve, maximum recorded plasma concentration, time to maximum plasma concentration, half-life and clearance, between the two groups. The multiple-dose study was conducted in 14 healthy elderly volunteers who received 50 mg of the drug twice daily for 28 days (Duphar, 1985a). The results showed that the area under the plasma concentration time curve on Day 28 was not significantly different from that on Day 14 and there were also no differences in maximum recorded plasma concentrations and time to maximum concentration on these two days. Pre-dose plasma concentrations were similar on Days 5, 10, 14 and 28, thus indicating that steady state is reached within five days. In addition, no difference was found when comparing these results with steady state pharmaco-kinetic data from younger subjects. Further support for a lack of any age-related pharmacokinetic changes comes from a retrospective com-parison of plasma fluvoxamine concentrations in patients aged over 60 compared to those under 60 (Duphar, 1985b). At daily doses of fluvox-amine of 100–300 mg, no significant differences in mean plasma drug concentrations were found. These results indicate that there are no pharmacokinetic reasons why the dose of fluvoxamine should be reduced in the elderly.

8.5.2 Mianserin

Shami *et al.* (1983) studied the pharmacokinetics of mianserin in elderly (age 64 to 90) and younger (age 19 to 31) subjects. They found that the terminal elimination half-life of the drug was prolonged from a mean of 9.6 h (range 7–10 h) to 27 h (range 13–58 h) and the apparent oral clearance was significantly reduced from 87.1 l/h to 38.1 l/h. These results confirm the findings with tricyclic antidepressants and other drugs that not only is metabolism impaired, but that variation in pharmacokinetic measurements is much greater in the elderly. It may take well over a week to reach steady state in some elderly patients. It should be noted that in this study the young group comprised healthy volunteers, whilst the elderly group were patients with depression. Altamura *et al.* (1982) studied two smaller groups of elderly and young patients with mild depression. Their findings were similar to those of Shami *et al.* (1983) with the elderly group having a longer elimination half-life, an increased area under the plasma concentration time curve and a slower clearance. On the other hand one study (Maguire *et al.*, 1983) concluded that there was no statistical difference in elderly subjects' half-life and clearance compared to young volunteers, al-though the area under the plasma concentration time curve was in-creased. However, in this study the mean half-life was increased by 50% over the younger group. These results indicate that mianserin should be given in reduced dose to the elderly.

The relationship between plasma concentration after a single oral dose of mianserin and that at steady state has been investigated by Dawling *et al.* (1987). They found that unlike amitriptyline the relationship was insufficiently robust to allow dosage prediction from single-dose plasma concentration data. Other workers have suggested that mianserin may in fact induce its own metabolism (Gram *et al.*, 1982) which may help to explain this anomaly.

8.5.3 Trazodone

Bayer, Pathy and Ankier (1983), have investigated the pharmacokinetics of orally-administered trazodone in young and elderly volunteers given the medication either fasting or with milk. There was no significant difference in maximum recorded plasma trazodone concentrations between the groups, but the elderly had higher plasma concentrations at 8, 24, 30, 36 and 48 h after dosing. The terminal elimination half-life was prolonged in the elderly (11.6 vs. 6.4 h), the area under the plasma concentration time curve was increased (18.0 vs. 10.1 µg/ml.h) and the clearance reduced (6.3 vs. 10.8 l/h). The numbers of men and women in the young and elderly groups in this study were not similar and it is possible that some of these changes may have been due to sex differences rather than to age. The influence of sex was investigated further by Miller *et al.* (1987) who compared the kinetics of oral and intravenous doses of trazodone in younger (18–40 years) and older (60–76 years) subjects. They found that the absolute bioavailability was 70–90% and was unaffected by age. Amongst men, half-life was increased from 4.7 h to 8.2 h. However, amongst women, although the distribution volume was increased, clearance was unaltered and the half-life was only slightly prolonged (5.9 h to 7.6 h).

8.5.4 Viloxazine

Viloxazine is metabolized by hydroxylation (Case and Reeves, 1975). Its pharmacokinetics in the elderly have been investigated by Altamura *et al.* (1983). In this study single doses of viloxazine were given to a group of young subjects (mean age 35 years) and a group of old (mean age 73.3 years) volunteers. The elderly group had a prolonged half-life (11.5 vs. 9.1 h), an increased area under the plasma concentration time curve (73.1 vs. 45.8 µg/l.h and a reduced clearance (6.0 vs. 7.7 l/kg/h). These results indicate that there are pharmacokinetic reasons that viloxazine should be given in reduced dosage to the elderly.

8.6 CONCLUSION

It is possible to make some general conclusions as to the clinical relevance of the age-related changes in pharmacokinetics reported above. Firstly, the dose of antidepressants should be reduced probably to a third but certainly not more than a half of the standard recommended adult dose. Secondly, therapeutic drug monitoring is useful and should be used in the following circumstances: changes in concomitant drug therapy, changes in the physical condition of the patient, excessive side-effects and inadequate response. In the future, it may be possible to use dose-prediction tests to determine more precisely the optimal dose to be prescribed. Finally, it needs to be emphasized that all patients are individuals. The elderly show a marked variation in pharmacokinetic measurements and although on average they require lower doses, some will need doses similar to, or even greater than, younger subjects.

REFERENCES

Abernethy, D.R., Greenblatt, D.J. and Shader, R.I. (1984) Trimipramine kinetics and absolute bioavailability: use of gas–liquid chromatography with nitrogen-phosphorus detection. *Clin. Pharmacol. Ther.*, **35**, 348–53.

Abernethy, D.R. and Todd, E.L. (1986) Doxepin-cimetidine interaction: increased doxepin bioavailability during cimetidine treatment. *J. Clin. Psychopharmacol.*, **6**, 8–12.

Alexanderson, B. (1972) Pharmacokinetics of nortryptyline in man after single and multiple doses: the predictability of steady state plasma concentrations from single dose plasma level data. *Eur. J. Clin. Pharmacol.*, **4**, 82–91.

Alexanderson, B. (1973) Prediction of steady state plasma levels of nortriptyline from single oral dose kinetics: a study in twins. *Eur. J. Clinc. Pharmacol.*, **6**, 44–53.

Altamura, A., Melorio, T., Invernizzi, G. and Gomeni, R. (1982) Influence of age on mianserin pharmacokinetics. *Psychopharmacol.*, **78**, 380–2.

Altamura, A.C., Melorio, T., Invernizzi, G. *et al.* (1983) Age-related differences in kinetics and side effects of viloxazine in man and their clinical implications. *Psychopharmacol.*, **81**, 281–5.

Ayesh, R., Dawling, S., Widdop, B. *et al.* (1988) Influence of quinidine on the pharmacokinetics of nortriptyline and desipramine in man. *Br. J. Clin. Pharmacol. Soc.*, September 1987.

Ballinger, B.R., Presly, A., Reid, A.H. and Stevenson, I.H. (1974) The effects of hypnotics on imipramine treatment. *Psychopharmacologia (Berl).*, **39**, 267–74.

Bayer, A.J., Pathy, M.S.J. and Ankier, S.I. (1983) Pharmacokinetic and pharmacodynamic characteristics of trazodone in the elderly. *Br. J. Clin. Pharmacol.*, **16**, 371–6.

Bertilsson, L., Braithwaite, R., Tybring, G. *et al.* (1979) Techniques for plasma protein binding of desmethylclomipramine. *Clin. Pharmacol. Ther.*, **26**, 265–71.

Bertilsson, L., Mellström, B. and Sjöqvist, F. (1979) Pronounced inhibition of noradrenaline uptake by 10–hydroxy metabolites of nortriptyline. *Life Sci.*, **25**, 1285–92.

Bickel, M.H. (1975) Binding of chlorpromazine and imipramine to red cells, albumin, lipoproteins and other blood components. *J. Clin. Pharmacol.*, **27**, 733–8.

Bjerre, M., Gram, L.F., Kragh-Sørensen, P. *et al.* (1981) Dose–dependent kinetics of imipramine in elderly patients. *Psychopharmacol.*, **75**, 354–7.

Braithwaite, R.A., Flanagan, R.J. and Richens, A. (1975) Steady state plasma nortriptyline concentrations in epileptic patients. *Br. J. Clin. Pharmacol.*, **2**, 469–71.

Braithwaite, R., Montgomery, S. and Dawling, S. (1978) Nortriptyline in depressed patients with high plasma levels (II) *Clin. Pharmacol. Ther.*, **23**, 303–8.

Braithwaite, R.A., Heard, R. and Snape, A. (1978) Plasma protein binding of maprotiline in geriatric patients – influence of alpha–1–acid glycoprotein. *Br. J. Clin. Pharmacol.*, **6**, 448–9.

Breyer-Pfaff, U., Gaertner, H.J., Kreuter, F. *et al.* (1982) Antidepressive effect and pharmacokinetics of amitriptyline with consideration of unbound drug and 10–hydroxynortriptyline plasma levels. *Psychopharmacol.*, **76**, 240–4.

Brøsen, K., Gram, L.F., Klysner, R. and Bech, P. (1986) Steady state levels of imipramine and its metabolites: significance of dose–dependent kinetics. *Eur. J. Clin. Pharmacol.*, **30**, 43–9.

Brunswick, D.J., Amsterdam, J.D., Mendels, J. and Stern, S. (1979) Prediction of steady state imipramine and desmethylimipramine plasma concentrations from single-dose data. *Clin. Pharmacol. Ther.*, **25**, 605–10.

Carr, A.C. and Hobson, F.P. (1977) High serum concentrations of antidepressants in elderly patients. *Br. Med. J.*, **2**, 1151.

Case, D.E. and Reeves, P.R. (1975) The disposition and metabolism of ICI 58,834 (viloxazine) in humans. *Xenobiotica*, **5**, 113–29.

Ciraulo, D.A., Barnhill, J. and Boxenbaum, H. (1985) Pharmacokinetic interaction of disulfiram and antidepressants. *Am. J. Psychiat.*, **142**, 1373–4.

Castleden, C.M. and George, C.F. (1979) The effect of ageing on the hepatic clearance of propranolol. *Br. J. Clin. Pharmacol.*, **7**, 49–54.

Cooke, R.G., Warsh, J.J., Stancer, H.C. *et al.* (1984) The nonlinear kinetics of desipramine and 2–hydroxydesipramine. *Clin. Pharmacol. Ther.*, **36**, 343–9.

Coppen, A. and Rama Rao, V.A. (1979) Amitriptyline and its demethylation-rate. *Lancet*, **i**, 49.

Crampton, E.L., Glass, R.C., Marchant, B. and Rees, J.A. (1980) Chemical ionization mass fragmentographic measurement of dothiepin plasma concentrations following single oral dose in man. *J. Chromatogr.*, **183**, 141–8.

Curry, S.H. (1980) *Drug Disposition and Pharmacokinetics*, 3rd edn, Blackwell Scientific Publications, Oxford, pp. 99–101.

Dawling, S. (1982) Monitoring of tricyclic antidepressant therapy. *Clin. Chem.*, **15**, 56–61.

Dawling, S., Braithwaite, R., McAuley, R. and Montgomery, S. (1979) Single oral dose pharmacokinetics of amitriptyline and maprotiline in depressed patients – prediction of steady state plasma concentrations. *Br. J. Clin. Prac. Suppl.*, **7**, 28–33.

Dawling, S., Crome, P., Braithwaite, R.A. and Lewis, R.R. (1980) Nortriptyline therapy in elderly patients: dosage prediction after single dose pharmacokinetic study. *Eur. J. Clin. Pharmacol.*, **18**, 147–50.

Dawling, S., Braithwaite, R., McAuley, R. and Montgomery, S. (1980a) Single oral dose pharmacokinetics of clomipramine in depressed patients. *Postgrad. Med. J.*, **56** (Suppl. 1) 115–16.

Dawling, S., Crome, P. and Braithwaite, R. (1980b) Pharmacokinetics of single oral doses of nortriptyline in depressed hospital patients and young healthy volunteers. *Clin. Pharmacol.*, **5**, 394–401.

Dawling, S., Crome, P., Heyer, E.J. and Lewis, R.R. (1981) Nortriptyline therapy in elderly patients: dosage prediction from plasma concentration at 24 hours after a single 50 mg dose. *Br. J. Psychiat.*, **139**, 413–16.

Dawling, S., Lynn, K., Rosser, R. and Braithwaite, R. (1982) Nortriptyline metabolism in chronic renal failure: metabolite elimination. *Clin. Pharmacol. Ther.*, **32**, 322–9.

Dawling, S., Ford, S., Rangedara, D.C. and Lewis, R.R. (1984) Amitriptyline dosage prediction in elderly patients from plasma concentrations at 24 hours after a single 100 mg dose. *Clin. Pharmacokin.*, **9**, 261–6.

Dawling, S., Ford, S., Ariyanayagam, P. *et al.* (1987) Plasma concentrations of mianserin after single dose and at steady state in depressed elderly patients. *Clin. Pharmacokin.*, **12**, 73–8.

de Vane, C.L., Savett, M. and Jusko, W.J. (1981) Desipramine and 2–hydroxy-desipramine pharmacokinetics in normal volunteers. *Eur. J. Clin. Pharmacol.*, **19**, 61–4.

Duphar Report No. H.114.621 (1984) Duphar, Weesp.

Duphar Report No. H.114.625 (1985a) Duphar, Weesp.

Duphar Report No. H.114.623 (1985b) Duphar, Weesp.

Garland, W.A., Min, B.H. and Birkett, D.J. (1978) The kinetics of amitriptyline following single oral dose administration to man. *Res. Commun. Chem. Pathol. Pharmacol.*, **22**, 475–84.

Gram, L.F. (1975) Effects of perphenazine on imipramine metabolism in man. *Psychopharmacol. Commun.*, **1**, 165–7.

Gram, L.F. and Overø, R.F. (1972) Drug interaction: inhibitory effect of neuroleptics on metabolism of tricyclic antidepressants in man. *Br. Med. J.*, **1**, 463–5.

Gram, L.F. and Christiansen, J. (1975) First-pass metabolism of imipramine in man. *Clin. Pharmacol. Ther.*, **17**, 555–63.

Gram, L.F., Pedersen, O.L., Kristensen, C.B. *et al.* (1982) Drug level monitoring in psychopharmacology: usefulness and clinical problems, with special reference to tricyclic antidepressants. *Ther. Drug Monitoring*, **4**, 17–25.

Heikkila, R.E., Goldfinger, S.S. and Orlansky, H. (1976) The effect of various phenothiazines and tricyclic antidepressants on the accumulation and release of (^{3}H) norepinephrine and (^{3}H) 5–hydroxytryptamine in slices of rat occipital cortex. *Res. Commun. Chem. Pathol. Pharmacol.*, **13**, 237–50.

Henry, J.F., Altamura, C., Gomeni, R. *et al.* (1981) Pharmacokinetics of amitriptyline in the elderly. *Int. J. Clin. Pharmacol. Ther. Toxicol.*, **19**, 1–5.

Hessauer, S.A. and Hollister, L.E. (1984) Cimetidine interaction with imipramine and nortriptyline. *Clin. Pharmacol. Ther.*, **35**, 183–7.

Hrdina, P.D., Rovei, V., Henry, J.F. *et al.* (1980) Comparison of single-dose pharmacokinetics of imipramine and maprotiline in the elderly. *Psychopharmacol.*, **70**, 29–34.

Jandhyala, B.S., Steenberg, M.L., Perel, J.M. *et al.* (1977) Effects of several tricyclic antidepressants on the haemodynamics and myocardial contractibility. *Eur. J. Pharmcol.*, **42**, 403–10.

John, V.A., Luscombe, D.K. and Kemp, H. (1980) Effects of age, cigarette smoking and the oral contraceptive on the pharmacokinetics of clomipramine and its desmethyl metabolite during chronic dosing. *J. Int. Med. Res.*, **8** (Suppl. 3) 88–95.

Jones, R.B. and Luscombe, D.K. (1976) Single-dose study with maprotiline in normal subjects. In: *Depression – the Biochemical and Physiological Role of Ludiomil* (ed. A. Jukes) Metropolis Press Ltd., London, pp. 135–43.

Joyce, P.R. and Sharman, J.R. (1985) Doxepin plasma concentrations in clinical practice. Could there be a pharmacokinetic explanation for low concentrations? *Clin. Pharmacokinetics*, **10**, 365–70.

Jungkunz, G. and Kus, H.J. (1980) On the relationship of nortriptyline: amitriptyline ratio to clinical improvement of amitriptyline treated depressive patients. *Pharmacopsychiat.*, **13**, 111–16.

Kitanaka, I., Ross, R.J., Cutler, N.R. *et al.* (1982) Altered hydroxydesipramine concentrations in elderly depressed patients. *Clin. Pharmacol. Ther.*, **31**, 51–5.

Kragh-Sørensen, P. and Larsen, N.E. (1980) Factors influencing nortriptyline steady state kinetics: plasma and saliva levels. *Clin. Pharmacol. Ther.*, **28**, 769–803.

Lieberman, J.A., Suckow, R.F., Borenstein, M. and Kane, J.M. (1985) Tricyclic antidepressants and metabolite levels in chronic renal failure. *Clin. Pharmacol. Ther.*, **37**, 301–7.

Linnoila, M., Seppala, T., Mattila, M.J. *et al.*(1980) Clomipramine and doxepin in depressive neurosis: plasma levels and therapeutic response. *Arch. Gen. Psychiat.*, **37**, 1295–9.

Linnoila, M., Insel, T., Kilts, C. *et al.* (1982) Plasma steady state concentrations of hydroxylated metabolites of clomipramine. *Clin. Pharmacol. Ther.*, **32**, 208–11.

Lynn, K., Braithwaite, R., Dawling, S. and Rosser, R. (1981) Comparison of serum protein binding of maprotiline and phenytoin in uraemic patients on haemodialysis. *Eur. J. Clin. Pharmacol.*, **19**, 73–7.

Madakasira, S. and Khazanie, P.G. (1985) Reliability of amitriptyline dose prediction based on single-dose plasma levels. *Clin. Pharmacol. Ther.*, **37**, 145–9.

Maguire, K., Norman, T.R., Burrows, G.D. and Scoggins, B.A. (1980) An evaluation of maprotiline: intravenous kinetics and comparison of two oral doses. *Eur. J. Clin. Pharmacol.*, **18**, 249–54.

Maguire, K.P., Burrows, G.D., Norman, T.R. and Scoggins, B.A. (1981) Metabolism and pharmacokinetics of dothiepin. *Br. J. Clin. Pharmacol.*, **12**, 405–9.

Maguire, K.P., McIntyre, I., Norman, T. and Burrows, G.D. (1983) The pharmacokinetics of mianserin in elderly depressed patients. *Psychiatry Research*, **8**, 281–7.

Mellström, B. and Tybring, G. (1977) Ion-pair liquid chromatography of steady state plasma levels of chlorimipramine and desmethyl-chlorimipramine. *J. Chromatogr.*, **143**, 597–605.

Miller, D.D., Sawyer, J.B. and Duffy, J.P. (1983) Cimetidine effect on steady state serum nortriptyline concentrations. *Drug. Intell. Clin. Pharm.*, **17**, 904–5.

Miller, L.G., Greenblatt, D.J., Friedman, H. *et al.* (1987) Trazodone kinetics in old age. *Clin. Pharm. Ther.*, **41**, 210.

Montgomery, S., McAuley, R., Montgomery, D.B., Dawling, S. and Braithwaite, R.A. (1980) Plasma concentration of clomipramine and desmethylclomipramine and clinical response in depressed patients. *Postgrad. Med. J.*, **56** (Suppl. 1) 130–3.

Moody, J.P., Whyte, S.F., MacDonald, A.J. and Naylor, G.J. (1977) Pharmacokinetic aspects of protriptyline plasma levels. *Eur. J. Clin. Pharmacol.*, **11**, 51–6.

Nelson, J.C. and Jatlow, P.I. (1987) Nonlinear desipramine kinetics: prevalence and importance. *Clin. Pharmacol. Ther.*, **41**, 666–70.

Nelson, J.C., Jatlow, P., Quinlan, D.M. and Bowers, M.B. (1982) Desipramine plasma concentration and antidepressant response. *Arch. Gen. Psychiat.*, **39**, 1419–22.

Nelson, J.C., Jatlow, P.I. and Mazure, C. (1987) Rapid desipramine dose adjustment using 24-hour levels. *J. Clin. Psychopharmacol.*, **7**, 72–7.

Nies, A., Robinson, D., Friedman, M.J. *et al.* (1977) Relationship between age and tricyclic antidepressant plasma levels. *Am. J. Psychiat.*, **134**, 790–3.

Perry, P.J., Browne, J.L., Alexander, B.A. *et al.* (1984) Two prospective dosing methods for nortriptyline. *Clin. Pharmacokinet.*, **9**, 555–63.

Perucca, E. and Richens, A. (1977) Interactions between phenytoin and imipramine. *Br. J. Clin. Pharmacol.*, **4**, 485–6.

Piafsky, K.M. and Borgå, O. (1977) Plasma protein binding of basic drugs. *Clin. Pharmacol. Ther.*, **22**, 545–9.

Potter, W.Z., Calil, H.M., Manian, A.A. *et al.* (1979) Hydroxylated metabolites of tricyclic antidepressants: preclinical assessment of activity. *Biol. Psychiat.*, **14**, 601–13.

Potter, W.Z., Zavadil, A.P., Kopin, I.J. and Goodwin, F.K. (1980) Single-dose kinetics predict steady state concentrations of imipramine and desipramine. *Arch. Gen. Psychiat.*, **37**, 314–20.

Rawlins, M.D., James, O.F.W., Williams, F.M. *et al.* (1987) Age and the metabolism of drugs. *Q. J. Med.*, **64**, 545–7.

Reidenberg, M.M. (1977) The binding of drugs to plasma proteins and the interpretation of measurements of plasma concentrations of drugs in patients with poor renal function. *Am. J. Med.*, **62**, 466–70.

Roy, D. and Dawling, S. (1987) Application of an individually predicted dosage of amitriptyline to the treatment of depression. *Int. J. Clin. Psychopharmacol.*, **2**, 307–16.

Schulz, P., Turner-Tamiyasu, K., Smith, G. *et al.* (1983) Amitriptyline disposition in young and elderly normal men. *Clin. Pharmacol. Ther.*, **33**, 360–6.

Shami, M., Elliott, H.L., Kelman, A.W., and Whiting, B. (1983) The pharmacokinetics of mianserin. *Br. J. Clin. Pharmacol.*, **15**, 313S–322S.

Spina, E. and Yoike, Y. (1986) Differential effects of cimetidine and randitidine on imipramine demethylation and desmethylimipramine hydroxylation by human liver microsomes. *Eur. J. Clin. Pharmacol.*, **30**, 239–42.

Swift, C.G. and Triggs, E.J. (1987) Clinical pharmacokinetics in the elderly. In: *Clinical Pharmacology in the Elderly* (ed. C.G. Swift), Marcel Dekker, New York and Basel, pp. 31–82.

Tollefson, G. and Lesar, T. (1984) Effect of propanolol on maprotilineclearance. *Am. J. Psychiat.*, **141**, 148–9.

Turbott, J., Norman, T.R., Burrows, G.D. and Maguire, K.P. (1980) Pharmacokinetics of nortriptyline in elderly volunteers. *Commun. Psychopharmacol.*, **4**, 225–31.

Young, R.C., Alexopoulos, G.S., Shamoian, C.A. *et al.* (1984) Plasma 10–hydroxynortriptyline in elderly depressed patients. *Clin. Pharmacol. Ther.*, **35**, 540–4.

Young, R.C., Alexopoulos, G.S., Shamoian, C.A., Kent, E., Dhar, A.K. and Kutt, H. (1985) Plasma 10–hydroxynortriptyline and ECG changes in elderly depressed patients. *Am. J. Psychiat.*, **142**, 866–8.

Yu, D.K., Dimmitt, D.C., Lanman, R.C. and Giesing, D.H. (1986) Pharmacokinetics of dothiepin in humans: a single dose-proportionality study. *J. Pharm. Sci.*, **75**, 582–5.

Ziegler, V.E., Biggs, J.T., Wylie, L.T. *et al.* (1978a) Protriptyline kinetics. *Clin. Pharmacol. Ther.*, **23**, 580–4.

Ziegler, V.E., Biggs, J.T., Wylie, L.T. *et al.* (1978b) Doxepin kinetics. *Clin. Pharmacol. Ther.*, **23**, 573–9.

Chapter Nine

Which antidepressant?

MALCOLM PEET

CONTENTS

9.1 INTRODUCTION

There are many reasons why depression is so common in the elderly. Loss of role, bereavement, physical deterioration and illness, social isolation, lack of money, and other factors combine to promote depression. There is a tendency for antidepressant drugs to be prescribed inappropriately under these circumstances, because communication problems and the relative immobility of the elderly make it difficult to offer other forms of help for which resources may be lacking. Conversely, treatable depressive illness in the elderly may be overlooked because it is seen as an unavoidable accompaniment of ageing. Though this review focuses on the use of antidepressant drugs in the elderly, other forms of intervention should always be considered in conjunction with, or in preference to, drug treatment.

The choice of an appropriate antidepressant depends upon finding the best fit between the therapeutic and side-effect profile of the drug relative to the patient characteristics.

9.2 EFFICACY OF ANTIDEPRESSANTS

9.2.1 Trials in depressive patients

The efficacy of antidepressant agents is normally first established in younger patients. Equivalent efficacy in the elderly cannot necessarily be assumed, particularly because of neurochemical and receptor changes in the ageing brain (Lal and Carroll, 1979). The severity and consequences of side-effects may also alter in the elderly. Relatively few controlled trials have been conducted in an elderly depressive population, and many of those have methodological defects such as inadequate patient selection criteria, small numbers of patients, inclusion of some younger patients, inadequate duration of treatment, and lack of a placebo-treated control group.

Placebo-controlled trials of currently available antidepressant agents in the elderly are shown in Table 9.1.

Gerner *et al.* (1980) treated 60 elderly out-patients having unipolar primary depression with trazodone, imipramine or a placebo for four weeks. There was a high dropout rate, particularly for the imipramine group in which 60% of patients failed to complete the study relative to 30% in each of the other two groups. Both active drugs showed a significant therapeutic advantage over placebo on the Hamilton Depression Scale, though this was not shown on the Beck Self-Rating Scale. Imipramine was less well tolerated than trazodone, with a significantly higher incidence of both anticholinergic and total side-effects. Cognitive function tests did not show any change during the study.

The same group (Jarvik *et al.*, 1982) reported on 32 geriatric out-patients with major depressive disorder who were treated with imipramine, doxepin, or placebo for up to 26 weeks. Patients who did poorly were withdrawn at various times during the study and the endpoint ratings on the Hamilton Depression Scale were used for group comparison. Percentage improvement was greater for imipramine (50%) and doxepin (52%) than for placebo (19%). These differences are not reported as statistically significant, not surprisingly in view of the methodological problems which include very small patient numbers, variable duration of treatment with half the placebo-treated patients withdrawing within the first month but three-quarters of the drug-treated patients continuing beyond eight weeks, and the recruitment of

Table 9.1 Controlled trials of antidepressants in the elderly versus placebo

Reference	n	Age	Duration (weeks)	Efficacy
Gerner (1980)	60	60–90	4	TRAZ = IMI>PLAC
Branconnier (1981a)	75	60+	5	MIAN = AMI>PLAC
Branconnier (1983)	63	55–80	5	BUP = IMI>PLAC
Meredith (1984)	61	mean 69	5	NOM = IMI>PLAC
Cooper (1980)	40	mean 79	6	TP = PLAC
Von Knorring (1980)	21	60–86	3	VIL>PLAC
Jarvik (1982)	32	55–81	up to 26	DOX = IMI>PLAC
Georgotas (1986)	75	mean 65	7	NOR = PH>PLAC
Wakelin (1986)	33	60–71	4	FLUV = IMI>PLAC

Table 9.2 Controlled trials of antidepressants in the elderly without placebo

Reference	n	Age	Duration (weeks)	Efficacy
Eklund (1985)	50	60–80	4	MIAN = IMI
Kretschmar (1980)	37	59–86	3	MIAN>AMI
Scardigli (1982)	87	n.s.	4	MIAN>NOM = TRAZ
Jessel (1981)	37	64–84	4	LOF = AMI
Dorn (1980)	60	36–89	6	LOF= AMI
Valle-Jones (1983)	143	60+	4	FLX>AMI
Middleton (1975)	28	65–83	4	MAP = IMI
Gwirtsman (1983)	49	55+	6	MAP>DOX
Khan (1981)	50	60+	4	DOTH>AMI
Nugent (1979)	48	60–89	4	VIL = AMI
Ather (1985)	149	59–85+	4	TRAZ = AMI = DIAZ
Ananth (1979)	30	65–80	8	DOX = AMI = CPX
Brodie (1975)	62	65+	4	FLU/NOR>PROM

Key to abbreviations (Tables 1 and 2)
TRAZ Trazodone, IMI Imipramine, AMI Amitriptyline, BUP Bupropion,
TP Tryptophan, VIL Viloxazine, DOX Doxepin, NOM Nomifensine,
PH Phenelzine, FLUV Fluvoxamine, MIAN Mianserin, LOF Lofepramine,
FLX Flupenthixol, MAP Maprotiline, DOTH Dothiepin,
FLU Fluphenazine, NOR Nortriptyline, PROM Promazine,
DIAZ Diazepam, CPX Chlordiazepoxide, PLAC Placebo.

patients into the study who were subsequently excluded from data analysis because they were found not to have met the stated entry criteria. In a parallel study, patients who were not suitable for the drug trial because of their medical condition or concomitant medication were treated with either cognitive–behavioural or psychodynamic group psychotherapy which brought about some apparent improvement.

Branconnier, Cole and Ghazvinian (1981a) gave mianserin* up to 60 mg daily, amitriptyline up to 150 mg daily, or placebo, to 75 elderly patients described as having mild to moderate depressive symptomatology and impaired cognitive function. On the Hamilton Depression Scale both drugs were more effective than placebo over the five-week treatment period. There were important qualitative differences in side-effect profiles between the two active agents. Dry mouth, constipation, and increased heart rate were greater with amitriptyline, whereas the commonest side-effect with mianserin was drowsiness. Cognitive function declined during amitriptyline treatment but improved during treatment with mianserin or placebo. In a later study, Branconnier *et al.* (1983) compared bupropion, imipramine and placebo, and again found that both drugs were effective, with imipramine having the higher incidence of side-effects. However, the performance of imipramine differed from that of amitriptyline in the previous study in that imipramine did not impair cognitive function.

Von Knorring (1980) compared viloxazine and placebo in 31 elderly patients with mixed depressive syndromes including some with organic cerebral pathology. The viloxazine-treated patients improved significantly more than the placebo group after three weeks. Two patients on viloxazine experienced nausea, which is the commonest side-effect of this drug. Because of the small numbers of patients and the heterogeneity of the patient sample, the results of this study cannot be generalized. One interesting feature of the study is that all patients were considered unsuitable for treatment with tricyclic antidepressants because of cardiac disorder, a tendency to urinary retention, or a previous history of confusion precipitated by tricyclic drugs.

Cooper and Datta (1980) conducted the only study of tryptophan in geriatric patients with 'mild to moderate depression of any presumed aetiology' and with a wide variety of physical pathologies. The study showed no advantage for tryptophan over placebo. Although the design of this study was less than ideal, the result is consistent with studies in younger patients in which tryptophan is of no practical value as the sole treatment for more severe degrees of depression (Mendels *et al.*, 1975) though it may have some antidepressant benefits in mildly depressed patients seen in general practice (Jaffe and Grimshaw, 1985). Tryptophan at least appeared to lack any serious unwanted effects in this group of patients with physical illnesses including myocardial infarction, atrial fibrillation, cardiac failure and cerebrovascular accidents.

In another study of imipramine, Meredith, Feighner and Hendrickson (1984) gave nomifensine, imipramine, or placebo to 61 elderly patients

* Not available in USA

with primary depressive illness of moderate to severe intensity, over a five-week period. Nomifensine is unfortunately no longer available because of an increased incidence of haemolytic anaemia, but the study did again demonstrate the efficacy of imipramine, the most prominent side-effect being drowsiness, nervousness and blurred vision.

Georgotas *et al.* (1986) compared nortriptyline (average dose 79 mg daily), phenelzine (average dose 54 mg daily) or placebo given for seven weeks to 75 patients aged 55–76 years (mean 65 years) suffering from major depressive disorder. The response rate was approximately 60% for the active drugs but only 13% for placebo. Significant antidepressant benefits were not observed until after five weeks of treatment. Anticholinergic side-effects were more common in the nortriptyline group.

Wakelin (1986) reported placebo-controlled trials of fluvoxamine*, a specific 5–hydroxytryptamine uptake inhibitor, in depressive patients aged 60–71 years. Data were pooled from three studies, one of them multicentre. It was found that fluvoxamine was as effective as imipramine, both drugs being superior to placebo. The most common side-effects were nausea with fluvoxamine and dry mouth with imipramine. Whilst the statistical validity of such pooled data can be questioned, the data provide some support for the efficacy of fluvoxamine in elderly depressive patients.

Other studies have compared active agents, usually including a standard tricyclic antidepressant, but with no placebo control. These studies are summarized in Table 9.2.

Eklund *et al.* (1985) compared mianserin and imipramine given for four weeks to elderly patients. The drugs were of similar efficacy but imipramine produced more side-effects, this difference being statistically significant for dry mouth, faintness, dizziness and weakness. Three patients from each treatment group developed confusional states. Kretschmar (1980) compared mianserin and amitriptyline in 37 elderly hospitalized patients with endogenous depression. The two drugs were of similar efficacy on the Hamilton Depression Scale but mianserin was rated more effective on a Clinical Global Impression Scale. Vegetative symptoms rated on the German AMP scale, including dry mouth, sweating and constipation which can be both symptoms of depression and side-effects of drugs, improved significantly more after mianserin treatment than after amitriptyline treatment.

Lofepramine*, the most recently introduced tricyclic antidepressant, has been compared with amitriptyline in two studies conducted in Germany. Dorn (1980) gave either lofepramine or amitriptyline to 60 patients in General Practice described as having depression of varying

---

* Not available in USA

degrees. Though the average age of patients was 67 years, some younger patients were included so that the age range was wide, from 36 to 89. The drugs were found to be of similar efficacy with amitriptyline producing somewhat more side-effects, particularly dry mouth. Jessel, Jessel and Wegener (1981) also found lofepramine and amitriptyline to be of similar efficacy in 37 female in-patients with 'depressive symptomatology of various genesis', half of whom were given concomitant medication including neuroleptics. Because of methodological deficiencies, these trials cannot be interpreted as demonstrating the efficacy of lofepramine in the elderly, though efficacy and a reduced incidence of anticholinergic side-effects has been well demonstrated in younger patients (Peet, 1984).

In a large multicentre General Practice study Valle-Jones and Swarbrick (1983) gave flupenthixol 0.5–1 mg in the morning or amitriptyline 25–50 mg in the evening to 143 elderly patients described as suffering from mild to moderately severe depressive disorder. On a self-rating visual analogue scale patients given flupenthixol consistently rated themselves as more improved than those given amitriptyline during the four-week treatment period, and this advantage to flupenthixol was reflected in the physicians' ratings in the middle period of treatment but not by week four. The very low and generally subtherapeutic dose of amitriptyline used renders the study virtually a placebo-controlled trial of flupenthixol, and it is therefore suggestive of flupenthixol having real antidepressant efficacy. Side-effects, particularly dry mouth, occurred more frequently in the amitriptyline group despite the small doses used. Two studies have compared maprotiline with tricyclic drugs. Middleton (1975) found maprotiline to be as effective as imipramine in a small group of 28 patients suffering from 'any form of depressive manifestation'. The author makes the valid point that any real difference in efficacy is unlikely to be apparent from such a small trial.

Gwirtsman et al. (1983) compared maprotiline and doxepin in 49 elderly patients suffering from primary major depression and found that maprotiline appeared to have a small but statistically significant advantage therapeutically over doxepin. The difference did not emerge until between four and six weeks of treatment during which time the doxepin-treated patients appeared to show some clinical deterioration. Both drugs produced similar side-effects.

Nugent (1979) compared viloxazine and amitriptyline in 48 elderly hospitalized female depressive patients. Two patients on viloxazine were withdrawn because of nausea and vomiting. There was no apparent difference in efficacy between the two drugs.

Scardigli and Jans (1982) compared trazodone, nomifensine and mianserin in 87 elderly patients with endogenous, reactive and involutional depression. Mianserin in a 60 mg daily dose was significantly more effective than nomifensine from days 14–28 over the study and the same trend was apparent on a physician's global evaluation and the Beck Self-Rating Scale. Trazodone and nomifensine were similar in efficacy. Mianserin tended to produce fewer side-effects though the differences were not statistically significant.

Brodie *et al.* (1975), in a General Practice study including elderly patients with mixed anxiety and depression, found that a combination of fluphenazine and nortriptyline was more effective than promazine but the choice of comparative agents makes the study uninterpretable.

Two further studies have used amitriptyline and a benzodiazepine as comparators for doxepin (Ananth *et al.*, 1979) and trazodone (Ather, Ankier and Middleton, 1985). The trial of Ananth *et al.* was conducted in a very small group of 30 patients poorly defined as 'manifesting psychiatric symptomatology'. Not surprisingly no difference in overall outcome was found between the groups. Ather, Ankier and Middleton (1985) used a larger population of 149 patients suffering from depressive illness with defined criteria, but even in this group no significant difference between treatments was found on the Hamilton Rating Scale for Depression, though by week 6 but not earlier, the antidepressant-treated group showed a greater percentage of patients than the diazepam-treated group rated as markedly improved on a physician's global rating. These studies illustrate the difficulty of interpreting trials comparing active agents with a placebo control. Non-specific drug effects and methodological deficiencies such as inadequate patient numbers or short duration of treatment, may obscure real differences between the drugs.

In summary, efficacy greater than placebo in elderly depressive patients has been shown for imipramine, amitriptyline, nortriptyline, trazodone, bupropion, phenelzine and mianserin, and less convincingly for viloxazine, fluvoxamine and doxepin. There is also evidence suggestive of benefit from flupenthixol. For other available antidepressants, evidence of efficacy in the elderly is lacking or inadequate, though common sense dictates that drugs known to be effective in younger patients will, with some reservations, also benefit the elder population. None of the available antidepressants has any advantage in terms of overall efficacy or speed of onset of action, and all give a similar profile of symptomatic improvement. There is therefore no reason for choosing one drug rather than another on ground of efficacy.

9.2.2 Additional therapeutic effects

Not all side-effects are unwanted. Antidepressant agents have a number of pharmacological properties which can be put to therapeutic advantage.

(a) Sedation

This is caused by many antidepressant agents, whether tricyclic (such as amitriptyline, doxepin and dothiepin) or a non-tricyclic (such as mianserin or trazodone). Agitation and anxiety are a common feature of depression in the elderly (Jacoby, 1981) and a sedative drug in divided doses during the day may help to calm such patients. Insomnia associated with depression can sometimes be alleviated by larger night-time doss of sedative tricyclic antidepressants (Ware, 1983) mianserin (Smith, Naylor and Moody 1978; Mendelwicz, Dunbar and Hoffman, 1985), or trazodone (Montgomery *et al.*, 1983; Wheatley, 1983). However, the practice commonly followed in younger patients of giving the total daily dosage as a single night-time dose is not usually appropriate in the elderly because of the increased susceptibility to side-effects associated with peak plasma levels. Tryptophan, used primarily as an adjunct to other antidepressant drugs, can also improve sleep when given in a night-time dose (Schneider-Helmert and Spinweber, 1986). The new agent fluvoxamine has no sedative properties (Curran, Shine and Lader, 1986).

(b) Pain relief

This is another property of tricyclic antidepressant agents. The most studied drugs have been amitriptyline, imipramine and clomipramine. Pain relief has been shown in a number of conditions pertinent to the elderly population such as post herpetic neuralgia, low back pain, arthritis and cancer (Walsh, 1983; Zorumski and Rubin, 1984). Pain relief may occur independently of antidepressant effect (Feinmann, 1985), so that it can be worth a trial of a tricyclic antidepressant in painful conditions even where the depression seems to be secondary to the pain rather than primary. The drugs may act through 5–hydroxytryptamine pathways which are probably involved in the genesis of both depression and pain. Antidepressant drugs have also been used in the treatment of pain and depression associated with cancer, but the side-effects of tricyclic antidepressants tend to be poorly tolerated in cancer patients who are already debilitated and suffering from the effects of cytotoxic drugs. It is therefore of interest that mianserin has been shown to be well tolerated and effective in the treatment of depression in women with cancer of various types who are receiving a variety of anti-tumour agents and radiotherapy (Costa, Mogos and Toma, 1985).

(c) Peptic ulceration

This has been successfully treated with antidepressant agents. In an open study using endoscopy to verify the healing of peptic ulceration, doxepin was found to be as effective as cimetidine (Hoff *et al.*, 1981). Trimipramine has been shown to be effective in promoting the healing of duodenal (Wetterhus *et al.*, 1977) and gastric (Valnes, Myren and Qvigstad, 1978) ulcers. This effect is not due to anticholinergic properties, as it has also been recently shown that mianserin promotes the healing of duodenal ulcers (Wilson, Boyd and Wormsley, 1985).

(d) Antiarrhythmic properties

Antiarrhythmic properties similar to those of type 1 antiarrhythmic drugs such as quinidine have been described for imipramine (Bigger *et al.*, 1977). Atrial and ventricular premature contractions are therefore not a contraindication to, and are likely to be supressed by, imipramine and related drugs. However, this property has not been exploited in the clinical treatment of non-depressed patients with cardiac arrhythmias. The main importance of this property is that the dosage of existing antiarrhythmic drug treatment may need to be reduced if treatment with imipramine and similar antidepressant agents is to be instituted. Any patient with a pre-existing cardiac arrhythmia would require careful ECG monitoring during tricyclic antidepressant treatment. It has been reported that trazodone may aggravate ventricular arrhythmia (Janowski *et al.*, 1983).

Other potentially useful though less well documented additional benefits from antidepressant agents include migraine prophylaxis with mianserin (Monro, Swade and Coppen, 1985) and amitriptyline (Gomersall and Stuart, 1973), weight reduction with fluvoxamine (Abell *et al.*, 1986), and improvement of irritable bowel syndrome with anticholinergic tricyclic agents.

9.3 ADVERSE EFFECTS OF ANTIDEPRESSANTS

Whilst the therapeutic side-effects of antidepressant agents may lead to a positive choice of a specific drug for a particular patient who is, for example, in pain or in suffering from peptic ulceration, antidepressants also have many unwanted side-effects. Intolerance of these unwanted effects may become apparent only after treatment has been started. However, there are a number of physical conditions from which intolerance can be predicted and which will influence the choice of antidepressants from the outset.

9.3.1 Cardiovascular disorders

These may preclude the use of certain antidepressant agents. Orthostatic hypotension is the commonest cardiovascular side-effect of tricyclic antidepressants. Though the incidence of this does not appear to increase with age, the elderly are more susceptible to its effects, particularly in the presence of cerebral or myocardial circulatory insufficiency. Falls resulting in fractures can occur. Blumenthal and Davie (1980) found that the combination of tricyclic antidepressants with other hypotensive agents such as diuretics and neuroleptics, was the commonest cause of falling in a group of elderly psychiatric outpatients. Glassman *et al.* (1979) found that the degree of orthostatic drop in blood pressure prior to treatment was the best predictor of orthostatic hypotension during treatment, though others (Thayssen *et al.*, 1981; Neshkes *et al.*, 1985) could not confirm this finding. Nevertheless, it would seem prudent not to give the more hypotensive antidepressant agents to patients with marked pre-treatment orthostatic blood pressure changes or with impaired circulation of the brain or myocardium. Patients should be warned against standing up too quickly, particularly when in a warm environment such as a hot bath. If orthostatic hypotension becomes a problem during treatment it may be necessary to change to a less hypotensive agent. Reducing the dosage of the existing drug whilst possibly reducing the severity of orthostatic hypotension, is likely to be associated with poor antidepressant efficiency because hypotension first appears at sub-therapeutic plasma levels (Thayssen *et al.*, 1981).

Of the drugs which have been studied adequately, those most likely to induce orthstatic hypotension are imipramine (Thayssen *et al.*, 1981), and amitriptyline (Christensen *et al.*, 1985). Mianserin causes less orthostatic hypotension than imipramine in younger patients (Pichot, Dreyfus and Pull, 1978), but was found to have effects on blood pressure almost as pronounced as imipramine in the elderly (Moller *et al.*, 1983). However, this last study used 60 mg daily doses of mianserin, which is double the dose usually necessary for therapeutic effect in the elderly. Lower doses may cause less problems with blood pressure. One tricyclic antidepressant drug less prone to induce orthostatic hypotension is nortriptyline (Thayssen *et al.*, 1981; Roose *et al.*, 1981; Roose *et al.*, 1987). Doxepin has also been shown to cause less postural change in blood presure than imipramine (Neshkes *et al.*, 1985). Amongst the newer antidepressants, trazodone appear less liable than standard tricyclic drugs to cause postural hypotension in the elderly (Gerner *et al.*, 1980; Himmelhoch, Schechtman and Auchenbach, 1984), though more studies are needed. Lofepramine induces less orthostatic blood pressure changes than amitriptyline in volunteers whether young (Stern *et al.*, 1985), or elderly (Ghose and Sedman, 1987). In depressive patients, lofepramine causes less orthostatic blood pressure changes than amitriptyline in the younger age group (Marneros, Philipp and Legeler, 1979) but there have been no systematic studies in elderly depressive patients. Fluvoxamine may produce less orthostatic hypotension than imipramine in older depressive patients (Wakelin, 1986). Viloxazine and flupenthixol also appear to be less liable to cause postural hypotension, though their antidepressant efficacy is less firmly established than for standard agents.

Patients with pre-existing conduction abnormalities are at risk of developing heart block during treatment with tricyclic antidepressants (Glassman and Bigger, 1981; Roose *et al.*, 1987). The effect may be less pronounced with doxepin (Ahles *et al.*, 1984) and dothiepin (Claghorn, Schroeder and Goldstein, 1984) which appear to have less effect on cardiac conducting systems. However heart block is rarely if ever induced by therapeutic concentrations of tricyclic antidepressants in patients with healthy conducting systems. A pre-treatment electrocardiogram is necessary to identify patients at risk. Such patients should be preferentially treated with a drug less likely to cause conduction abnormalities, such as mianserin (Moller *et al.*, 1983), trazodone (Himmelhoch, Schechtman and Auchenbach, 1984), or fluvoxamine (Roos, 1983). However, even these drugs cannot be regarded as entirely without effect on conduction; there are now individual case reports on patients who have developed heart block during treament with trazodone (Rausch, Pavlinac and Newman, 1984). Careful electrocardiographic monitoring is therefore necessary.

Heart failure should be adequately controlled prior to antidepressant treatment. Earlier studies suggesting that tricyclic antidepressants can significantly impair myocardial contractility have been criticized on methodological grounds and it is now apparent that tricyclic antidepressants at therapeutic doses do not have any significant detrimental effect. Glassman *et al.* (1983) gave imipramine to elderly patients with congestive heart failure and found no change in myocardial contractility using sophisticated radionuclide technology. However, these patients seem to be at particular risk of developing severe orthostatic hypotension (Glassman *et al.*, 1982; Roose *et al.*, 1987) and so the more hypotensive drugs should be avoided in patients with heart failure.

It is generally advised that antidepressant treatment should be avoided during the first month following acute myocardial infarction. Thereafter, the choice of antidepressant agent depends upon the functional state of the heart though in general one of the newer, less cardiotoxic drugs would clearly be preferable. Patients with angina should not be given drugs which cause marked hypotension or tachycardia which can exacerbate angina by increasing myocardial oxygen demand. Drugs most likely to cause tachycardia are the tricyclic antidepressants, though the newer agent lofepramine may be less troublesome in this regard (Warrington, 1984). The newer non-tricyclic agents mianserin, trazodone and fluvoxamine do not cause tachycardia (Hayes *et al.*, 1983; Moller *et al.*, 1983; Roos, 1983).

It has been shown that untreated or inadequately treated depressive illness is associated with increased mortality not only from suicide but also from cardiovascular causes (Avery and Winokur, 1976). This risk should be weighed against the potential cardiotoxic effects of anti-depressant drugs. It must be said that these effects have in the past been exaggerated and that many patients with chronic heart disease can be successfully treated with tricyclic antidepressant agents without serious adverse consequences (Veith *et al.*, 1982). Nevertheless, it would be prudent to avoid the more cardiotoxic tricyclic drugs in patients with more severe degrees of cardiovascular disorder, and use instead the less toxic newer agents such as trazodone, mianserin and lofepramine.

9.3.2 Organic brain syndromes

These commonly have a significant depressive component, and depressive illness in the elderly is not uncommonly misdiagnosed as dementia (Ron *et al.*, 1979). Though most antidepressant drugs produce significant impairment of cognitive function in healthy volunteers, there is in patients an interaction between cognitive improvement due to lessening of depression and possible cognitive impairment due to the antidepressant agent (Thompson and Trimble, 1982). A number of studies have been carried out in elderly patients. Branconnier and Cole (1981b) showed that a single 50 mg dose of amitriptyline impairs memory function in the normal elderly. In a clinical study of elderly mild depressive patients with impaired cognitive function, amitriptyline was found to significantly increase cognitive impairment relative to mianserin and placebo which were both associated with improved intellectual function as the depression ameliorated (Branconnier, Cole and Ghazvinian, 1981a). Imipramine and trazodone do not appear to impair cognitive function relative to placebo in elderly depressed non-demented patients (Gerner *et al.*, 1980; Branconnier *et al.*, 1983; Glass *et al.*, 1981). Doxepin has been reported to improve cognitive performance relative to placebo in geriatric patients with memory deficits (Goldberg, Finnerty and Cole, 1975).

The elderly are particularly prone to develop overt confusional states with tricyclic antidepressants particularly when plasma levels are high (Livingstone *et al.*, 1983). This may be partly caused by a central anticholinergic effect, but drugs with virtually no anticholinergic effects such as mianserin (Eklund *et al.*, 1985) and trazodone (Gerner *et al.*, 1980) can also induce confusional states though with an apparently lower incidence than seen with tricyclic agents (Schmidt *et al.*, 1986). Fluvoxamine also appears less likely to induce confusional states in older patients (Wakelin, 1986). These newer non-tricyclic drugs should therefore be tried if confusion is a problem during tricyclic antidepressant treatment.

Patients with chronic organic brain syndrome and secondary depression can be successfully treated with tricyclic antidepresssants (Cole *et al.*, 1983). As Branconnier, Cole and Ghazvinian (1981a) found deterioration of cognitive function with amitriptyline it would seem wise to avoid this drug. Imipramine has been successfully used in the treatment of emotional disturbances associated with multi-infarct dementia (Lawson and MacLeod, 1969), but in these patients it would seem preferable to use a drug with less propensity to cause hypotension. Lipsey *et al.* (1984) have shown in a placebo-controlled trial that nortriptyline is effective in the treatment of depression following a stroke. Furthermore, it appears that the presence of depression following a stroke is associated with a greater degree of intellectual impairment which might therefore improve with antidepressant treatment (Robinson *et al.*, 1986).

In open studies, trazodone has also been shown to improve mood and organicity in chronic organic brain syndrome (Nair *et al.*, 1973) and following acute stroke (Allori, Cioli and Silvestrini, 1975).

9.3.3 Prostatic enlargement

Tricyclic antidepressant drugs, because of their anticholinergic effect, can precipitate acute retention of urine in patients who are predisposed, for example due to prostatic enlargement in the elderly. In the presence of symptoms of urinary tract obstruction or the finding of an enlarged prostate on examination, or in patients who develop disorders of micturition during tricyclic antidepressant treatment, then a non-anticholinergic drug such as mianserin or trazodone should be used in preference.

9.4 PHARMACOKINETIC CONSIDERATIONS

The pharmacokinetics of antidepressant drugs are altered in the elderly with practical implications for the prescriber (Norman *et al.*, 1979). Liver enzyme activity is reduced, so that drug metabolism is slower. Plasma protein binding is reduced, so that more free drug is available. Body fat increases with age, so that antidepressants, which are fat-soluble, have an increased distribution volume. Renal function deteriorates, so that antidepressant metabolites may accumulate. These and other changes result in a decreased rate of drug elimination in the elderly and increased availability of drugs at the receptor sites. Standard doses of amitriptyline and imipramine produce higher blood levels at steady state in the elderly than in younger patients (Nies *et al.*, 1977). In contrast, plasma levels and elimination half-life of nortriptyline in the elderly are similar to those of younger patients (Kumar *et al.*, 1987). The newer antidepressants trazodone (Bayer, Pathy and Ankier, 1983) and mianserin (Shami *et al.*, 1983; Montgomery, McAuley and Montgomery, 1978) have also been shown to have slower elimination and therefore higher blood levels in the elderly. These increased blood levels, together with possible increased receptor sensitivity in the elderly, lead to increased side-effects.

There are several practical implications of these pharmacokinetic changes in the elderly. First, dosage will in general need to be reduced to one-third or a half of that normally used in younger patients. However, there is a great variability between patients so that some will require substantially higher doses than others. Secondly, elderly patients will take longer than the young, perhaps up to three weeks, before reaching steady state blood levels. Thus toxic effects may first become apparent relatively late in treatment. Also, drugs may need to be tried for longer in the elderly before the level of therapeutic efficacy can be judged.

9.5 DRUG INTERACTIONS

The possibility of drug interactions should always be considered before prescribing an antidepressant to an elderly patient. The main interactions are listed elsewhere (Blackwell, 1981). Some are specially pertinent to the elderly. Antiparkinsonian drugs may interact with tricyclic antidepressants. The absorption of l–dopa is reduced by concomitant treatment with a tricyclic antidepressant. There is an additive anticholinergic effect between anticholinergic agents and the tricyclic antidepressants, with a consequently increased liability to confusion.

The antihypertensive effects of guanethidine, bethanidine, clonidine and methyldopa are antagonized by tricyclic antidepressants. Patients on these drugs should either be re-established on an alternative antihypertensive agent (such as betablockers or diuretics) prior to antidepressant therapy, or treated with the non-tricyclic antidepressant mianserin which does not appear to interact with adrenergic neurone blocking agents (Burgess, Turner and Wadsworth, 1978) or centrally active antihypertensive agents (Elliott, Whiting and Reid, 1983).

Concurrent treatment with neuroleptic drugs leads to increased blood levels of tricyclic antidepressants with possible increased toxicity. Thioridazine, commonly prescribed for the elderly, shares the cardiotoxic properties of the tricyclic antidepressants and combination may increase the risk of arrhythmias.

Other interactions include potentiation of the central depressant effect of alcohol and other sedative agents; potentiation of the hypertensive effect of sympathomimetic agents such as noradrenaline and phenyl-ephrine; and the well known potentially fatal interaction with mono-amine oxidase inhibitors.

This list is not exhaustive and the clinician should be alert for hitherto unexpected interactions, particularly with the newer agents.

9.6 TYPES OF DEPRESSION

Patients with the typical endogenous symptom pattern, including 'biological' features such as early morning wakening, diurnal variation of mood, loss of appetite and disturbance of psychomotor activity, are those most likely to need antidepressant medication (Bielski and Friedal, 1976). Symptomatic improvement may also occur with the less severe depressive reactions including those related to psychosocial problems, but it is generally preferable to first seek other methods of helping rather than to give potentially dangerous medication.

Delusional depression is reported to respond relatively poorly to antidepressant drug treatment (Charney and Nelson, 1981), though Howarth and Grace (1985) have suggested that the use of high doses of tricyclic antidepressants for periods of at least six weeks is associated with a better response rate. Brown *et al.* (1984) treated a group of elderly delusional depressive patients with high-dose tricyclic antidepressants, but not surprisingly found that side-effect problems, particularly post-ural hypotension, were severe. Spiker *et al.* (1985), in a group of younger patients, showed that a combination of amitriptyline with neuroleptic perphenazine was superior to either drug alone in the treatment of delusional depression. An antidepressant neuroleptic combination may therefore also be effective in the elderly delusional depressive, though again side-effect problems may be increased by adding a neuroleptic drug (Nelson *et al.*, 1982). Also, a long-term neuroleptic drug treatment should be avoided if possible in the elderly because of the increased risk of tardive dyskinesia. Because of these problems, many psychogeria-tricians would feel that electroconvulsive therapy (ECT) is the treatment of choice for the elderly delusional depressive patients. However, this remains a matter of clinical judgment because there are no adequate clinical trials demonstrating that ECT is preferable to an antidepressant neuroleptic combination in this group of patients. Electroconvulsive therapy may give a rapid response, but it is associated with a high relapse in subsequent months (Post, 1985). Drug treatment may give a slower response, but there is then more certainty that the drug will also be effective for continuation treatment in subsequent months.

Suicidal impulses are a common feature of depressive illness. Older depressive patients are at increased risk of suicide, particularly if they live alone and have painful physical illnesses. In addition to deliberate overdosage, the elderly patient who is cognitively impaired is also at risk of accidental overdose. Even moderate overdosage of the older tricyclic drugs such as imipramine and amitriptyline can cause serious problems in the elderly. Dothiepin, though widely regarded by clinicians as less toxic than most tricyclic drugs, ranks with amitriptyline as a cause of death by tricyclic overdose (OPCS, 1984). Some newer agents appear to be less toxic in overdosage and are therefore preferable where intentional or accidental overdosage is a possibility. Reduced toxicity in overdosage, particularly with respect to the cardiovascular system, has been described for mianserin (Shaw, 1980), lofepramine (Heath and Hulten, 1983), and trazodone (Henry *et al.*, 1984).

One of the newer agents should therefore be the choice for patients treated outside hospital who are at some risk of deliberate or accidental overdosage.

9.7 CHOICE OF ANTIDEPRESSANT FOR THE INDIVIDUAL PATIENT

Many patients requiring antidepressant treatment have suffered previous episodes of depressive illness. Their previous response to treatment will give a valuable guide to the most appropriate drug to use for the current episode, provided that other factors such as the physical state of the patient have not changed in the meantime.

For the patient at the younger end of the psychogeriatric age range in whom there are no complicating factors such as physical illness or potential interactions with other medication, many psychiatrists would still choose one of the standard tricyclic antidepressants such as amitriptyline or imipramine despite their list of side-effects. The reason for this is that these drugs have been well tried and tested, their efficacy both in the short term and in the long term is clearly established, and their side-effects are well known and can be monitored. The confidence which comes from familiarity with a drug has been underlined by recent unexpected side-effects which have caused some of the newer drugs to be taken off the market. Treatment with imipramine or amitriptyline would begin at lower dosages than used in younger patients. In general, dosages would be about half of those used in younger patients or even lower in the very elderly. Nevertheless, it should be emphasized that the elderly, like younger patients, show a very wide range of blood levels of antidepressant drugs on standard dosages, so that while some elderly patients may only be able to tolerate 30 mg daily of a tricyclic antidepressant, others may require 150 mg or occasionally even more to get full therapeutic benefit.

For patients in whom the standard tricyclic drugs are contraindicated, and for those who are frail, or who cannot tolerate these drugs, a choice must be made of one of the other antidepressants. The specialist treating depression in the elderly will wish to choose from the whole range of available drugs. The non-specialist is unlikely to retain details of the whole range of available antidepressants, and will wish to choose perhaps two of the relatively non-toxic drugs and be aware in some detail of the practical clinical use of these drugs. Which drugs to choose is a contentious issue. It is unfortunately true that the drugs which so far appear to lack some of the more serious toxic efects of the older tricyclic antidepressants are new drugs which have not themselves been tested as fully as one would wish before recommending them. Nevertheless, it is necessary to make some specific recommendations, whilst recognizing that these will change as knowledge grows.

In choosing two drugs, it is logical that one of them should be more sedative and therefore perhaps preferred in the more agitated or insomniac patient, whilst the other should be relatively non-sedative.

Furthermore, it would be preferable for one drug to be tricyclic in structure and for the other to be different chemically and pharmacologically, so that the second drug can be tried if the first fails. Both drugs should be relatively non-toxic, both to the cardiovascular system and in overdosage; both should have a lesser incidence of anticholinergic effects which are troublesome in the elderly; and both should be free from troublesome new side-effects of their own.

Among the non-tricyclic antidepressants, only mianserin and trazodone have adequate demonstration of efficacy in the elderly, though fluvoxamine is also rapidly gaining popularity. Both have a much reduced incidence of anticholinergic side-effects, appear to have less effect on cardiac conduction (though heart block has been reported with trazodone), and to be safer in overdosage than standard tricyclic drugs. Both can produce postural hypotension. Mianserin in 60 mg doses appears to cause almost as much postural hypotension as imipramine though smaller doses may be less troublesome in this regard. Trazodone has not been adequately investigated in properly-designed studies to assess effects on blood pressure in the elderly, but clinical trial data indicate that it probably is less prone to the phenomenon. Both drugs have rare idiosyncratic side-effects. Trazodone has been reported to cause priapism (Scher, Krieger and Juergens, 1983), though this can also occur with other psychotropic drugs which block alpha adrenoreceptors (Kogeorgos and de Alwis, 1986). Mianserin has an increased incidence of agranulocytosis (Clink, 1983). Recently a recommendation has been put out by the manufacturers of mianserin that white cell count should be monitored every month for the first three months of treatment with mianserin. Clinicians may find this a disincentive to using the drug. The choice therefore tends towards trazodone whilst accepting that more data need to be generated, particularly on the cardiovascular effects of this drug in the elderly.

This leaves the choice of a suitable tricyclic antidepressant to partner trazodone. As trazodone is sedative, we should seek a relatively non-sedative tricyclic drug. Choices might include nortriptyline, desipramine, protriptyline or lofepramine. Nortriptyline causes less orthostatic hypotension than standard tricyclics, but shares the other anticholinergic and cardiac effects. A further complication of using nortriptyline is that there appears to be a therapeutic window of blood levels, so that too high a blood level, just as too low a blood level, is associated with a poor therapeutic outcome. This can make dosage difficult to adjust unless plasma level monitoring is available. Desipramine, which had previously gained a reputation for relative cardiac safety, has more recently been shown to produce potentially clinically significant electrocardiographic changes (Kutcher *et al.*, 1986). Protriptyline, though non-sedative, shares all other tricyclic antidepressant side-effects and is little investigated and little used clinically. It has a particularly long plasma half-life which makes it less attractive for use in the elderly (Moody, Whyte and MacDonald, 1977). Lofepramine, one of the newer tricyclic antidepressants, appears to have real differences from amitriptyline and imipramine. The incidence of anticholinergic effects is about half that seen with imipramine and amitriptyline (Peet, 1984). Blood pressure effects appear from rather limited current data to be less marked than with older drugs. Though more detailed data are again needed, it appears that on present knowledge lofepramine goes some way to meeting the needs of the elderly depressive patient. If the discussion were not limited to non-sedative tricyclic drugs, then the more sedative agents dothiepin and doxepin would be considered. Dothiepin is widely used in the elderly, perhaps surprisingly so as there is virtually no documented evidence from adequately conducted studies relating to either the therapeutic effect or the side-effect profile of dothiepin in the elderly population. This drug does seem to have slightly fewer side-effects in therapeutic doses in younger patients but is known to be toxic in overdosage in the same way as other tricyclic drugs. Doxepin has been shown to cause less postural hypotension in the elderly and therefore might be used to advantage if this side-effect is problematic, but other than this and a possibly reduced incidence of anticholinergic side-effects, the drug appears to have no other particular strengths in relation to other tricyclic agents (Pinder *et al.*, 1977; Luchins, 1983).

9.8 GUIDELINES FOR TREATING THE ELDERLY DEPRESSIVE

1. The diagnosis should be carefully confirmed taking into account all physical, social, pharmacological and other factors which may be contributing to the mental disorder. Full physical examination and investigation is necessary, particularly to identify physical disorders which may be contributing to the depression or which would complicate antidepressant therapy.
2. The physical state of the patient should be optimized, for example by treating any intercurrent anaemia or heart failure, before anti-depressant therapy is instituted. Treatment of the physical disorder may in itself improve mental state. Drugs used for such treatment should be chosen with an eye to the possible use of antidepressant drugs in the future so that the potential for drug interactions can be minimized.
3. The medication which the patient may already be taking should be reviewed, and the total number of drugs reduced to the minimum possible in the simplest dosage regime that can be achieved, again with particular reference to the possibility of interactions with anti-depressant agents.
4. Before choosing an antidepressant drug, the following points should be considered:
   (a) Previous antidepressant response
   (b) Associated physical conditions which may be aggravated or alleviated by antidepressant treatment
   (c) Type of depressive symptomatology (e.g. presence of delusions: suicidal impulses or the possibility of accidental overdosage)
   (d) Possible drug interactions.
5. Use a lower dosage range than that used in younger patients and a slower incremental rate. The dosage schedule should be kept as simple as possible, particularly if the patient is taking several different medications.
6. There should be careful monitoring for known side-effects. This may include monitoring of orthostatic blood pressure changes, and electrocardiography.
7. The chosen antidepressant, if it is tolerated by the patient, should be tried for at least six weeks. Though antidepressant benefits are commonly seen after two to three weeks of treatment, there is

significant additional therapeutic gain between four and six weeks (Quitkin *et al.*, 1984).

9.9 FURTHER TREATMENT

Patients who respond to initial acute treatment with an antidepressant should receive the same drug as continuation treatment for a period of six to eight months in order to reduce the risk of relapse. Patients who have recurrent episodes of affective disorder should be considered for prophylactic treatment in order to prevent future episodes of depression or mania.

If patients cannot tolerate the chosen antidepressant then an alternative more suitable agent can be chosen on the basis of its side-effect profile. Patients who fail to respond to a six-week course of treatment with adequate doses of a suitable antidepressant should be tried on an alternative drug with a differing pharmacology. Thus, a patient who failed to respond to nortriptyline or lofepramine might be tried on trazodone or mianserin. Patients who have failed to respond to two different antidepressants given each for six weeks can be catagorized as treatment-resistant. They may be considered for treatment with ECT or with less conventional antidepressants such as lithium or monoamine oxidase inhibitors, and combinations of drugs. Such treatment requires supervision by a psychiatrist with expertise in the pharmacotherapy of resistant depression.

REFERENCES

Abell, C.A., Farquhar, D.L., Galloway, S.McL. *et al.* (1986) Placebo-controlled double-blind trial of fluvoxamine maleate in the obese. *J. Psychosom. Res.*, **30**, 143–6.

Ahles, S., Gwirtsman., Halavis, A. *et al.* (1984) Comparative cardiac effects of maprotiline and doxepin in elderly depressed patients. *J. Clin. Psychiat.*, **45**, 460–5.

Allori, L., Cioli, V. and Silvestrini, B. (1975) Experimental and clinical data indicating a potential use of trazodone in acute stroke. *Curr. Therap. Res.*, **18**, 410–16.

Ananth, J.V., Sohn, J.H., Ban, T.A. and Lehmann, H.E. (1979) Doxepin in geriatric patients. *Curr. Therap. Res.*, **25**, 133–8.

Ather, S.A., Ankier, S.L. and Middleton, R.S.W. (1985) A double-blind evaluation of trazodone in the treatment of depression in the elderly. *Brit. J. Clin. Pract.*, **39**, 192–9.

Avery, D. and Winokur, G. (1976) Mortality in depressed patients treated with electroconvulsive therapy and antidepressants. *Arch. Gen. Psychiat.*, **33**, 1029–37.

Bayer, A.J., Pathy, M.S.J. and Ankier, S.L. (1983) Pharmacokinetic and pharmacodynamic characteristics of trazodone in the elderly. *Brit. J. Clin. Pharm.*, **16**, 371–6.

Bielski, R.J. and Friedel, R.O. (1976) Prediction of tricyclic antidepressant response: a critical review. *Arch. Gen. Psychiat.*, **33**, 1479–89.

Bigger, J.T., Giardina, E.G.V., Perel, J.M. *et al.* (1977) Cardiac antiarrhythmic effects of imipramine hydrochloride. *N. Engl. J. Med.*, **296**, 206–8.

Blackwell, B. (1981) Adverse effects of antidepressant drugs. Part 1: monoamine oxidase inhibitors and tricyclics. *Drugs*, **21**, 201–19.

Blumenthal, M.D. and Davie, J.W. (1980) Dizziness and falling in elderly psychiatric out-patients. *Am. J. Psychiat.*, **137**, 203–6.

Branconnier, R.J., Cole, J.O. and Ghazvinian, S. (1981a) The therapeutic profile of mianserin in elderly depressives. *Psychopharmacol. Bull.*, **17**, 129–31.

Branconnier, R.J. and Cole, J.O. (1981b) Effects of acute administration of trazadone and amitriptyline on cognitive, cardiovascular function and salivation in the normal geriatric subject. *J. Clin. Psychopharmacol.*, **1**, 835–85.

Branconnier, R.J., Cole, J.O., Ghazvinian, S. *et al.* (1983) Clinical pharmacology of bupropion and imipramine in elderly depressives. *J. Clin. Psychiat.*, **44**, 130–3.

Brodie, N.H., McGhie, R.L., O'Hara, H.*et al.* (1975) Anxiety/depression in elderly patients. A double-blind comparative study of fluphenazine/nortriptyline and promazine. *Practitioner*, **215**, 660–4.

Brown, R.P., Kocsis, J.H., Glick, I.D. and Dhar, A.K. (1984) Efficacy and feasibility of high-dose tricyclic antidepressant treatment in elderly delusional depressives. *J. Clin. Psychopharmacol.*, **4**, 311–14.

Burgess, C.D. Turner, P. and Wadsworth, J. (1978) Cardiovascular responses to mianserin hydrochloride: a comparison with tricyclic antidepressant drugs. *Brit. J. Clin. Pharmacol.*, **5** (Suppl. 1) 21S–28S.

Charney, D.S. and Nelson, J.C. (1981) Delusional and nondelusional unipolar depression: further evidence for distinct subtypes. *Am. J. Psychiat.*, **138**, 328–33.

Christensen, P., Thomsen, H.Y., Pederson, O.L. *et al.* (1985) Cardiovascular effects of amitriptyline in the treatment of elderly depressed patients. *Psychopharmacol.*, **87**, 212–15.

Claghorn, J.L., Schroeder, H. and Goldstein, B.J. (1984) Comparison of the electrocardiographic effect of dothiepin and amitriptyline. *J. Clin. Psychiat.*, **45**, 291–3.

Clink, H.M. (1983) Mianserin and blood dyscrasias. *Brit. J. Clin. Pharmacol.*, **15** (Suppl. 2), 291S–293S.

Cole, J.O., Branconnier, R., Salomon, M. and Dessain, E. (1983) Tricyclic use in the cognitively impaired elderly. *J. Clin. Psychiat.*, **44**, 14–19.

Cooper, A.J. and Datta, S.R. (1980) A placebo-controlled evaluation of l–tryptophan in depression in the elderly. *Can. J. Psychiat.*, **25**, 386–90.

Costa, D., Mogos, L. and Toma, T. (1985) Efficacy and safety of mianserin in the treatment of depression of women with cancer. *Acta Psychiat. Scand.*, **72** (Suppl. 320) 85–92.

Curran, H.V., Shine, P. and Lader, M. (1986) Effects of repeated doses of fluvoxamine, mianserin and placebo on memory and measures of sedation. *Psychopharmacology*, **89**, 360–63.

Dorn, M. (1980) Comparative trial between lofepramine and amitriptyline. *Z. Allg. Med.*, **56**, 133–9.

Eklund, K., Dunbar, G.C., Pinder, R.M. and Steffensen, K. (1985) Mianserin and imipramine in the treatment of elderly patients. *Acta. Psychiat. Scand.*, **72** (Suppl. 320) 54–9.

Elliott, H.L., Whiting, B. and Reid, J.L. (1983) Assessment of the interaction between mianserin and centrally-acting antihypertensive drugs. *Brit. J. Clin. Pharmacol.*, **15** (Suppl. 2) 323S–328S.

Feinmann, C. (1985) Pain relief by antidepressants: possible modes of action. *Pain*, **23**, 1–8.

Georgotas, A., McCue, R.E., Hapworth, W. *et al.* (1986) Comparative safety and efficacy of MAOIs versus TCAs in treating depression in the elderly. *Biol. Psychiat.*, **21**, 1155–66.

Gerner, R., Estabrook, W., Steuer, J. and Jarvik, L. (1980) Treatment of geriatric depression with trazodone, imipramine and placebo: a double-blind study. *J. Clin. Psychiat.*, **41**, 216–20.

Ghose, K. and Sedman, E. (1987) A double-blind comparison of the pharmaco-dynamic effects of single doses of lofepramine; amitriptyline and placebo in elderly subjects. *Eur. J. Clin. Pharmacol.*, **33**, 505–9.

Glass, R.M., Uhlenhuth, E.H., Hartel, F.W. *et al.* (1981) Cognitive dysfunction and imipramine in outpatient depressives. *Arch. Gen. Psychiat.*, **38**, 1048–51.

Glassman, A.H., Giardina, E.V., Perel, J.M. *et al.* (1979) Clinical characteristics of imipramine-induced orthostatic hypotension. *Lancet*, **i**, 468–72.

Glassman, A.H., Walsh, B.T., Roose, S.P. *et al.* (1982) Factors related to orthostatic hypotension associated with tricyclic antidepressants. *J. Clin. Psychiat.*, **43**, 35–8.

Glassman, A.H. and Bigger, J.T. (1981) Cardiovascular effects of therapeutic doses of tricyclic antidepressants: a review. *Arch. Gen. Psychiat.*, **38**, 815–20.

Glassman, A.H., Johnson, L.L., Giardina, E.G.V. *et al.*, (1983) The use of imipramine in depressed patients with congestive heart failure. *J. Am. Med. Ass.*, **250**, 1997–2001.

Goldberg, H.L., Finnerty, R.J. and Cole, J.O. (1975) The effects of doxepin in the aged: interim report on memory changes and electrocardiographic findings. In: *Senequan (Doxepin HCL): a Monograph of Clinical Studies* (ed. J. Mendels), Exerpta Medica, Amsterdam.

Gomersall, J.D. and Stuart, A. (1973) Amitriptyline in migraine prophylaxis: change in pattern of attacks during a controlled clinical trial. *J. Neurol. Neurosurg. Psychiat.*, **36**, 684–90.

Gwirtsman, H.E., Ahles, S., Halaris, A. *et al.* (1983) Therapeutic superiority of maprotiline versus doxepin in geriatric depression. *J. Clin. Psychiat.*, **44**, 449–53.

Hayes, R.L., Gerner, R.H., Fairbanks, L. *et al.* (1983) ECG findings in geriatric depressives given trazodone, placebo or imipramine. *J. Clin. Psychiat.*, **44**, 180–3.

Heath, A. and Hulten, B.A. (1983) Lofepramine toxicity in overdose. Presented at *VII World Congress of Psychiatry, Vienna.*

Henry, J.A., Ali, C.J., Caldwell, R. and Flanagan, R.J. (1984) Acute trazodone poisoning: clinical signs and plasma concentrations. *Psychopathol.*, **17** (Suppl. 2) 77–81.

Himmelhoch, J.M., Schechtman, K. and Auchenbach, R. (1984) The role of trazodone in the treatment of depressed cardiac patients. *Psychopathol.*, **17** (Suppl. 2) 51–63.

Hoff, G.S., Ruud, T.E., Tonder, M. and Holter, O. (1981) Doxepin in the treatment of duodenal ulcer. *Scand. J. Gastroenterol.*, **16**, 1041–2.

Howarth, B.G. and Grace, M.G.A. (1985) Depression drugs and delusions. *Arch. Gen. Psychiat.*, **42**, 1145–7.

Jacoby, R.J. (1981) Depression in the elderly. *Brit. J. Hosp. Med.*, **25**, 40–7.

Jaffe, G. and Grimshaw, J.J. (1985) A placebo-controlled comparison of l–tryptophan and amitriptyline in the treatment of depressive illness in general practice. *Brit. J. Clin. Social Psychiat.*, **3** (Suppl. 3) 51–5.

Janowski, D., Curtis, G., Zisook, S. *et al.* (1983) Ventricular arrhythmias possibly aggravated by trazodone. *Amer. J. Psychiat.*, **140**, 796–7.

Jarvik, L.F., Mintz, J., Stever, J. and Gerner, R. (1982) Treating geriatric depression: a 26-week interim analysis. *J. Am. Geriatr. Soc.*, **30**, 713–17.

Jessel, H.J., Jessel, I. and Wegener, G. (1981) Therapie von alteren depressiven patienten: lofepramin und amitriptylin unter doppelblindbedingungen. *Z. Allg. Med.*, **57**, 784–8.

Khan, A.U. (1981) A comparison of the therapeutic and cardiovascular effects of a single nightly dose of dothiepin and sustained–release amitriptyline in depressed elderly patients. *J. Brit. Med. Res.*, **9**, 108–12.

Kogeorgos, J. and de Alwis, C. (1986) Priapism and psychotropic medication. *Brit. J. Psychiat.*, **149**, 241–3.

Kretschmar, J.H. (1980) Mianserin and amitriptyline in elderly hospitalized patients with depressive illness: a double-blind trial. *Curr. Med. Res. Opin.*, **6** (Suppl. 7) 144–51.

Kumar, V., Smith, K., Reed, J. and Ledavathi, D.E. (1987) Plasma levels and effects of nortriptyline in geriatric depressed patients. *Acta. Psych. Scand.*, **75**, 20–8.

Kutcher, S.P., Reid, K., Dubbin, J.D. and Shulman, J.I. (1986) Electrocardiogram changes and therapeutic desipramine and 2–hydroxydesipramine concentrations in elderly depressives. *Brit. J. Psychiat.*, **148**, 676–9.

Lal, H. and Carroll, P.T. (1979) Alterations in brain neurotransmitter systems related to senescence. In: *Geriatric Psychopharmacology: Developments in Neurology Vol. 3* (ed. K. Nandy) Elsevier, New York, pp. 3–9.

Lawson, L.R. and MacLeod, R.D. (1969) The use of imipramine (Tofranil) and other psychotropic drugs in organic emotionalism. *Brit. J. Psychiat.*, **115**, 281–5.

Lipsey, J.R., Robinson, R.G., Pearlson, G.D. *et al.* (1984) Nortriptyline treatment of post stroke depression. *Lancet*, **i**, 297–300.

Livingstone, R.L., Zucker, D.K., Isenberg, K. and Wetzel, R.D. (1983) Tricyclic antidepressants and delirium. *J. Clin. Psychiat.*, **44**, 173–6.

Luchins, D.J. (1983) Review of the clinical and animal studies comparing the cardiovascular effects of doxepin and other tricyclic antidepressants. *Amer. J. Psychiat.*, **140**, 1006–9.

Marneros, A., Philipp, M. and Legeler, H.J. (1979) A double-blind trial with amitriptyline and lofepramine in the treatment of endogenous depression. *Int. Pharmacopsychiat.*, **14**, 300–4.

Mendels, J., Stinnett, J.K., Burns, D. and Frazer, A. (1975) Amine precursors and depression. *Arch. Gen. Psychiat.*, **32**, 22–30.

Mendlewicz, J., Dunbar, G.C. and Hoffman, G. (1985) Changes in sleep EEG architecture during the treatment of depressed patients with mianserin. *Acta. Psychiat. Scand.*, **72** (Suppl. 320) 26–9.

Meredith, C.H., Feighner, J.P. and Hendrickson, G. (1984) A double-blind comparative evaluation of the efficacy and safety of nomifensine, imipramine and placebo in depressed geriatric outpatients. *J. Clin. Psychiat.*, **45**, 73–7.

Middleton, R.S.W. (1975) A comparison between maprotiline (ludiomil) and imipramine in the treatment of depressive illness in the elderly. *J. Int. Med. Res.*, **3**, 79–83.

Moller, M., Thayssen, P., Kragh-Sorensen, P. *et al.* (1983) Mianserin: cardiovascular effects in elderly patients. *Psychopharmacol.*, **80**, 174–7.

Monro, P., Swade, C. and Coppen, A. (1985) Mianserin in the prophylaxis of migraine: a double-blind study. *Acta. Psychiat. Scand.*, **72** (Suppl. 320) 98–103.

Montgomery, I., Oswald, I., Morgan, K. and Adam, K. (1983) Trazodone enhances sleep in subjective quality but not in objective duration. *Brit. J. Clin. Pharmacol.*, **16**, 139–142.

Montgomery, S., McAuley, R. and Montgomery, D.B. (1978) Relationship between mianserin plasma levels and antidepressant effect in a double-blind trial comparing a single night-time and divided daily dose regimes. *Brit. J. Clin. Pharmac.*, **5** (Suppl. 1) 71S–76S.

Moody, J.P., Whyte, S.F. and MacDonald, A.J. (1977) Pharmacokinetic aspects of protriptyline plasma levels. *Eur. J. Clin. Pharmac.*, **11**, 51–6.

Nair, N.P.V., Ban, T.A., Hontella, S. and Clarke, R. (1973) Trazodone in the treatment of organic brain syndromes, with special reference to geriatrics. *Curr. Therap. Res.*, **15**, 769–75.

Nelson, J.C., Jatlow, P.L., Bock, J. *et al.* (1982) Major adverse reactions during desipramine treatment: relationship to plasma drug concentrations, concomitant antipsychotic treatment, and patient characteristics. *Arch. Gen. Psychiat.*, **39**, 1055–61.

Neshkes, R.E., Gerner, R., Jarvick, L.F. *et al.* (1985) Orthostatic effect of imipramine and doxepin in depressed geriatric patients. *J. Clin. Psychopharmacol.*, **5**, 102–6.

Nies, A., Robinson, D.S., Friedman, M.J. *et al.* (1977) Relationship between age and tricyclic antidepressant plasma levels. *Am J. Psychiat.*, **134**, 790–3.

Norman, T.R., Burrows, G.D., Scoggins, B.A. and Davies, B. (1979) Pharmacokinetics and plasma levels of antidepressants in the elderly. *Med. J. Aust.*, **1**, 273–4.

160

Nugent, D. (1979) A double-blind study of viloxazine (Vivalan) and amitriptyline in depressed geriatric patients. *Clin. Trials J.*, **16**, 13–17.

Office of Population and Censuses Survey (1984) *Deaths from solid and liquid poisoning 1982*. DH4 No. 8, Table 10.

Peet, M. (1984) The clinical profile of lofepramine. *Internat. Med.* (Suppl. **10**) 8–10.

Pichot, P., Dreyfus, J.F. and Pull, C. (1978) A double-blind multicentre trial comparing mianserin with imipramine. *Brit. J. Clin. Pharmacol.*, **5** (Suppl. 1) 87S–90S.

Pinder, R.M., Borgden, R.N., Speight, T.M. and Avery, G.S. (1977) Doxepin up-to-date: a review of its pharmacological properties and therapeutic efficacy with particular reference to depression. *Drugs*, **13**, 161–218.

Post, F. (1985) Psychotherapy, electroconvulsive treatments and long-term management of elderly depressives. *J. Aff. Dis.* (Suppl. 1) 41S–45S.

Quitkin, F.M., Rabkin, J.G., Ross, D. and McGrath, P.J. (1984) Duration of antidepressant drug treatment. *Arch. Gen. Psychiat.*, **41**, 238.

Robinson, R.G., Bolla Wilson, K., Kaplan, E. *et al.* (1986) Depression influences intellectual impairment in stroke patients. *Brit. J. Psychiat.*, **148**, 541–7.

Rausch, J.L., Pavlinac, D.M. and Newman, P.E. (1984) Complete heart block following a single dose of trazodone. *Am. J. Psychiat.*, **141**, 1472–3.

Ron, M.A., Toone, B.K., Garralda, M.E. and Lishman, W.A. (1979) Diagnostic accuracy in presenile dementia. *Brit. J. Psychiat.*, **134**, 161–8.

Roos, J.C. (1983) Cardiac effects of antidepressant drugs. A comparison of the tricyclic antidepressants and fluvoxamine. *Br. J. Clin. Pharmacol.*, **15**, 439S–445S.

Roose, S.P., Glassman, A.H., Siris, S.G. *et al.*, (1981) Comparison of imipramine and nortriptyline induced orthostatic hypotension: a meaningful difference. *J. Clin. Psychopharmacol.*, **1**, 316–19.

Roose, S.P., Glassman, A.H., Giardina, E.G.V. *et al.*, (1987) Tricyclic antidepressants in depressed patients with cardiac conduction disease. *Arch. Gen. Psychiat.*, **44**, 273–5.

Scardigli, G. and Jans, G. (1982) Comparative double-blind study on efficacy and side-effects of trazodone, nomifensine, mianserin in elderly patients. In: *Typical and Atypical Antidepressants: Clinical Practice* (eds. E. Costa and G. Racagni), Raven Press, New York, pp. 229–36.

Scher, M., Krieger, J.N. and Juergens, S. (1983) Trazodone and priapism. *Am. J. Psychiat.*, **140**, 1362–4.

Schmidt, L.G., Grohmann, R., Muller-Oerlinghausen, B. *et al.* (1986) Adverse drug reactions to first and second generation antidepressants: a critical evaluation of drug surveillance data. *Brit. J. Psychiat.*, **148**, 38–43.

Schneider-Helmert, D. and Spinweber, C.L. (1986) Evaluation of l–tryptophan for treatment of insomnia: a review. *Psychopharmacol.*, **89**, 1–7.

Shami, M., Elliott, H.L., Kelman, A.W. and Whiting, B. (1983) The pharmacokinetics of mianserin. *Brit. J. Clin. Pharmac.*, **15**, 313S–322S.

Shaw, W.L. (1980) The comparative safety of mianserin in overdose. *Curr. Med. Res. Opin.*, **6** (Suppl 7) 44–51.

Smith, A.H.W., Naylor, G.S. and Moody, J.P. (1978) Placebo-controlled double-blind trial of mianserin hydrochloride. *Br. J. Clin. Pharmacol.*, **5** (Suppl. 1) 67S–70S.

Spiker, D.G., Weiss, J.C., Dealy, R.S. *et al.*, (1985) The pharmocological treatment of delusional depression. *Am. J. Physchiat.*, **142**, 430–36.

Stern, H., Konestchny, J., Herrmann, L. *et al.*, (1985) Cardiovascular effects of single doses of the antidepressants amitriptyline and lofepramine in healthy subjects. *Pharmacopsychiat.*, **78**, 272–7.

Thayssen, P., Bjerre, M., Kragh-Sorensen, P. *et al.*, (1981) Cardiovascular effects of imipramine and notriptyline in elderly patients. *Psychopharmacol.*, **74**, 360–4.

Thompson, P.J. and Trimble, M.R. (1982) Non-MAOI antidepressant drugs and cognitive functions: a review. *Psychol. Med.*, **12**, 539–48.

Valle-Jones, J.C. and Swarbrick, D.J. (1983) A comparative study of once daily flupenthixol and amitriptyline in the treatment of elderly depressed patients: a multicentre trial in general practice. *J. Internat. Biomed. Inf. Data.*, **4**, 29–35.

Valnes, K., Myren, J. and Qvigstad, T. (1978) Trimipramine in the treatment of gastric ulcer. *Scand. J. Gastroenterol.*, **13**, 497–500.

Von Knorring, L. (1980) A double-blind trial: vivalan against placebo in elderly depressive patients. *J. Int. Med. Res.*, **8**, 18–21.

Veith, R.C., Raskind, M.A., Caldwell, J.H. *et al.* (1982) Cardiovascular effects of tricyclic antidepressants in depressed patients with chronic heart disease. *N. Engl. J. Med.*, **306**, 954–9.

Wakelin, J.S. (1986) Fluvoxamine in the treatment of the older depressed patient: double-blind, placebo-controlled data. *Int. Clin. Psychopharmacol.*, **1**, 221–30.

Walsh, T.D. (1983) Antidepressants in chronic pain. *Clin. Neuropharmacol.*, **6**, 271–95.

Ware, J.C. (1983) Tricyclic antidepressants in the treatment of insomnia. *J. Clin. Psychiat.*, **44**, 25–8.

Warrington, S. (1984) Cardiovascular effects of lofepramine. *Internat. Med.*, (Suppl. 10) 23–6.

Wetterhus, S., Aubert, E., Berg, C.E. *et al.*, (1977) The effect of trimipramine (Surmontil) on symptoms and healing of peptic ulcer: a double-blind study. *Scand. J. Gastroenterol.*, **12** (Suppl. 43) 33–8.

Wheatley, D. (1983) Effects of two dose regimens of trazodone on sleep. In: *Trazodone: Second Clinical Workshop*, Medicine Publishing Foundation, Oxford, pp. 4–5.

Wilson, J.A., Boyd, E.J.S. and Wormsley, K.G. (1985) Effects of some polycyclic drugs on gastric secretion and on the healing of duodenal ulcers. *Acta. Psychiat. Scand.*, **72** (Suppl. 320) 93–7.

Zorumski, C.F. and Rubin, E.H. (1984) Psychopharmacologic and behavioral approaches to chronic arthritic pain. *Compr. Ther.*, **10**, 35–9.

Chapter Ten

Cardiovascular effects of tricyclic antidepressants in elderly people

JILA DANA-HAERI and STEVEN J. WARRINGTON

CONTENTS

10.1 INTRODUCTION

During the last twenty years or so psychiatrists have shown a preoccupation with the cardiovascular effects of antidepressants which has become almost obsessional. Their concern may well be unnecessary in the case of younger patients taking therapeutic doses of these drugs, but they are probably right to be anxious about their elderly patients. Unfortunately, it is not possible to relieve this anxiety by prescribing only drugs which are known to be safe in the elderly, since there is no drug which is known to be completely safe even in younger patients, and there is every reason to suppose that the elderly are especially susceptible to the adverse cardiovascular effects of these drugs.

10.2 POSSIBLE CARDIOVASCULAR ADVERSE EFFECTS

The possible cardiovascular adverse effects of antidepressant drugs may be summarized as follows:-

1 changes in blood pressure
2 impairment of cardiac contractility
3 intracardiac conduction disturbances
4 arrhythmias
5 sudden death (presumably due to arrhythmia)

The evidence that antidepressants impair cardiac contractility or cause sudden death is weak, but there is no doubt that, in therapeutic doses, they can cause troublesome falls in blood pressure; there is also no doubt that they can cause chaotic blood pressure regulation and arrhythmias after overdosage (Glassman and Bigger, 1981). Of all these possible adverse effects, a reduction in blood presure on standing seems particularly likely to be a problem in the elderly; their homeostatic mechanisms are inferior to those of younger patients and the presence of cerebrovascular disease might accentuate the effects of any fall in blood pressure. Furthermore, the elderly tend to be unsteady on their feet, which perhaps increases the risk of falls during episodes of postural hypotension. The consequences of falls can be particularly serious in older patients; some may simply be unable to get up again and others may suffer fractures in their osteoporotic bones, with subsequent high morbidity and mortality. Doctors hoping to mitigate these effects by instructing patients to take their treatment last thing at night should remember that many old people have nocturia and may therefore have to rise from their warm beds and stagger across dark, obstacle-strewn rooms just as their plasma concentrations of antidepressant reach a peak.

10.3 SPECIAL PROBLEMS IN THE ELDERLY

Depression is common in the elderly and since it is reasonable to suppose that antidepressants might have important cardiovascular toxicity in the elderly, one might expect that there would be numerous published reports of studies designed to assess the size of this problem and to compare the toxicity of the available antidepressant drugs. In fact, few studies have addressed this question, and those that have should be interpreted with caution. Most studies of antidepressants in the elderly have been designed to assess therapeutic efficacy rather than toxicity and the observations made have been unlikely to detect cardio-vascular toxicity even when it is present. Numbers of patients studied may have been adequate to detect therapeutic effects, which are found in 60–70% of patients, but insufficient to show cardiovascular toxicity, which is likely to affect a much smaller proportion. Even if toxicity can be detected, very large numbers of patients may be needed to allow a useful comparison of the cardiovascular toxicity of two or more anti-depressant drugs. If the aim of a study is to show that a drug has no cardiovascular toxicity, then a small, badly designed trial is the kind most likely to yield the desired results.

In papers describing studies of antidepressant treatment in the elderly, the cardiovascular tolerability data should be viewed with circumspection. For example, presentation of mean blood pressure results is often unhelpful, since postural hypotension may affect one or two patients very severely, but the others not at all; means may be meaningless. Full details should be given of patients who have with-drawn from the study; some of these may have dropped out because of dizziness or faintness caused by low blood presure, but they may well be omitted from the final analysis because they did not participate in the study for long enough to have any cardiovascular measurements made.

Since the existing reports of the efficacy and tolerability of anti-depressants in the elderly do not allow the prescriber to assess fully the risks and benefits of treatment with each drug, it is tempting to rely upon the results of the studies carried out in younger patients. This should be done with extreme caution; only the unfavourable results of treatment in the young can safely be extrapolated to the elderly. Adverse effects of antidepressant drugs seem more likely to occur in the elderly than in the young because of both pharmacodynamic and kinetic factors. The elderly have impaired hepatic and, particularly, renal clearance of drugs leading to higher steady state plasma concentrations at any given dose. They are also very likely to have pre-existing cardiovascular disease such as hypertension, coronary artery obstruc-tion, degenerative changes in the cardiac conduction system and ortho-static hypotension. A final complication is that the elderly are much more likely than the young to be taking other medication which might interact with their antidepressant therapy.

We now review the available evidence that antidepressant drugs given to the elderly in therapeutic doses can have important effects on blood pressure or on the mechanical or electrophysiological performance of the heart. We also consider the evidence that they can cause sudden death, and review the evidence for their safety or otherwise in overdosage. In general, we have tried to limit our review to studies in the elderly, but for most drugs the studies performed in the elderly are not adequate to make a full assessment and there is no alternative but to extrapolate from unfavourable results of studies in younger patients.

10.4 ORTHOSTATIC HYPOTENSION

10.4.1 Background

A fall in blood pressure on standing seems to be the most common and troublesome cardiovascular effect of antidepressants (Glassman and Bigger, 1981). In a review of 148 patients who were receiving imipramine at a mean dose of 225 mg daily, Glassman *et al.* (1979) found that 20% of patients had symptoms of orthostatic hypotension sufficient to interfere with their participation in the study and 4% actually sustained physical injuries attributable to postural hypotension. This study was retrospective, but orthostatic hypotension has been reported in prospective studies of amitriptyline (Kopera, 1978), imipramine (Roose *et al.*, 1981), desmethylimipramine (Nelson *et al.*, 1982), doxepin (Vohra, Burrows and Sloman, 1975) and trazodone (Van de Merwe, Silverstone and Ankier, 1984). All these drugs should be assumed to be capable of causing postural hypotension in the elderly until proved otherwise.

10.4.2 Studies in the elderly

The expectation that imipramine should cause postural hypotension in elderly patients has been amply confirmed by Muller, Goodma and Bellet (1960) who studied 82 depressed patients, 41 of whom were elderly and had underlying cardiovascular diseases. Seventy-eight percent of the older patients had a significant postural fall in blood pressure compared with 37% of the younger patients. Two of the elderly patients developed myocardial infarction which the authors attributed to orthostatic hypotension. Similar but less catastrophic results were reported by Neshkes *et al.* (1985). They studied 36 'elderly' depressed patients aged 55–81 years who were receiving conventional doses of either imipramine, doxepin or placebo. Three out of 14 patients receiving imipramine had severe orthostatic hypotension and their medication had to be changed; the effects of doxepin on blood pressure were similar to those of placebo.

Amitriptyline was reported by Christensen *et al.* (1985) to cause orthostatic hypotension in patients aged 60–82 years who were receiving the drug in a fixed daily dose of 100 mg in a sustained release preparation. In contrast, Khan (1981) found no postural changes in pulse rate or blood pressure in 50 elderly depressed patients who were receiving therapeutic doses of amitriptyline or dothiepin.

Nortriptyline treatment did not cause any change in orthostatic blood pressure response in 10 elderly depressed patients (Thayssen *et al.*, 1981); in the same study, imipramine caused marked postural hypotension.

Conflicting results have been obtained with doxepin, which was associated with orthostatic hypotension in the elderly patients of Veith and co-workers (1982), but not in those of Neshkes *et al.* (1985; see above) and Ahles and colleagues (1984); in a double-blind study of 49 elderly patients receiving treatment with maprotiline or doxepin, Ahles *et al.* (1984) reported no significant difference in orthostatic blood pressure responses between treatment and non-treatment phases or between the two drugs.

Mianserin caused orthostatic dizziness and a significant reduction in systolic blood pressure upon standing in 10 elderly depressed patients (Moller *et al.*, 1983); there were no significant changes in supine blood pressure or in heart rate upon standing.

In a double-blind placebo-controlled study in 60 elderly patients, trazodone was better tolerated than imipramine, with fewer cardiovascular unwanted effects (Gerner *et al.*, 1980). However, experience in younger patients suggests that trazodone can indeed cause orthostatic hypotension (Van de Merwe, Silverstone and Ankier, 1984).

If we allow ourselves to extrapolate to the elderly from unfavourable results in younger patients, we can be fairly confident that imipramine, desmethylimipramine, amitriptyline, doxepin, mianserin and trazodone are all capable of causing postural hypotension in a proportion of elderly depressed patients. The encouraging negative results with dothiepin (Khan, 1981) and maprotiline (Ahles *et al.*, 1984) should be interpreted very cautiously, since in these studies negative reults were also obtained for amitriptyline and doxepin respectively, both of which have been found to cause postural hypotension on other studies. Data is lacking for lofepramine.

10.5 EFFECTS ON VENTRICULAR MECHANICAL FUNCTION

10.5.1 Background

Antidepressant drugs can cause severe hypotension when taken in overdose and a smattering of case reports have described heart failure occurring in patients taking therapeutic doses of some of these drugs. Many studies have attempted to show whether therapeutic doses of antidepressants systematically depress left ventricular contractility; in these studies, contractility has usually been assessed by serial measurement of systolic time intervals (STI) or radionuclide left ventricular angiography.

Measurement of STI in volunteers and patients receiving antidepressants has been claimed to show drug-induced reduction in contractility (Burckhardt *et al.*, 1978; Taylor and Braithwaite, 1978; Burgess *et al.*, 1979; Guerra and Melina, 1980). In all these studies, however, the STI were corrected for heart rate using the regression equations described by Weissler, Harris and Schoenfeld (1968) and it is now clear that these equations over-correct for changes in heart rate which occur following the administration of a drug with, for example, anticholinergic activity (Johnson *et al.*, 1981). Hence, the observation that some antidepressants prolong the STI may simply have been an artifact, since most of the drugs studied also caused a substantial increase in heart rate.

There are two other problems in the interpretation of STI. Firstly, the tricyclic antidepressant drugs may slow intracardiac electrical conduction, which will inevitably prolong the STI independently of any effect on contractility. Secondly, the STI are infuenced by changes in peripheral resistance and venous return, upon which the tricyclic antidepressants undoubtedly have an effect.

Support for the view that therapeutic doses of antidepressants have little effect on cardiac contractility in younger depressed patients comes from studies using radionuclide left ventricular angiography to assess cardiac function (Veith *et al.*, 1982; Glassman *et al.*, 1983).

10.5.2 Studies in the elderly

Since we have disciplined ourselves not to extrapolate favourable or equivocal results from younger patients to the elderly population, we have to rely on only three studies in elderly patients to assess whether these drugs have a greater adverse effect on ventricular mechanical function in this age group. Thayssen and colleagues (1981) reported significant prolongation of STI in elderly patients receiving nortriptyline; these findings are the more persuasive because there were negligible changes in STI in patients receiving imipramine treatment in the same study. However, these workers did not measure any ECG intervals as indicators of delay in intracardiac conduction which might have accounted for the prolongation in STI. Amitriptyline prolonged the STI in elderly patients studied by Christensen and co-workers (1985). Moller and colleagues (1983) studied ten elderly patients aged 60–77 years who were receiving mianserin treatment and found prolongation of STI suggestive of reduced left ventricular contractility; however, these workers did measure the ECG intervals and found increases in PR and QRS duration indicating delayed intracardiac conduction, which could have accounted at least in part for the observed prolongation of STI.

Overall, the evidence that antidepressants cause important depression of left ventricular contractility in young or elderly patients is equivocal. The number and quality of studies so far reported do not allow any firm conclusions, particularly in the elderly. Tricyclic antidepressants, especially imipramine, do have quinidine-like (Class 1 antiarrhythmic) activity on the heart and would, therefore, be expected to have at least minor depressant effects on contractility, which might be enough to precipitate heart failure in patients with already compromised ventricular function.

10.6 ELECTROPHYSIOLOGICAL EFFECTS

10.6.1 Background

Tricyclic antidepressant drugs, particularly imipramine, may have antiarrhythmic effects at therapeutic doses (Bigger *et al.*, 1977; Giardina, Bigger and Johnson, 1981). Imipramine and nortriptyline can prolong PR interval, QRS duration and QT interval to a similar extent as procainamide or quinidine (Giardina *et al.*, 1979; Giardina and Bigger, 1982; Barnard, Giardina and Bigger, 1982). The observations have important clinical implications. First, the concurrent administration of quinidine-like (Class 1 antiarrhythmic) drugs and tricyclic antidepressants such as imipramine could lead to cardiac toxicity and it might be appropriate to reduce the dose of Class 1 antiarrhythmic drugs when they are given to patients receiving tricyclic antidepressants (Kantor *et al.*, 1978). Secondly, treatment with tricyclic antidepressants might be useful in suppressing arrhythmias; indeed, Glassman and Bigger (1981) have suggested that imipramine might be a valuable antiarrythmic drug. Thirdly, the tricyclic antidepressants would be expected to precipitate or worsen cardiac arrhythmias in some patients, since this phenomenon is well recognized with other antiarrhythmic drugs. Not surprisingly, studies in young or elderly depressed patients have not been large or detailed enough to confirm these predictions. Most studies have concentrated upon more easily measured variables such as heart rate and intracardiac conduction times.

Imipramine, nortriptyline, amitriptyline and doxepin all increase heart rate in patients with or without heart disease (Vohra, Burrows and Sloman, 1985; Bigger *et al.*, 1978; Veith *et al.*, 1982). Edwards and Goldie

(1983) found similar results with maprotiline, but mianserin did not increase heart rate.

Electrophysiological effects of antidepressant drugs have been compared using the surface ECG and intracardiac electrography. The ECG effects of imipramine at therapeutic plasma concentrations were studied by Giardina and co-workers (1979) in 44 patients, including 10 who had ECG evidence of disease in the cardiac conduction system. Imipramine signficantly increased heart rate and PR, QRS and QTC intervals. In a study of 35 depressed patients, Edwards and Goldie (1983) compared the cardiovascular effects of mianserin with those of placebo; maprotiline significantly increased PR interval and decreased QTC, whereas mianserin was not significantly different from placebo.

His bundle electrography has been used to study the effects of some tricyclic antidepressants upon intracardiac conduction in depressed patients. Vohra, Burrows and Sloman (1975) studied 12 patients before and during nortriptyline treatment; they found that nortriptyline prolonged H–V interval (conduction time from His bundle to ventricles) in five patients, while A–H (atrium to His bundle conduction time) was unaffected. Broadly similar results have been obtained for doxepin (Burrows *et al.*, 1977) and imipramine (Kantor *et al.*, 1978; Glassman and Bigger, 1981). Overall, these results confirm the quinidine-like action of tricyclic antidepressants on the intracardiac conduction system.

The importance of the effects of antidepressant drugs on the intracardiac conduction system remains the subject of debate. There is no doubt that tricyclic antidepressants can cause severe conduction defects and ventricular arrhythmias when taken in overdose (Smith and Rusbach, 1967; Kantor *et al.*, 1975; Ramanathan and Davidson, 1975; Todd and Faber, 1983) and can suppress ventricular extrasystoles when given in therapeutic doses (Bigger *et al.*, 1977; Giardina, Bigger and Johnson, 1981), but it remains uncertain whether the electrophysiological effects of these drugs confer a net benefit or hazard upon depressed patients, whatever their ages. The majority view in the UK seems to be that the electrophysiological effects of antidepressants are a greater potential hazard than benefit and there is considerable interest in identifying antidepressant drugs which have negligible cardiac electrophysiological effects.

10.6.2 Studies in the elderly

Drugs which increase heart rate are in principle undesirable in the elderly, since they increase myocardial oxygen consumption and reduce the proportion of the cardiac cycle available for diastolic coronary blood flow; the elderly are more likely than younger patients to have pre-existing coronary artery disease and so are at higher risk of drug-induced myocardial ischaemia or infarction. On the other hand, one might expect the anticholinergic effects of antidepressant drugs to be less noticeable in the elderly, who have lower vagal tone to the heart. This latter expectation was to some extent confirmed in a study of 27 elderly depressed patients by Thayssen *et al.* (1981), who found that nortriptyline treatment significantly increased heart rate, but imipramine treatment did not. This negative result for imipramine is encouraging, but too much reliance should not be placed on it since the study was of parallel group design in a very modest number of patients. Amitriptyline does increase heart rate in the elderly (Christensen, *et al.*, 1985). Mianserin, on the other hand, was without significant effect on heart rate in 10 elderly depressed patients, compared with placebo (Moller *et al.*, 1983).

There have been no studies in the elderly of the effects of antidepressants on intracardiac electrography, but several studies in the elderly have included examination of the 12-lead ECG and, in some cases, continuous ambulatory ECG monitoring. Christensen *et al.* (1985) reported increases in PR and QRS intervals in 13 elderly patients who had received amitriptyline treatment for five weeks. In contrast, Thayssen and co-workers (1981) observed no arrhythmias and no impairment of intracardiac conduction in any of 27 elderly patients receiving either imipramine or nortriptyline treatment for six weeks. Ahles and co-workers (1984) treated 49 elderly depressed patients with either maprotiline or doxepin and the patients underwent both standard 12-lead ECG recording and continuous ECG monitoring. Both drugs significantly increased heart rate and prolonged the PR interval; doxepin decreased, and maprotiline increased, QRS duration. Maprotiline decreased ventricular extrasystoles (VEs) in patients who had had a high pre-treatment frequency of VEs, whereas doxepin actually increased VEs.

On the basis of these reports it is probably safe to assume that all the standard tricyclic antidepressants, and the closely-related drug maprotiline, may have quinidine-like effects on the heart in elderly depressed patients. The negative results for imipramine and nortriptyline in the study of Thayssen *et al.* (1981) are not particularly reassuring, since contrary results have been obtained in studies which included elderly patients with pre-existing heart disease. Kantor and colleagues (1978) observed delays in intracardiac conduction in seven elderly depressed patients receiving imipramine treatment; four of these patients had evidence of underlying heart disease, including three with pre-existing bundle branch block. Young and co-workers (1985) studied 18 elderly depressed patients before and during nortriptyline administration; ten patients had a history of coronary heart disease and eight had ECG abnormalities, including right bundle branch block, evidence of myocardial infarction and non-specific ST segment and T wave changes. During nortriptyline treatment, PR interval increased in six patients and one patient developed right bundle branch block; QTC interval was increased in one patient. No clinically important adverse cardiovascular events were noted in these studies, but this is perhaps to be expected in view of the small number of patients included.

Insufficient data is available to allow assessment of the cardiac electrophysiological effects of the newer antidepressant drugs in elderly patients, but because the newer drugs generally have negligible quinidine-like effects they would be expected to have lesser effects on the ECG. This expectation has been confirmed to a very limited extent in a prospective study of 10 elderly depressed patients receiving mianserin treatment; no cardiac conduction defect or arrhythmias were observed during 24 h ECG monitoring (Moller *et al.*, 1983). Trazodone is supposed to have little effect on cardiac conduction (Himmelhoch, Schechtman and Auchenbach, 1984), but there is insufficient evidence to confirm this supposition in the elderly. Individual case reports of first degree heart block in a 74-year-old man (Irwin and Spar, 1983), junctional rhythm of 53 beats/min in a 50-year-old woman (Lippman *et al.*, 1983) and ventricular ectopics in two patients with pre-existing cardiac disease (Janowsky *et al.*, 1983) serve only to raise suspicions which may ultimately prove to be unjustified.

10.7 SUDDEN DEATH

10.7.1 Background

The evidence that tricyclic antidepressants in therapeutic doses can cause sudden death in young or elderly patients is far from convincing. The only support for this possibility comes from the studies of the Aberdeen General Hospitals Group (Coull *et al.*, 1970; Moir *et al.*, 1972; Moir, Dingwall-Fordyce and Weir, 1973) and relates to the increased incidence of 'sudden unexpected death' in patients receiving amitriptyline, and sudden death in a much smaller group of patients receiving imipramine. The findings with amitriptyline are greatly weakened by the fact that the study was not designed to test the hypothesis that the drug caused sudden death, and the analysis was retrospective and used rather odd criteria to distinguish between 'sudden unexpected death' and other kinds of death. In the case of imipramine, four sudden deaths were reported in a group of 89 patients receiving the drug, compared with two in a control group – a suggestive result, but hardly conclusive. The Boston Collaborative Drug Surveillance Program (1972) found no evidence of increased risk of sudden death in recipients of tricyclic anti-depressants, but the duration of treatment was short; on average, about two weeks. Eighty-nine percent of patients in this study were receiving either amitriptyline or imipramine. In a sub-group of 80 patients who had previous evidence of cardiovascular disease, there was no difference in incidence of arrhythmia, heart block, hypotension, syncope, shock, heart failure or sudden death compared with a control group.

10.7.2 The elderly

No data is available on the risk of sudden death during treatment of the elderly with antidepressant drugs. If we accept that the pharmacology of antidepressant drugs is such that they would be expected to cause sudden death in younger patients, we should also expect them to cause sudden death with similar or greater frequency in elderly patients, who are more likely to have pre-existing cardiac disease. We may perhaps draw some comfort from the fact that, even when many psychiatrists are gathered together, there are few anecdotal reports of sudden and unexpected death in the elderly. Although no formal analysis can be made, it seems unlikely that the risk of sudden death associated with therapeutic doses of these drugs is of the same order as the mortality from overdosage, or the morbidity and mortality which might result from postural hypotension.

10.8 OVERDOSE

Overdosage with tricyclic antidepressants often causes hypotension, prolongation of PR, QRS and QT intervals and severe arrhythmias, including cardiac arrest in ventricular fibrillation or asystole; cardiovascular toxicity in overdosage is a very important hazard of treatment with these drugs. No studies of this problem have considered the elderly as a separate group and this approach is probably reasonable since one would expect the drugs to have similar but more serious toxicity in the elderly than in younger patients. The circumstances of overdosage prevent the direct comparison of different drugs, but some tentative conclusions can be drawn.

A survey of 489 patients who had taken overdoses of tricyclic anti-depressants showed that hypotension occurred in 6.3% (Shaw, 1980). Shaw also reported on 75 patients who had taken maprotiline overdose and hypotension occurred in 2.7% of these. Maprotiline overdosgae seems to cause cardiovascular toxicity at least as severe as that associated with the classical tricyclic antidepressants; in a personal series, hypotension (systolic blood pressure less than 90 mmHg) was observed in 8 out of 41 patients (Knudsen and Heath, 1984). Langou and co-workers (1980) in a retrospective analysis of 35 patients who had taken amitriptyline or imipramine overdose, found that 18 patients had systolic blood pressures of less than 80 mmHg; amitriptyline overdose was associated with hypotension in 65% compared with 16% of patients who had taken imipramine. This does not however mean that imipramine is safer than amitriptyline in overdose, because the 'treatment' groups were not matched for age, pre-existing illness or size of overdose. Strom and colleagues (1984) reviewed 295 patients with severe tricyclic antidepressant poisoning and found a 35% incidence of hypotension. This contrasts quite markedly with the 6.3% incidence of hypotension reported by Shaw (1980) and indicates the extreme difficulty of assessing relative toxicity of the drugs in overdosage.

The newer antidepressant drugs do seem to be somewhat safer in overdose. Mianserin in overdosage seems to have relatively mild effects on blood pressure (Crome and Newman, 1977), but certainly can cause hypertension and, less commonly, hypotension (Shaw, 1980). Thirteen patients who had taken lofepramine overdose were studied by Heath (1984); one patient had sinus tachycardia and another patient had a wide QRS complex, but there were no arrhythmias or major changes in blood pressure. The lack of any other reports describing severe cardiovascular effects or death after lofepramine overdose is encouraging and is particularly interesting, since lofepramine is metabolized to desmethylimipramine which would be expected to have deleterious cardiovascular effects similar to those of imipramine. Possible explanations for the apparently low toxicity of lofepramine in overdose include rate-limited metabolism of lofepramine to desmethylimipramine or, more fancifully, a protective effect of lofepramine itself against the cardiovascular toxicity of its main metabolite (Warrington, 1984).

It has been suggested that prolongation of QRS interval greater than 100 milliseconds on the standard 12-lead ECG is a good indication of severity of overdose with the classical tricyclic antidepressants (Hulten and Heath, 1983; Boehnert and Lovejoy, 1985). Seizures and ventricular arrhythmias occur most frequently when plasma concentrations of tricyclic antidepressant drugs exceed 1000 ng/ml, and at these concentrations the QRS duration is over 100 ms (Bigger *et al.*, 1977; Spiker *et al.*, 1975). In a prospective study of 49 patients with acute overdosage of tricyclic antidepressants, Boehnert and co-workers (1985) confirmed that increased QRS duration is predictive both of seizures and ventricular arrhythmias; patients with QRS duration greater than 100 ms had a 34% incidence of seizures and 14% incidence of ventricular arrhythmias, whereas patients with QRS duration less than 100 ms had neither seizures nor arrhythmias.

Overall, the pernicious nature of tricyclic antidepressants in overdose was confirmed by the study of Strom and colleagues (1984) who studied 295 patients. Forty-three percent showed widening of QRS complexes with supraventricular and ventricular arrhythmias and 14 patients had cardiac arrest. The evidence so far available, although scanty, does suggest that the newer drugs lofepramine (Heath, 1984) mianserin (Chand, Crome and Dawling, 1981) and trazodone (Crome and Ali, 1986) may be safer in overdose.

10.9 CONCLUSION

The available evidence does not allow us to identify any single antidepressant drug which is particularly free from cardiovascular effects, and which might be ideal for the treatment of elderly patients with or without heart disease. However, there are some special circumstances in which one drug, or group of drugs, might seem more appropriate than others.

Patients with ventricular arrhythmias requiring treatment could be given long-term therapy with imipramine, since this drug is effective against both depression and ventricular arrhythmias. Use of imipramine would have the advantage of avoiding the use of a combination of antidepressants and antiarrhythmic drugs, with its attendant problems of poor compliance and possible interactions.

Elderly patients with coronary heart disease might be best treated with drugs which do not cause an increase in heart rate in therapeutic doses, and mianserin and trazodone are probably better than the older tricyclic drugs in this respect.

Patients who are receiving treatment with drugs which can cause postural hypotension, such as diuretics, adrenergic neurone blockers, organic nitrates or calcium antagonists, should be treated with drugs which have the smallest effects on blood pressure. Unfortunately, no drug seems to be entirely blameless in this respect, but imipramine seems to be especially hazardous. More studies are needed to show whether dothiepin, doxepin, lofepramine, mianserin, nortriptyline or trazodone have any advantage over each other.

Elderly patients with heart failure can probably be treated with the same drugs as patients without heart disease, but the cautious prescriber might choose one of the newer drugs which is without quinidine-like activity, such as mianserin or trazodone.

In the great majority of elderly depressed patients there are no special cardiovascular features which might lead the psychiatrist to choose one drug rather than another. Many doctors still favour the use of the classical tricyclic antidepressants such as amitriptyline or imipramine on

175

the grounds that they are of a proven efficacy and, while they are not free of adverse effects such as postural hypotension, they are highly unlikely to have any adverse effects which we have not yet discovered – such as those that led to the withdrawal of nomifensine and zimelidine. Other doctors may be particularly concerned about the risk of postural hypotension in the elderly and for that reason might favour nortriptyline or one of the newer drugs, in spite of the rather scanty evidence that they differ from the other available drugs in their effects on blood pressure. A final option, which is favoured, is to choose a drug which is likely to be relatively safe in overdosage, and here lofepramine, mianserin and trazodone seem to have a real advantage over the classical tricyclics and maprotiline. The final choice depends, as is so often the case, on the nice clinical judgement of the prescriber.

REFERENCES

Ahles, S., Gwirtsman, H., Halaris, A. *et al.* (1984) Comparative cardiac effects of maprotiline and doxepin in elderly depressed patients. *J. Clin. Psychiat.*, **45**, 460–5.

Barnard, J.T., Giardina, E.G.V. and Bigger, J.T. (1982) The antiarrhythmic and chronotropic effects of nortriptyline in cardiac patients (abst.) *Circulation*, **66**, 143.

Bigger, J.T., Giardina, E.G.V., Perel, J.M. *et al.* (1977) Cardiac antiarrhythmic effect of imipramine hydrochloride. *New Engl. J. Med.*, **296**, 206–8.

Bigger, J.T., Kantor, S.J., Glassman, A.H. *et al.* (1978) Cardiovascular effects of tricyclic antidepressant drugs. In: *Psychopharmacology: A Generation of Progress* (eds. M.A. Lipton, A. Di Mascio and K.F. Killam), Raven Press, New York, pp. 1033–46.

Boehnert, M.T. and Lovejoy, F.H. Jr. (1985) Value of the QRS duration versus the serum drug level in predicting seizures and ventricular arrhythmias after an acute overdose of tricyclic antidepressants. *New Engl. J. Med.*, **313**, 474–9.

Boston Collaborative Drug Surveillance Program (1972) Adverse reactions to tricyclic antidepressant drugs: report from Boston Collaborative Drug Surveillance Program. *Lancet*, **1**, 529–31.

Burckhardt, D., Raeder, E., Muller, V. *et al.* (1978) Cardiovascular effects of tricyclic and tetracyclic antidepressants. *J. Am. Med. Assoc.*, **239**, 213–16.

Burgess, C.D., Montgomery, S.A., Turner, P. and Wadsworth, J. (1979) Cardiovascular effects of amitriptyline, mianserin, zimelidine and nomifensine in depressed patients. *Postgrad. Med. J.*, **55**, 704–8.

Burrows, G.D., Vohra, J., Dumovic, P. *et al.* (1977) Tricyclic antidepressant drugs and cardiac conduction. *Prog. Neuropsychopharmacology*, **1**, 329–34.

Chand, S., Crome, P. and Dawling, S. (1981) One hundred cases of acute intoxication with mianserin hydrochloride. *Pharmacopsychiatry*, **14**, 15–17.

Christensen, P., Thomsen, H.Y., Pedersen, O.L. *et al.* (1985) Cardiovascular effects of amitriptyline in the treatment of elderly depressed patients. *Psychopharmacology*, **87**, 212–15.

Coull, D.C., Crooks, J., Dingwall-Fordyce, I. *et al.* (1970) Amitriptyline and cardiac disease: risk of sudden death identified by monitoring system. *Lancet*, **ii**, 590–1.

Crome, P. and Newman, B. (1977) Poisoning with maprotiline and mianserin. *Brit. Med. J.*, **2**, 260.

Crome, P. and Ali, C. (1986) Clinical features and management of self-poisoning with newer antidepressants. *Med. Toxicol.*, **1**, 411–20.

Edwards, J.G. and Goldie, A. (1983) Mianserin, maprotiline and intracardiac conduction. *Brit. J. Clin. Pharmacol.*, **15**, 249S–254S.

Gerner, R., Estabrook, W., Steuer, J. and Jarvik, L. (1980) Treatment of geriatric depression with trazodone, imipramine and placebo: a double-blind study. *J. Clin. Psychol.*, **41**, 216–20.

Giardina, E.G.V., Bigger, J.T., Glassman, A.H. *et al.* (1979) The electrocardiographic and antiarrhythmic effects of imipramine hydrochloride at therapeutic plasma concentrations. *Circulation*, **60**, 1045–52.

Giardina, E.G.V., Bigger, J.T. and Johnson, L.L. (1981) The effect of imipramine and nortriptyline on ventricular depolarization and left ventricular function. *Circulation*, **64**, 316.

Giardina, E.C. and Bigger, J.T. (1982) Antiarrhythmic effect of imipramine hydrochloride in patients with ventricular premature complexes without psychological depression. *Am. J. Cardiol.*, **50**, 172–9.

Glassman, A.H., Bigger, J.T., Giardina, E.V. *et al.* (1979) Clinical characteristics of imipramine-induced orthostatic hypotension. *Lancet*, **i**, 468–72.

Glassman, A.H. and Bigger, J.T. (1981) Cardiovascular effects of therapeutic doses of tricyclic antidepressants: a review. *Arch. Gen. Psychiat.*, **38**, 815–20.

Glassman, A.H., Johnson, L.L. and Giardina, E.G.V. (1983) The use of imipramine in depressed patients with congestive heart failure. *J. Am. Med. Assoc.*, **250**, 1997–2001.

Guerra, G. and Melina, D. (1980) Effetti cardiaci degli antidepressivi tricidici somministati dosi therapeutiche. *Minerva Cardioangiol.*, **28**, 743–52.

Heath, A. (1984) Suicidal overdoses of antidepressants, with special reference to lofepramine. *Internat. Med.* (Suppl. 10), 27–30.

Himmelhoch, J.M., Schechtman, K. and Auchenbach, R. (1984) The role of trazodone in the treatment of depressed cardiac patients. *Psychopathology*, **17** (Suppl. 2) 51–63.

Hulten, B.A. and Heath, A. (1983) Clinical aspects of tricyclic antidepressant poisoning. *Acta. Med. Scand.*, **213**, 275–8.

Irwin, M. and Spar, J.E. (1983) Reversible cardiac conduction abnormality associated with trazodone administration. *Am. J. Psychiat.*, **140**, 945–6.

Janowsky, D., Curtis, G., Zisook, S., Kuhn, K. *et al.* (1983) Ventricular arrhythmias possibly aggravated by trazodone. *Am. J. Psychiat.*, **140**, 769–7.

Johnson, B.F., Meeran, M.K., Frank, A. and Taylor, S.H. (1981) Systolic time intervals in measurement of inotropic response to drugs. *Brit. Heart J.*, **46**, 513–21.

Kantor, S.J., Bigger, J.T., Glassman, A.H. *et al.* (1975) Imipramine-induced heart block. A longitudinal case study. *J. Am. Med. Assoc.*, **231**, 1364–6.

Kantor, S.J., Glassman, A.H., Bigger, J.T. *et al.* (1978) The cardiac effects of therapeutic plasma concentrations of imipramine. *Am. J. Psychiat.*, **135**, 534–8.

Khan, A.U. (1981) Comparison of the therapeutic cardiovascular effects of a single nightly dose of Prothiaden (dothiepin, dosulepin) and Lentizol (sustained-release amitriptyline) in depressed elderly patients. *J. Int. Med. Res.*, **9**, 108–12.

Knudsen, K. and Heath, A. (1984) Effect of self-poisoning with maprotiline. *Brit. Med. J.*, **288**, 601–2.

Kopera, H. (1978) Anticholinergic and blood pressure effects of mianserin, amitriptyline and placebo. *Brit. J. Clin. Pharmacol.*, **5**, 29S–34S.

Langou, R.A., Van Dyke, C., Tahan, S.R. and Cohen, L.S. (1980) Cardiovascular manifestations of tricyclic antidepressant over-dose. *Am. Heart. J.*, **100**, 458–64.

Lippman, S., Bedford, P., Manshadi, N. and Mather, S. (1983) Trazodone cardiotoxicity. *Am. J. Psychiat.*, **140**, 1383.

Moir, D.C., Crooks, J., Cornwall, W.B. *et al.* (1972) Cardiotoxicity of amitriptyline. *Lancet*, **ii**, 561–4.

Moir, D.C., Dingwall-Fordyce, I. and Weir, R.D. (1973) Medicines evaluation and monitoring group: a follow-up study of cardiac patients receiving amitriptyline. *Eur. J. Clin. Pharmacol.*, **6**, 98–101.

Moller, M., Thayssen, P., Kragh-Soerensen, P. *et al.* (1983) Mianserin: cardiovascular effects in elderly patients. *Psychopharmacol.*, **80**, 174–7.

Muller, O.F., Goodma, N. and Bellet, S. (1960) The hypotensive effect of imipramine hydrochloride in patients with cardiovascular disease. *Clin. Pharmacol. Ther.*, **2**, 300–7.

Nelson, J.C., Jatlow, P.I., Bock, U. *et al.* (1982) Major adverse reactions during desipramine treatment: relationship to plasma drug concentration, concomitant antipsychotic treatment and patient characteristics. *Arch. Gen. Psychiat.*, **39**, 1055–61.

Neshkes, R., Gerner, R., Jarvik, L. *et al.* (1985) Orthostatic effect of imipramine and doxepin in depressed geriatric out-patients. *J. Clin. Psychopharmacol.*, **5**, 102–6.

Ramanathan, K.B. and Davidson, C. (1975) Cardiac arrhythmia and imipramine therapy. *Brit. Med. J.*, **1**, 661–2.

Roose, S.P., Glassman, A.H., Siris, S.G., Walsh, T. *et al.* (1981) Comparison of imipramine- and nortriptyline-induced orthostatic hypotension: A meaningful difference. *J. Clin. Psychopharmacol.*, **1** (5), 316–19.

Shaw, W.L. (1980) The comparative safety of mianserin in overdose. *Curr. Med. Res. Opinion*, **6** (Suppl. 7) 44–51.

Smith, R.B. and Rusbatch, B.J. (1967) Amitriptyline and heart block. *Brit. Med. J.*, **3**, 311.

Spiker, D.G., Weiss, A.N., Chang, S.S. *et al.* (1975) Tricyclic antidepressants overdose: clinical presentation and plasma levels. *Clin. Pharmac. Ther.*, **18**, 539–46.

Strom, J., Madsen, P.S., Nielsen, N.N. and Sørensen, M.B. (1984) Acute self-poisoning with tricyclic antidepressants in 295 consecutive patients treated in an ICU. *Acta Anaesth. Scand.*, **28**(6), 666–70.

Taylor, D.J.E. and Braithwaite, R.A. (1978) Cardiac effects of tricyclic antidepressant medication. A preliminary study of nortriptyline. *Brit. Heart. J.*, **40**, 1006–9.

Thayssen, P., Bjerre, M., Kragh-Soerensen, P. *et al.* (1981) Cardiovascular effects of imipramine and nortriptyline in elderly patients. *Psychopharmacol.*, **74**, 360–4.

Todd, R.D. and Faber, R. (1983) Ventricular arrhythmias induced by doxepin and amitriptyline: case report. *J. Clin. Psychiat.*, **44**, 423–5.

Van de Merwe, T.J., Silverstone, T. and Ankier, S.I. (1984) Electrophysiological and haemodynamic changes with trazodone, amitriptyline and placebo in depressed out-patients. *Current Med. Res. Opinion*, **9**, 339–52.

Veith, R.C., Raskind, M.A., Caldwell, J.H. *et al.* (1982) Cardiovascular effects of tricyclic antidepressants in depressed patients with chronic heart disease. *New Engl. J. Med.*, **306**, 954–9.

Vohra, J., Burrows, G.D. and Sloman, J.G. (1975) Assessment of cardiovascular side effects of therapeutic doses of tricyclic antidepressant drugs. *Aust. NZ. J. Med.*, **5**, 7–11.

Warrington, S. (1984) Cardiovascular effects of lofepramine. *Int. Med.* (Suppl. 10) 23–6.

Weissler, A.M., Harris, W.S. and Schoenfeld, C.D. (1968) Systolic time intervals in heart failure in man. *Circulation*, **37**, 149–59.

Young, R.C., Alexopoulos, G.S., Shamoian, C.A. *et al.* (1985) Plasma 10–hydroxynortriptyline and ECG changes in elderly depressed patients. *Am. J. Psychiat.*, **142**, 866–8.

Chapter Eleven

Side-effects of tricyclic and related antidepressants

KARABI GHOSE

CONTENTS

11.1 INTRODUCTION

Hospital admissions due to adverse drug reactions have been shown to be higher in patients aged sixty years or over than in any other age group (Caranasos, Stewart and Cluff, 1974). It is now well recognized that the elderly are particularly sensitive to most drugs acting at the central nervous system and tend to suffer from serious side-effects more frequently. Age-related deterioration in physiological functions is considered to be responsible for altered sensitivity to drugs. Apart from the various factors known to influence pharmacokinetics of drugs in the elderly, as discussed in Chapter 8, other physical or mental illnesses and some social factors probably also contribute to this increased incidence of adverse effects.

Drugs used in the treatment of acute episodes of depression fall mainly into two categories, monamine oxidase inhibitors and tricyclic

Table 11.1 Tricyclic and related antidepressant drugs marketed between 1989 and 1989 in the UK

| Approximate year of marketing | Generic name | Chemistry | | UK proprietary name(s) |
		Derivative	*Structure	
1958	Imipramine	Dibenzazepine	TCA (T)	Imipramine, Praminil, Tofranil
1961	Amitriptyline	Dibenzocycloheptadiene	TCA (T)	Amitriptyline, Domical, Elavil, Lentizol, Tryptizol
1962	Desipramine	Dibenzazepine	TCA (S)	Pertofran
1962	Trimipramine	Dibenzazepine	TCA (T)	Surmontil
1963	Nortriptyline	Dibenzocycloheptadiene	TCA (S)	Allegron, Aventyl
1966	Chlorimipramine	Dibenzazepine	TCA (T)	Anafranil
1966	Protriptyline	Dibenzocycloheptadiene	TCA (S)	Concordin
1968	Iprindol	Indenopyran	TCA (T)	Prondol
1968	Doxepin	Dibenzoxepine	TCA (T)	Sinequan
1969	Dothiepin	Dibenzothiazepine	TCA (T)	Prothiaden
1972	Maprotiline	Dibenzobicyclooctadiene	Non TCA	Ludiomil
1974	Viloxazine	Ethoxy–phenoxy–methyl–tetra–hydroxine	Non TCA	Vivalan
1974	Butriptyline	Dibenzocycloheptadiene	TCA (T)	Evadyne
1975	Mianserin	Piperazino-azepine	Non TCA	Bolvidon, Norval
1976	†Nomifensine	Tetrahydroisoquinoline	Non TCA	Merital
1977	Lofepramine	Dibenzazepine	TCA (S)	Gamanil
1978	Trazodone	S–Triazolopyridine	Non TCA	Molipaxin
1981	†Zimeldine	Alkylamine	Non TCA	Zelmid
1987	Fluvoxamine	Valerophenone	Non TCA	Feverin
1989	Fluoxetine	Benzene propanamine	Non TCA	Prozac
1989	Amoxapine	Dibenzoxazepin	Non TCA	Asendis

* Tricyclic (TCA): tertiary (T) and secondary (S) amines; Second generation antidepressants (non TCA).
† Withdrawn from the market for toxicity.

compounds. Tricyclic antidepressants possess three ring structures and have several common pharmacological properties. In the seventies, second generation antidepressants were introduced which though structurally different, appear to have pharmacological and antidepressant activities similar to tricyclics. Both tricyclic and second generation antidepressants possess a broad spectrum of pharmacological properties and are known to produce many side-effects in all age groups. As they all appear to possess comparable antidepressant activity, the incidence and severity of side-effects should be given consideration prior to prescribing.

Table 11.1 lists the approximate date of marketing of various antidepressants available in the UK. It will be seen that although a large number of drugs have been introduced since 1958, there has been a progressive decline in the number since the mid-seventies. Several new antidepressants are at various stages of development, but they are unlikely to be granted marketing permission without evidence of long-term safety and tolerance. Demonstration of efficacy alone is not enough.

In general, second generation antidepressants produce a relatively fewer number of side-effects, but clearly information regarding long-term toxicity of newer drugs has yet to be evaluated. Recently, two antidepressants have been withdrawn from the market for toxicity.

Patients over the age of 65 previously used to be systematically excluded from most drug trials. As a result, information regarding safety and tolerance in this age group is not available for many antidepressants marketed earlier. In this chapter, pharmacological properties of the antidepresant drugs currently available in the UK and their side-effects and tolerance in the elderly are discussed briefly.

11.2 CHEMICAL STRUCTURES

Iminodibenzyl was first synthesized in 1889 by Thiele and Holzinger, but its pharmacological activities were not studied until 1948 (Hafliger, 1959). Imipramine, an iminodibenzyl, is the first of the basic alkylated tricyclic compounds in this series, and was first synthesized in 1948 by Schindler and Hafliger (Hafliger, 1959). Structurally these drugs are similar to antihistamines and phenothiazines as shown in Fig. 11.1.

A classical tricyclic antidepressant possesses two benzene rings fused to a central seven-numbered ring. According to their side chains, they can be subdivided into a dimethylated compound or tertiary amine (such as imipramine, amitriptyline) or a monomethylated compound or secondary amine (such as desipramine or nortriptyline). Although second generation antidepressants have pharmacological resemblance

183

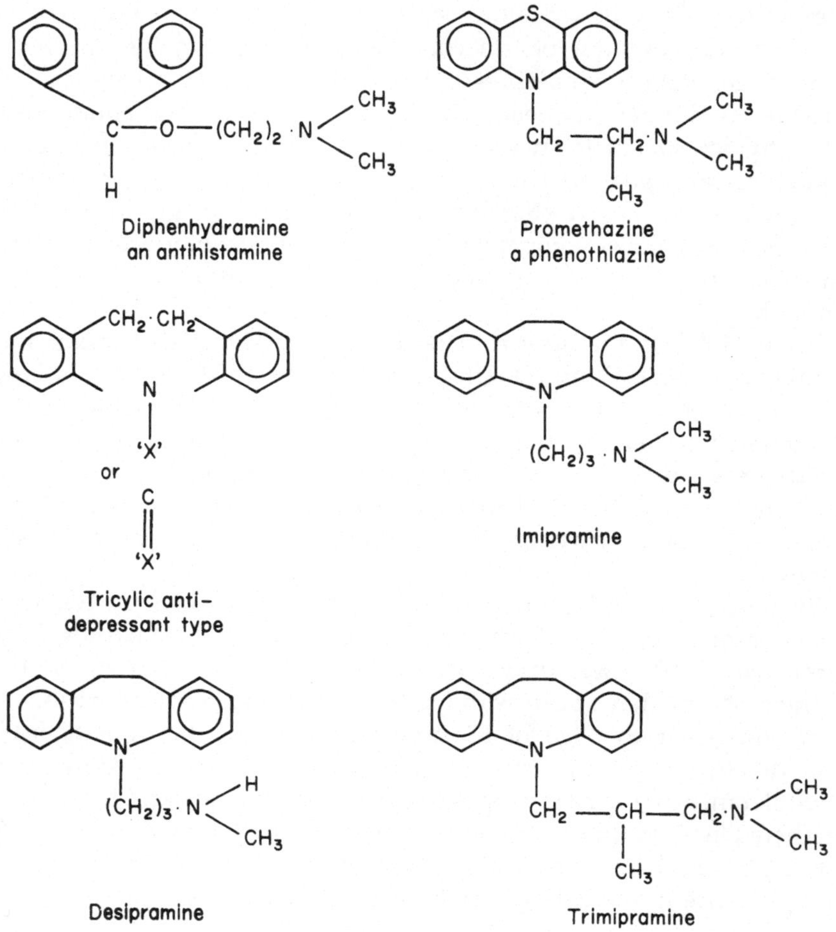

Fig. 11.1 Chemical structures of tricyclic-type antidepressants.

to tricyclic antidepressants, many of them possess novel structures, such as tetracyclic (maprotiline) or bicyclic (viloxazine), as shown in Fig. 11.2.

DeVane suggested that they should be called cyclic antidepressants (as shown in Table 11.2), but agrees that no classification is likely to cover all drugs (DeVane, 1987).

11.3 GENERAL PHARMACOLOGICAL PROPERTIES RELEVANT TO SIDE-EFFECTS

Tricyclic and related antidepressants, in addition to their expected ability to alleviate depressive symptoms, possess many other pharma-

Table 11.2 Classification of cyclic (tricyclic and related) antidepressants available for prescription in the UK according to their structure (after DeVane, 1987)

Structure	Drug
Monocyclic	Fluvoxamine
Bicyclic	Viloxazine
Tricyclic	Amitriptyline
	Clomipramine
	Desipramine
	Doxepin
	Imipramine
	Nortriptyline
	Protriptyline
	Trimipramine
	Lofepramine
Tetracyclic	Maprotiline
Heterocyclic	Mianserin
	Trazodone

cological activities. As stated above they resemble antihistamines and phenothiazines structurally (Fig. 11.1) and have weak antihistaminic and anxiolytic properties. They interact with biogenic amines and the cholinergic system, and produce many central effects. A brief summary of pharmacological effects is given in Table 11.3.

11.3.1 Effect on central nervous system

(a) Behavioural effects
In animals, classical tricyclic antidepressant drugs are known to prolong hexobarbital sleeping times, alcohol narcosis and cause decrease in body temperature. These drugs produce ataxia, sedation and catalepsy in a dose-dependent manner. Animals may also show signs of increased irritability and aggressive behaviour. It has been suggested that at lower doses, they have a stimulating effect and exhibit inhibitory effects at higher doses.

Imipramine and related drugs are known to reverse reserpine-induced sedation in laboratory animals. Reserpine depletes the tissue stores of biogenic amines. Tetrabenzine is pharmacologically similar to reserpine, but it is a short acting drug. Tricyclic antidepressants also abolish the tetrabenzine-induced sedation, catalepsy and ptosis in rats

Table 11.3 General pharmacological properties and side-effects of tricyclic and related drugs

Drugs	Pharmacological effects					Comments (Reference)
	Initial sedation	Anti-cholinergic	Re-uptake blockade	Epileptogenic activity	Psychiatric	
A. TRICYCLIC TERTIARY AMINES						
Imipramine Amitriptyline	+++	+++	5-HT and NA weak DA	Present	Confusion Psychosis	5-HT blocker but their metabolites TCA (S) block NA
Trimipramine	+++	+++	Mainly 5-HT Less NA			Activity very similar to IP/AT (Skaug, 1975)
Dothiepin	++	++	Mainly NA, less 5-HT, weak DA	Low incidence		(Lipsedge et al., 1971)
Doxepin	++	++	NA, 5-HT			Uptake blocking less than IP/AT (Pinder et al., 1977a)
Chlorimipramine	+++	+++	Mainly 5-HT weak NA and DA			Predominant 5-HT blocker (Beaumont, 1979)
Lofepramine	+	+	Mainly NA			TCA(T) but predominant NA blockers (more than DP) (Siwers et al., 1977)
Iprindol	+	+	No blocking effect	Less		No adrenergic interactions (Fann et al., 1974)
Butriptyline	++	+	No blocking effect			No adrenergic interactions (Ghose et al., 1977)

B. TRICYCLIC SECONDARY AMINES

Drug						
Desipramine / Nortriptyline	++	++	Selective NA	As IP/AT		No effect on 5-HT
Protriptyline	++	++	Selective NA	As IP/AT		More potent than DP/NT (Whyte et al., 1976)

C. NON TRICYCLICS

Drug						
Maprotiline	++	+	Selective NA			No effect on other amines (Pinder et al., 1977b)
Viloxazine	Almost negligible	nil	No significant effect	Unlikely	Stimulant effect	Pinder et al., 1977c
Mianserin	+++	nil	No blocking effect		Confusion	More sedation than IP/AT. No autonomic effect (Ghose et al., 1976)
Trazodone	+	+				
Fluvoxamine	+	nil	Predominant 5-HT			No significant effect on other amines
Fluoxetine	–		Selective 5-HT	Probable	?	Side-effects are nausea and headaches
Amoxapine	+	++	NA, 5-HT weak DA	Present	Possible	Rapid anti-depressant effect

+++ = severe
++ = moderate
+ = mild

DA = dopamine	SE = side-effects
NA = noradrenaline	IP = imipramine
5-HT = 5-hydroxytryptamine	AT = amitriptyline
DP = desipramine	NT = nortriptyline

and counteract the hypothermia in mice. These blocking effects are used as an animal screening test for antidepressant activity of a drug.

In man, tricyclic antidepressants alleviate symptoms of depression, but have no stimulant or mood-elevating property in normal subjects. They are known to precipitate mania only in susceptible subjects (i.e. in a patient with bipolar affective disorders treated with this drug during a depressive phase). They may produce sedation even in pharmacological doses but psychotomimetic effects usually occur at higher or toxic doses.

(b) Electroencephalographic (EEG) changes
In laboratory animals, tricyclic antidepressants may produce various EEG changes. Slow waves with increased amplitude at cortical leads may be seen in small doses. High doses usually produce spikes and dysrhythmia and may even provoke seizure discharges.

In man, these drugs decrease total electrical activity and increase delta, beta and burst activities. These drug-induced EEG changes are considered to be characteristic of an antidepressant drug (Fink, 1969). In a susceptible subject, especially following an overdose, some antidepressants may produce convulsions (Table 11.3).

(c) Effect on sleep
In animals, tricyclic antidepressants are shown to increase total sleeping time, decrease the number of rapid eye movement (REM) periods and decrease the number of waking periods per night. Similar shortening of REM sleep and prolongation of Stage 2 sleep have been observed in man. A longer latent period between the onset of sleep and the first REM phase also occurs in man.

11.3.2 Interactions with biogenic amines

(a) Re-uptake blocking activity
Almost all tricyclic and some second generation drugs influence the uptake and release of biogenic amines. The amines which have received most attention are noradrenaline, 5–hydroxytryptamine (5–HT) and dopamine. Tricyclic antidepressants block the neuronal re-uptake of these neurotransmitters and increase the functional amines at the postsynaptic receptor sites. Second generation antidepressants are usually devoid of these interactions (Rundrup and Braestrup, 1977).

(b) Effect on receptors
Tricyclic antidepressants, in addition to re-uptake blocking activity, may also possess, usually at higher concentrations, postsynaptic alpha adrenoceptor blocking activity (Ghose, 1980). They may also have effect

on the presynaptic receptors. In animals, chronic medication has been shown to reduce the density of postsynaptic beta adrenoceptors. They may also reduce the functional sensitivity of alpha and beta adrenergic receptors.

(c) Influence on turnover and synthesis
Some tricyclic antidepressants may influence the synthesis and turnover of biogenic amines. This may be independent of their effect on re-uptake mechanism. Metabolites of noradrenaline and 5–HT in the CSF were found to be low in some patients receiving chronic antidepressant therapy (Risby *et al.*, 1987).

11.3.3 Cholinergic interactions
The central anticholinergic effects of these drugs are well established. A typical antidepressant produces an inhibitory effect on acetylcholine-induced contraction of the isolated guinea-pig intestine, and increases blood pressure and heart rate in rats. In man, common symptoms of peripheral anticholinergic effects are dry mouth, tachycardia and visual difficulties. Their central effects may produce confusional states and psychosis. Most second generation antidepressants are devoid of anticholinergic effects.

11.4 UNWANTED EFFECTS

Enzyme inductions, biochemical and metabolic changes are responsible for most unwanted effects and interactions of a drug, but the mechanisms of many reactions and interactions are complex.

11.4.1 Adverse reactions

Adverse reactions usually indicate noxious changes produced by a drug which was administered at a dosage normally tolerable to man. The condition may require treatment and further exposure to the same drug carries unusual risk for that particular patient. Hypersensitivity and drug rash may occur with tricyclic and related drugs, but severe anaphylactoid reaction is rare. Reversible agranulocytosis and the cholestatic type of hepatitis during imipramine therapy, and jaundice with eosinophilia associated with amitriptyline therapy have been reported.

During recent years, two second generation antidepressants (nomifensine and zimeldine) were withdrawn from the market for adverse effects. Leucopenia and related blood disorders are now known to occur during mianserin therapy but the incidence is low.

11.4.2 Side-effects

Side-effects of a drug usually indicate therapeutically undesired but unavoidable effects, such as dry mouth (anticholinergic effect) observed during antidepressant therapy. These symptoms are due to other pharmacological properties of a drug and could be a desired effect in another condition. For example, anticholinergic effects of imipramine may be helpful in urinary incontinence. Common side-effects of various anti-depressants are summarized in Table 11.3.

Most side-effects are worse during the initial period of therapy. These can be minimized by starting treatment with a small dose which can be increased slowly to achieve the recommended therapeutic dose within a period of 5–14 days depending on the tolerance. Dosage adjustment is frequently required for elderly patients.

(a) Psychiatric symptoms

Tricyclic antidepressant drugs are known to produce (or aggravate) agitation, delusion, hallucination and excitement, usually during the initial period of treatment; these symptoms may also occur during chronic medication. In severe cases, it may be necessary to discontinue therapy. Such symptoms are frequently associated with drugs which preferentially increase the functional noradrenaline (Lehmann, Cahn and de Vertouil, 1958), and are also related to the central anticholinergic activity of a drug. Elderly patients are particularly susceptible to these psychotomimetic effects. These drugs may precipitate confusional state in a patient with early dementia.

(b) Sedation

Drowsiness is one of the most common central effects and although the severity may vary, it is associated with most antidepressant drugs. This is more pronounced with drugs which increase the concentration of central 5–HT. This symptom is usually troublesome only during the initial phase of therapy and becomes tolerable during continued medication. Besides, drowsiness may be a symptom of depressive illness *per se*, and it may sometimes be difficult to differentiate this symptom from drug-induced sedation in severely depressed patients (Abou-Saleh and Coppen, 1983). An inverse correlation between the subjective feelings of drowsiness and clinical improvement during amitriptyline therapy was observed, but there was no relationship with the plasma drug concentrations (Coppen and Ghose, 1976). Elderly patients are usually less bothered by this symptom.

(c) Convulsions or epileptic seizures

These may occur even in therapeutic doses. Convulsions are usually grand mal seizures, but myoclonus is also common. Attacks may be precipitated in patients with a history of convulsions, or in patients with a low convulsive threshold. However, they may also occur in an apparently non-susceptible subject. Seizures were reported to be more frequent with imipramine, amitriptyline, chlorimipramine, and less commonly associated with maprotiline, viloxazine, mianserin and trazodone.

(d) Other neurological effects
A persistent fine tremor, especially in elderly patients, and occasionally a reversible Parkinsonian syndrome, may occur. Hypokinetic disorders of speech and motion and tonic–atonic disturbances during antidepressant drug therapy have also been reported (Boning, 1978). Rarely, there may be symptoms of peripheral neuritis and weakness of the proximal muscles. Tardive or orofacial dyskinesia is also known to occur (Yassa, Camille, and Belzile, 1987).

(e) Anticholinergic effects
Manifestations of central anticholinergic effects are described in section 11.3.3. Like drowsiness, peripheral symptoms such as dry mouth, excessive sweating, constipation, visual difficulties and urinary retention are usually worse at the beginning of therapy. Many old people are unable to tolerate these drugs because of these symptoms. Cardiovascular complications are particularly hazardous in the elderly and are discussed in Chapter 10. Special precautions should be taken while prescribing these drugs in patients with glaucoma and prostatic hypertrophy. However, many second generation antidepressants, such as mianserin and trazodone (Table 11.3) are relatively free from anticholinergic effects and should be selected for an elderly patient.

(f) Effects on appetite and weight
Depressed patients are known to have appetite disturbances (usually poor appetite). However, although these drugs suppress appetite in normal subjects, they are known to increase body weight in depressed patients.

11.4.3 Interactions with other drugs

A drug–drug interaction may occur if both act on the same target site, producing synergism, potentiation or antagonism of a particular pharmacological effect (pharmacodynamics). The effect of a drug may also be modified by another drug which interacts indirectly from a remote site by altering the plasma concentrations (pharmacokinetics).

Tricyclic antidepressants in combination with a monoamine odixase inhibitor or lithium were observed to be more beneficial than a tricyclic alone in patients with resistant depression. The effects of central depressant drugs, such as morphine, pethidine and other narcotics, and sedative drugs including alcohol, may be potentiated by a tricyclic antidepressant. The elderly are particularly vulnerable to the central depressant effects of drugs and serious complications (for example, respiratory depression) may occur, especially during an overdose. Phenothiazines and benzodiazepines are less hazardous but should also be prescribed with caution.

Addition of a stimulant drug is likely to potentiate central effects and may precipitate convulsions and psychosis.

The pharmacological effects of most directly-acting sympathomimetic amines (noradrenaline, adrenaline) are potentiated, and those of indirectly-acting amines (ephedrine, tyramine and amphetamine) are diminshed, by a typical tricyclic antidepressant drug which inhibits re-uptake blocking activity. The effect of local anaesthetics is also potentiated by some tricyclic antidepressants.

Severe adrenergic stimulation leading to cardiac arrhythmia and death has been reported following isopranaline aerosol in an asthmatic patient who was receiving amitriptyline (Kadar, 1975). Although such serious reactions are rare, these drugs should be prescribed with caution in elderly patients with asthma.

Tricyclic antidepressants reverse the antihypertensive effects of adrenergic neurone blocking drugs, but the latter drugs are not commonly used now. Combination with an anticholinergic drug may potentiate the central and peripheral anticholinergic effects and may precipitate a toxic confusional state.

11.5 SOME SECOND GENERATION ANTIDEPRESSANTS AND THE ELDERLY

As discussed above, second generation antidepressants usually possess relatively fewer clinically significant side-effects. Most drugs in this group were first marketed in the mid- and late seventies (Table 11.1), but a small number of drugs, sometimes referred to as third generation antidepressants, were introduced in the 1980s. Several other drugs are also currently undergoing clinical investigation.

11.5.1 Maprotiline

This is a tetracyclic compound (Fig. 11.2 and Table 11.1) which selectively blocks the neuronal noradrenalin re-uptake mechanism. Maprotiline has no significant effect on the 5–HT uptake mechanism and is considered to possess less anticholinergic property than amitriptyline or imipramine. The antidepressant activity of maprotiline has been shown to be equal to imipramine in elderly patients (Khan, 1978; Middleton, Rahman and Lloyd, 1979). Its side-effects profile is also considered to be similar to imipramine.

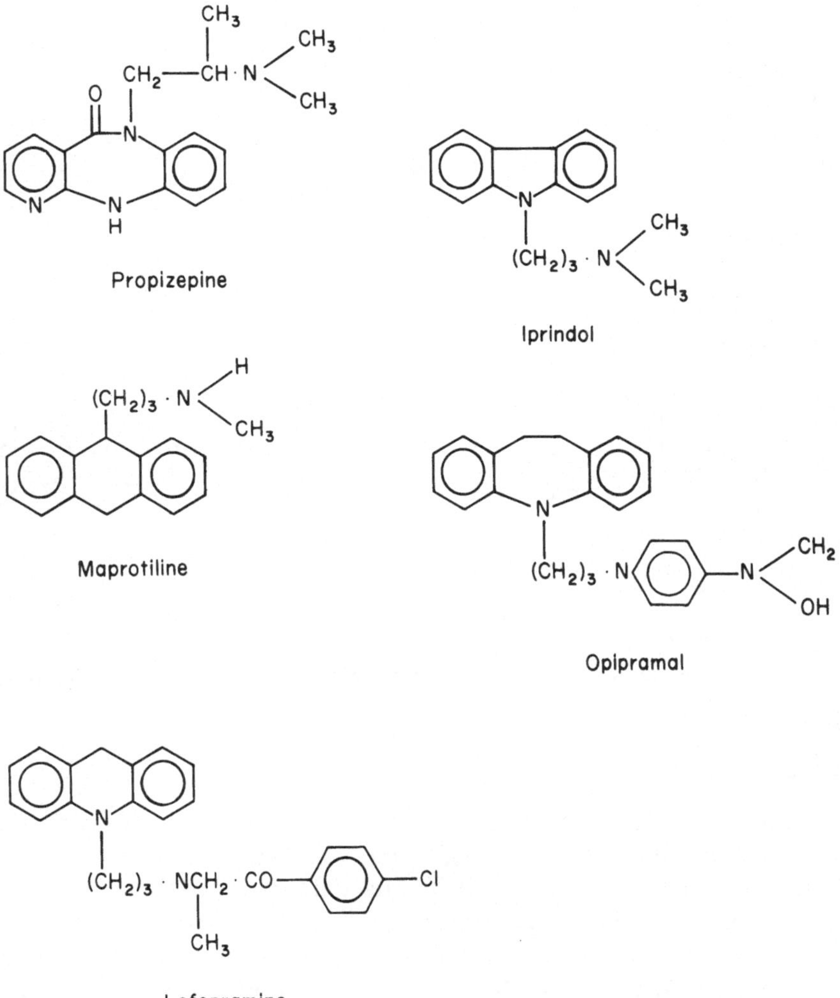

Fig. 11.2 Chemical structures of some newer antidepressants: nomifensine and zimeldine are withdrawn from the market; propizepine and opipramal are not available in the UK.

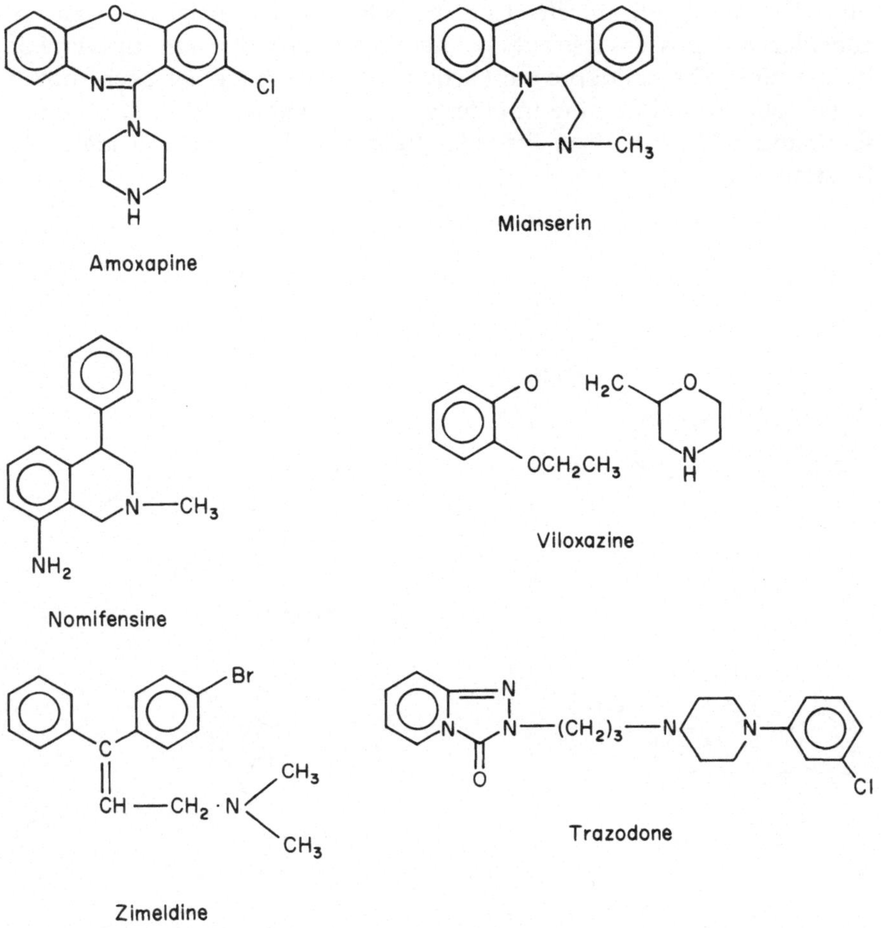

Amoxapine

Mianserin

Nomifensine

Viloxazine

Zimeldine

Trazodone

Fig. 11.2 Chemical structures of a new generation of non-tricyclic anti-depressants.

11.5.2 Mianserin

Structurally this is a novel compound and is the first antidepressant drug without any anticholinergic effect or adrenergic interactions (Ghose, Coppen and Turner, 1976). Its efficacy and tolerance in the elderly population have been investigated in a number of studies. In view of this drug's lack of anticholinergic effects and reduced profile of cardiotoxicity, mianserin is clearly one of the antidepressants of choice in the elderly. Its sedative effect is usually not a serious problem in these patients. Although blood dyscrasia associated with mianserin is uncommon and is probably related to high blood levels, it is important to monitor patients' progress at regular intervals.

11.5.3 Trazodone

Trazodone is a new generation non-tricyclic antidepressant (Fig. 11.3) with a reduced profile of side-effects. Its antidepressant activity in the geriatric population is comparable to imipramine (Gerner *et al.*, 1980), but it has no significant anticholinergic effects. Its cardiotoxicity is comparable to mianserin (Bucknell *et al.*, 1988). On the whole this drug is tolerated well by elderly patients and should be considered in patients with glaucoma or prostatic hypertrophy.

11.5.4 Lofepramine

Although structurally this is a tertiary tricyclic compound which possesses antidepressant activity similar to imipramine, pharmacologically it is not a typical tricyclic antidepressant. It is a noradrenaline re-uptake inhibitor, which is probably related to its desmethyl metabolite (desipramine). It has been suggested that lofepramine's antidepressant activity is independent of this metabolite (Leonard, 1986). Lofepramine is effective in elderly patients with depression and has less sedative and anticholinergic effects than amitriptyline (Ghose and Sedman, 1987).

11.5.5 Fluvoxamine

This is a new non-tricyclic antidepressant with selective 5–HT uptake inhibiting activity. Its pharmacology and clinical effects have been reviewed by Benfield and Ward (1986). Fluvoxamine appears to possess antidepressant activity comparable to imipramine and chlorimipramine. It has fewer anticholinergic and cardiovascular side-effects than these drugs, but, like other 5–HT uptake inhibitor antidepressants, nausea, vomiting, and other gastric disturbances are common. Its efficacy in elderly patients with depression has also been demonstrated in a double-blind study (Wakelin, 1986). The elderly tolerated this medication well and they experienced no significant side-effect apart from mild nausea.

However, it should be emphasized that fluvoxamine has only recently been granted marketing permission and further postmarketing surveillance is necessary before making any definite comment regarding its safety. This is particularly necessary as another drug (zimeldine) with similar 5–HT uptake inhibiting activity was withdrawn because of toxicity within a year of marketing.

11.6 PRESCRIBING IN THE ELDERLY

Clearly, tricyclic antidepressants possess a broad spectrum of pharmacological activities and produce many side-effects. The elderly are particularly sensitive to these drugs. The incidence and severity of side-effects are often dose related and an appropriate dosage reduction is recommended for this age group. Tricyclic and related (second generation) antidepressants appear to possess comparable antidepressant activity. Therefore, the incidence and severity of side-effects of a drug should be taken into account during prescribing. A drug with cardiotoxicity and articholinergic effects should preferably be avoided. In general second generation antidepressants are safer but the long-term side-effects of many new drugs are still to be evaluated.

Prior to the initiation of therapy, the patient's general physical condition should be assessed. It may be necessary to carry out certain routine laboratory investigations. The benefits should be considered against the risks. At present several antidepressants are available for clinical use. Each drug has its special advantages and disadvantages and a particular patient may benefit from a specific drug. Therefore, choice of an antidepressant, depending on a patient's particular situation (i.e. physical condition, mental state, other concomitant drug therapy and social circumstances) is important.

It is advisable to initiate therapy with approximately one-third to one-quarter of the recommended adult dose, if no dosage guidance is available for elderly patients. The dose may then be cautiously increased, according to a patient's tolerance, to achieve the 'therapeutic' dose within the next 3–10 days. Further dosage adjustment may also be required depending on the clinical response. The aim is to administer the minimum effective dose.

In order to avoid serious side-effects, close supervision is required for patients with multiple pathology who require polypharmacy. Routine monitoring of drug level is unnecessary, but it should be considered in patients with poor response despite receiving an adequate dose, and also prior to further dosage increment. Low levels may, however, be due to noncompliance. In patients suffering from toxicity or severe symptoms of a side-effect, in view of wide individual variations in antidepressant drug levels, measurement of a single plasma level is unlikely to be helpful in diagnosing toxicity or evaluating symptoms of side-effects.

Therefore, suspicion of side-effects is made mainly on clinical grounds. Most side-effects pose no diagnostic problem, but in elderly patients some neurological features may be difficult to interpret. In such patients dosage reduction may reduce or abolish the symptoms. Dosage reduction should be considered in all patients presenting with serious side-effects.

During long-term therapy, side-effects should be monitored at frequent intervals as some side-effects, such as tardive dyskinesia or cardiovascular problems, may develop later during long-term therapy.

REFERENCES

Abou-Saleh, M.T. and Coppen, A. (1983) Subjective side-effects of amitriptyline and lithium in affective disorders. *Brit. J. Psychiat.*, **142**, 391–7.

Beaumont, G. (1979) Side-effects and toxicity of clomipramine. *Brit. J. Clin. Pract.* (Suppl. 3) pp. 51–3.

Benfield, P. and Ward, A. (1986) Fluvoxamine: a review of its pharmacodynamic and pharmacokinetic properties and therapeutic efficacy in depressive illness. *Drugs*, **32**, 313–34.

Boning, J. (1978) Side-effects and complications of antidepressant drugs. *Arzneimittel-Forschung*, **28**, 1284.

Bucknell, C., Brooks, D., Currey, P.K. *et al.* (1988) Mianserin and trazodone for cardiac patients with depression. *Eur. J. Pharmacol.*, **33**, 565–9.

Caranasos, G.J., Stewart, R.B. and Cluff, E. (1974) Drug-induced illness leading to hospitalization. *J. Am. Med. Assoc.*, **228**, 713–18.

Coppen, A. and Ghose, K. (1976) Do tricyclic antidepressants work? *Lancet*, **i**, 913–14.

DeVane, C.L. (1987) Naming the cyclic antidepressants. *J. Clin. Psychopharmacol.*, **7**, 285–6.

Fann, W.E., Davies, J.M., Janowsky, D.S. *et al.* (1974) Effect of antidepressant and antimanic drugs on amine uptake in man. *J. Ner. Ment. Diseas.*, **158**, 361–71.

Fink, M. (1969) EEG and human psychopharmacology. *A Review of Pharmacology*, **9**, 241.

Gerner. R., Estabrook, W., Steuer, J. and Jarvik, L. (1980) Treatment of geriatric depression with trazodone, imipramine and placebo; a double-blind study. *J. Clin. Psychiat.*, **14**, 216–20.

Ghose, K. (1980) Biochemical assessment of antidepressive drugs. *Brit. J. Clin. Pharmacol.*, **10**, 539–50.

Ghose, K., Coppen, A. and Turner, P. (1976) Autonomic actions and inter-actions of mianserin hydrochloride (Org GB94) in patients with depressive illness. *Psychopharmacology*, **49**, 201–4.

Ghose, K., Huston, G., Kirby, K. *et al.* (1977) Clinical pharmacology of butriptyline. *Brit. J. Clin. Pharmacol.*, **4**, 91–3.

Ghose, K. and Sedman, E. (1987) A double comparison of the pharmacodynamic effect of single doses of lofepramine, amitriptyline and placebo in elderly subjects. *Eur. J. Clin. Pharmacol.*, **33**, 505–9.

Hafliger, F. (1959) Chemistry of tofranil. *Canad. Psychiat. Assoc. J.* (Suppl. 4) 69–74.

Kadar, D. (1975) Amitriptyline and isoproternal: fatal drug combination. *Canad. Med. Assoc. J.*, **112**, 556–60.

Khan, A. (1978) Maprotiline vs. imipramine in depression in the elderly. *Brit. J. Clin. Pract.*, **32**, 42–6.

Lehmann, H.E., Cahn, C.H. and de Vertouil, R.L. (1958) The treatment of depressive conditions with imipramine. *Canad. Psychiat. Assoc. J.*, **3**, 155.

Leonard, B.E. (1986) Antidepressants: current concepts of mode of action. *Inter. Med.* (Suppl. 11), 2–5.

Lipsedge, M.S., Rees, W.L. and Pike, D.J. (1971) A double-blind comparison of dothiepin and amitriptyline for the treatment of depression with anxiety. *Psychopharmacol. (Berl.)*, **19**, 153.

Middleton, R.S.W., Rahman, A.F.M.M. and Lloyd, A.H. (1979) Maprotiline vs. imipramine in depression of old age. *Brit. J. Clin. Pract.* (Suppl. 2), 56–63.

Pinder, R.M., Brogden, R.N., Speight, T.M. and Avery, G.S. (1977a) Doxepin: up-to-date. A review of its pharmacological properties and therapeutic efficacy with particullar reference to depression. *Drugs*, **13**, 161–73.

Pinder, R.M., Brogden, R.N., Speight, T.M. and Avery,, G.S. (1977b) Maprotiline: a review of its pharmacological properties and therapeutic efficacy in mental depressive illness. *Drugs*, **13**, 321–34.

Pinder, R.M., Brogden, R.N. and Avery, G.S. (1977c) Viloxazine: a review of its pharmacological properties and therapeutic efficacy in depressive illness. *Drugs*, **13**, 401–11.

Risby, E.D., Hsiao, J.K., Sunderland, T. *et al.* (1987) The effects of antidepressants on the cerebrospinal fluid homovanillic acid/5–hydroxyindoleacetic acid ratio. *Clin. Pharmacol. Ther.*, **42**, 547–54.

Rundrup, A. and Braestrup, C. (1977) Uptake inhibition of biogenic amines by newer antidepressant drugs. Relevance to the dopamine hypothesis of depression. *Psychopharmacology*, **53**, 309–14.

Siwers, B., Borg, S., d'Elia, G. *et al.* (1977) Comparative clinical evaluation of lofepramine and imipramine *Acta. Psychiat. Scand.*, **55**, 21.

Skaug, O.E. (1975) Serum concentration of trimipramine in healthy subjects. *Nord. Psykiat. Tidssk.*, **29**, 453.

Wakelin, J. (1986) Fluvoxamine in the treatment of the older depressed patient: double-blind, placebo-controlled data. *Int. Clin. Psychopharmac.*, **1**, 221–30.

Whyte, S.F., MacDonald, A.J., Naylor, G.F. and Moody, J.P. (1976) Plasma concentrations of protriptyline and clinical effects in depressed women. *Brit. J. Psychiat.*, **128**, 384.

Yassa, R., Camille, Y. and Belzile, L. (1987) Tardive dyskinesia in the course of antidepressant therapy: a prevalence study and review of the literature. *J. Clin. Psychopharmacol.*, **7**, 243–6.

FOUR

Monoamine Oxidase Inhibitor Antidepressants

Chapter Twelve

Efficacy and problems of MAO inhibitor antidepressants

DIANA CODY and COSMO HALLSTROM

CONTENTS

12.1 INTRODUCTION

Monoamine oxidase inhibitors (MAOIs) are effective in the treatment of depression. However, despite some notable exceptions, there are few adequate studies as to their efficacy and their associated problems in the elderly. This review therefore examines not only those studies which address themselves particularly to the treatment of the elderly, but also those which provide information on the use of MAOIs in general, and will attempt, where possible, to draw conclusions of relevance to the elderly. We will examine not only the existing MAOIs but also look at the new generation of MAOIs which may prove to be as effective and safer as antidepressants than their parent drug and therefore of particular use in the treatment of the elderly depressed patient.

12.2 GENERAL BACKGROUND

The mood-elevating effects of the MAOIs were first observed by Bosworth (1959) as an incidental finding during clinical trials of iproniazid in the treatment of tuberculosis. This led to their use in the treatment of depressed, anergic patients, at a time when the only other effective antidepressant drugs were the amphetamines. Early trials by West and Dally (1959) and Sargant and Dally (1962) demonstrated their efficacy in the treatment of anxiety and phobic states as well as depression.

MAOIs fell into disrepute following Blackwell's recognition (1963) of the 'cheese reaction', a hypertensive crisis resulting from the interaction of MAOIs and tyramine-containing foods. Because of this MAOIs have generally been avoided in the elderly, and have been considered less safe than tricyclic antidepressants (TCAs) (Fann, 1976). Hepatotoxicity and toxic interactions with other drugs (Pare, 1964; Sjoqvist, 1965) led to further disillusionment with MAOIs, and TCAs were generally used in their place.

Interest was rekindled in 1968 when different MAO subtypes, termed A and B, were identified (Johnstone, 1968). In humans MAO–A preferentially deaminates noradrenalin (NA) and serotonin (5–HT), and MAO–B deaminates dopamine (DA) and phenylethylamine (Glover *et al.*, 1977). MAO–A is predominantly found in the gut whilst MAO–B is found in platelets and human brain.

The development of a simple direct method of monitoring platelet MAO inhibition *in vivo* has shown that there is an association between the degree of platelet MAO inhibition and clinical efficacy (Robinson *et al.*, 1978). This leads to the possibility of determining optimal dosage on an individual basis.

Depression in the elderly patient poses a pharmacological challenge. Physical diseases such as prostatic hypertrophy, ischaemic heart disease, hypertension, glaucoma or diabetes may co-exist, and polypharmacy is common. The ageing process can also cause alterations in drug absorption, distribution, biotransformation and excretion.

In general the absorption capacity is diminished. However, this is related to the reduction in metabolism and excretion, so that smaller doeses of drugs are usually required in the elderly patient.

The elderly tend to be more sensitive to the side-effects of drugs, particularly the anticholinergic ones, and because of this tricyclic antidepressants are often contraindicated.

The rationale for considering MAOIs for the treatment of depression in the elderly is based, in addition to their mechanism of action (inhibition of the breakdown of catecholamines and serotonin), on the finding of increased MAO activity in the brain and other organs, predominantly MAO–B (Robinson, Sourkes and Nies, 1977).

12.3 MAO PHYSIOLOGY

Current therapeutic MAOIs are for the most part non-selective irreversible inhibitors. They may be of the hydrazine group of which phenelzine is an example; from the hydrazid group, for example isocarboxazide; or the non-hydrazines such as tranycypromine which is a reversible inhibitor. The non-hydrazine MAOIs are structurally related to the amphetamines and also appear to have amphetamine-like actions (Costa *et al.*, 1980). The hydrazines and acetylenic agents (deprenyl) exert their effect by inactivating the MAOIs' prosthetic group, having themselves been oxidated by MAO to reactive intermediates. The mode of inhibition by tranylcypromine is less certain but does involve the reaction of a sulphhydryl group in the active centre of the enzyme (Goodman *et al.*, 1985).

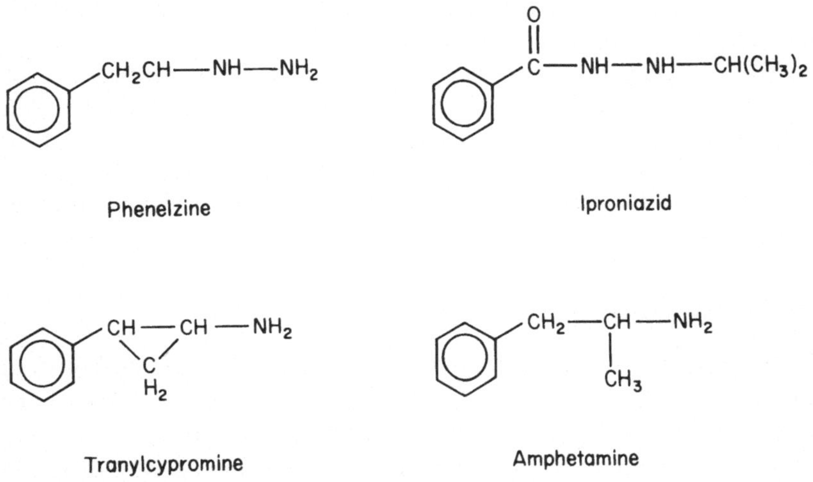

Phenelzine

Iproniazid

Tranylcypromine

Amphetamine

Fig. 12.1 Chemical structures of some MAO inhibitor antidepressants and the structure of amphetamine.

Human brain MAO is almost completely associated with mitochondrial function, and is probably located on the outer mitochondrial membrane. It is a relatively non-specific enzyme, capable of deaminating many amines with the formula $R–CH_2–NHS$, where R is a substituted alkyl or aryl group. In physiological terms the substrates are the biogenic amines, 5–HT, NA, adrenalin, DA and tyramine.

MAO–A and MAO–B may represent two independent types of substrate binding site on the same protein molecule (White and Stine, 1982). Clorgyline selectively inhibits MAO–A, whilst MAO–B is inhibited by deprenyl. The original hypothesis, that MAO–A acts on noradrenalin and 5–HT, and MAO–B on DA and phenylethylamine, is an oversimplification. Recent work suggests that substrates are able to interact with both forms of the enzyme, but do so preferentially with one of the two sub-types (Fowler and Tipton, 1982; Youdim, 1983).

The roles of MAO–A and MAO–B are still incompletely understood but may well be important in developing a new generation of safer MAOIs which do not carry the risk of the 'cheese reaction'. A number of compounds have been identified which are reversible selective MAOIs for example cimoxatone, toloxatone and CGP-11305A. These drugs may have a clinical advantage over the irreversible selective MAOIs, in that tyramine in the gut would be able to displace the reversible MAOI from its site. Since MAO–B, although less plentiful in the gut, would remain intact, it would then be able to deaminate tyramine, theoretically reducing the risk of a hypertensive reaction. *In vivo* studies to date have however failed to demonstrate this 'safety valve' effect (Strolin-Bennedetti *et al.*, 1983).

MAO–B inhibitors, which are currently used as an adjunct to L-dopa in the management of Parkinson's disease, are being evaluated. They show no increase in tyramine sensitivity, and patients who had been treated with L-deprenyl for up to 18 months showed no increase in the risk of hypertensive reactions (Elsworth *et al.*, 1978). Their efficacy as antidepressants is less clear.

12.3.1 Acetylator status

MAOIs are absorbed after oral ingestion and metabolized by acetylation (Johnstone, 1976). Acetylator status is genetically determined (Evans, 1968). It might be expected that slow acetylators would show a better clinical response than fast acetylators (which metabolize the drug more rapidly). Johnstone and Marsh (1973) have shown a better therapeutic response in slow acetylators but others (Tyrer *et al.*, 1980; Tyrer *et al.*, 1981) have failed to show any difference. The question remains open. Paykel *et al.* (1982) have suggested that a slow acetylator effect is most evident in the early weeks of treatment and in patients on lower doses of phenelzine.

Even whether phenelzine is metabolized by acetylation remains in dispute. Cooper *et al.* (1984), using radioactive isotopes of phenelzine, have failed to detect any acetylated phenelzine in urine or plasma samples 24 h post-drug.

12.3.2 Dosage

Lower doses of MAOIs are thought to be inadequate (Pare, 1985). Post-mortem studies of the brains of 76 elderly patients who had died whilst taking MAOIs showed that there was considerable individual variation in pharmacological response, and that 60 mg of isocarboxazid was frequently required before a good response was achieved. This is approximately equivalent to 20–30 mg of tranylcypromine (Bevan Jones *et al.*, 1972). To achieve 80% inhibition of platelet MAOI, 60–75 mg of phenelzine is required daily (Robinson *et al.*, 1973). This also applies to the elderly (Georgotas, Mann and Friedman, 1981). Plasma concentrations of phenelzine tend to be higher than in younger patients during the first two weeks of treatment, presumably from an age-related decrease in the apparent volume of distribution of phenelzine. This may also reflect a slower rate of phenelzine metabolism and elimination (Salzman, 1985). Clinical improvement in depression has been shown to occur when REM sleep is abolished (Akindele, Evans and Oswald, 1970), and this requires high doses of MAOIs.

12.4 CLINICAL STUDIES

Fourteen elderly depressed patients, some of whom suffered from associated senile dementia, were studied in an open trial of tranylcypromine (20–30 mg/day for 11–43 days) or phenelzine (30–60 mg/day for 7–43 days) (Ashford and Ford, 1979). Depressive symptoms improved, but memory or other cognitive functions remained unchanged. Patients suffering from primary affective disorders also responded poorly. The results might have been different if higher doses and longer treatment periods had been used.

Georgotas *et al.* (1983) studied the effects of phenelzine on 30 elderly patients (mean age 68). All patients suffered from a 'resistant depression' of a mean duration of five years, and met the Research Diagnostic Criteria (RDC) for major depressive illness. They had all previously been treated with TCAs in doses of 150–300 mg daily. One third of the group had been treated with between seven and twelve sessions of ECT, one had undergone psychosurgery, and nearly half had been treated with psychotherapy either alone or in conjunction with antidepressants. All patients had also been given nortriptyline 50–125 mg daily for a period of two to eight weeks, again without benefit. A two-week placebo washout period preceded phenelzine treatment. Placebo responders were excluded.

The initial phenelzine dose was 15 mg b.d. (twice daily), and the dose was gradually increased in weekly increments at the discretion of the investigator. Depression was rated weekly using the Hamilton Depression Scale (HAM–D), Beck Self Rating Scale and Clinical Global Impression. Cognitive function was measured pre and post treatment by a battery of psychological tests, and platelet MAO activity was measured weekly.

Of the 30 patients who entered the trial, 20 completed between two and seven weeks of treatment. Of those not included two were placebo responders and one was non-compliant, and seven withdrew because of a poor therapeutic response during the first four weeks of treatment. Analysis of the results showed that there were 13 responders, scoring less than ten on the HAM–D, and seven non-responders. There were no changes in cognitive test scores, which suggests a possible advantage of MAOIs over TCAs, which can impair memory function in the elderly because of their sedative and anticholinergic effects.

The most frequently reported side-effects were dizziness, weight gain and orthostatic hypotension. One patient developed anorexia and another ejaculatory impotence. These side-effects (apart from the impotence) subsided with a reduction of the dose. No hypertensive episodes occurred.

The majority of the responders achieved a >80% platelet MAO inhibition, whilst 70% of the non-responders showed a <80% rate of inhibition. This substantiates the view that 80% platelet MAO inhibition is needed for optimal clinical response (Georgotas, Mann and Friedman, 1981; Robinson *et al.*, 1978). The 65% response rate in elderly patients with resistant depression was regarded as excellent and the authors concluded that MAOIs should be considered as alternative treatments in the elderly depressed patient.

Phenelzine, nortriptyline and placebo were compared in a carefully designed double-blind trial in the elderly depressed (Georgotas *et al.*, 1986). Ninety patients with RDC major depressive illness and a score of 16 or more on the HAM–D, entered the double-blind treatment phase. Fifteen patients were excluded from the final data analysis because of inadequate data, early withdrawal or non-compliance. Of the remaining 75 patients who were included in the efficacy analysis, 56 had seven weeks of active treatment. Eleven of the 19 who withdrew early because of clinical deterioration were in the placebo group. Five had responded at the time of withdrawal, and four dropped out because of side-effects. Blood concentrations of nortriptyline and platelet MAO activity were measured. Patients treated with nortriptyline generally reached the optimal therapeutic blood concentration in the first week, but the phenelzine-treated patients did not reach the acceptable level of inhibition (>70%) until the third week. The nortriptyline and phenelzine-treated patients showed significantly higher responses (65% and 61%) than the placebo group (13%). Nortriptyline-treated patients responded after the fifth week, whereas most of the phenelzine-treated patients did not respond until the seventh week.

Side-effects reported most frequently by the phenelzine-treated patients included drowsiness and nasal congestion. Orthostatic symptoms were reported with similar frequency in both the nortriptyline and phenelzine groups. There were no significant differences in the frequencies of cardiovascular side-effects such as palpitations, dizziness, or tachycardia. No hypertensive reactions were reported. Nine of the 90 patients (five on placebo) withdrew early because of side-effects. Otherwise the drugs were well tolerated and MAO dietary restrictions were generally not a problem.

The indications for choosing an MAOI over a TCA are unclear. In the United Kingdom MAOIs have traditionally been used in the treatment of atypical or non-endogenous depression, with symptoms such as initial insomnia, hyperphagia, mood reactivity and p.m. diurnal variation (Ravaris *et al.*, 1980; Nies, 1984).

Georgotas *et al.* (1987) also examined which symptoms responded best to MAOIs or TCA antidepressant treatment. Using a multiple regression analysis of HAM–D items, no significant differences between the placebo and treatment groups emerged for initial insomnia, retardation weight loss and p.m. diurnal variation. When the responses to nortriptyline and phenelzine were compared only middle/late insomnia responded better to nortriptyline. The other items responded equally to either drug. Significant improvements did not emerge until the fourth week of treatment.

The chronological order of symptom resolution was the same for both antidepressants. Differences between drugs and placebo began to appear after about two weeks of treatment, but some symptoms such as agitation were not significantly improved until the sixth or seventh week of treatment.

These results show that the traditional four-week antidepressant therapeutic trial is probably too short, and overall nortriptyline and phenelzine appeared to be equally effective in the general treatment of major depression in the elderly.

12.5 UNWANTED EFFECTS

12.5.1 The 'cheese' reaction

Van Praag (1977) has suggested that 'MAOIs are better not prescribed for elderly out-patients' and Rice and Aire (1981) wrote that 'MAOIs should only be used rarely in the treatment of the elderly patient'. The main reason for the reluctance to prescribing MAOIs is the risk of the 'cheese reaction'.

Tyramine is normally metabolized by MAO as it passes through the gut mucosa. MAOIs inhibit this protective mechanism and allow a large and sudden influx of tyramine into the systemic circulation. This is then taken into adrenergic nerve endings displacing NA, resulting in a hypertensive crisis. Although the majority of the noradrenalin is inactivated by reabsorption into the neurones, the released noradrenalin is metabolized more slowly because of the inhibition of neuronal MAO which prolongs and accentuates the crisis (Reigle *et al.*, 1980). In the elderly this hypertensive reaction may be particularly hazardous because of the fragile and atherosclerotic cerebral blood vessels (Salzman, 1982).

Controlled studies (Robinson *et al.*, 1978; Georgotas *et al.*, 1986) have however shown that the occurrence of side-effects was no higher in patients treated with phenelzine compared to patients treated with TCAs, both in the younger age groups and the elderly.

Studies of the use of MAOIs in the elderly reported no single case of a hypertensive. The relative safety of MAOIs may lie in them only being prescribed to patients who are capable of observing the dietary and drug restrictions (Pare, 1985). Patients should have the restrictions explained to them carefully and be given a large print card with the instructions. These dietary and drug restrictions were not regarded as being too onerous in the study by Georgotas *et al.* (1986).

Although Ashford (1979) found that MAOIs were effective in the treatment of depressive symptoms with co-existing dementia, particular care should be taken with these patients who should only be treated under close supervision, since their memory and concentration difficulties make them unreliable.

A hypertensive crisis may also be caused by the interaction of MAOIs and sympathomimetic drugs (ephedrine, pseudoephedrine, phenylephrine, phenylpropanolamine and amphetamine). These are found in 'over the counter' cold remedies, and patients should be warned against them.

The number of reported deaths occurring in association with tranylcypromine, the MAOI most frequently implicated in hypertensive reactions, is one death per 14 000 patient years (Pare, 1985). Thus the overall risk of using MAOIs would appear justified. The treating doctor should however be prepared to deal with a potential hypertensive crisis by giving an alpha blocking drug such as chlorpromazine (25 mg) if mild or a slow intravenous injection of 5 mg phentolamine if more severe hypertension occurs.

12.5.2 Interactions with other drugs

The interaction between MAOIs and narcotic analgesics has been recognized since the 1950s, but advice on the use of these drugs has often been conflicting, both in the young and the elderly. Patients on MAOIs may occasionally require narcotic analgesics for emergency surgery or the relief of severe pain. The interaction takes two forms, either an excitatory form which is characterized by the sudden onset of agitation, headaches, rigidity, hyperpyrexia, convulsions, hyper or hypotension and possibly coma. This reaction is presumably due to central 5–HT overactivity (Browne and Linter, 1987). The depressive form with respiratory depression, hypotension and eventually coma, results from inhibition of hepatic microsomal enzymes by MAOIs leading to the accumulation of unmetabolized narcotic.

Pethidine and possibly dextromethorphan can result in the excitatory form and are absolutely contraindicated in patients on MAOIs. Morphine does not block the re-uptake of 5–HT, but impaired metabolism may result in potentiation of its narcotic effects. If emergency pain relief is required, small doses of intravenous morphine may be given. Should an interaction occur, naloxone can be given to reverse respiratory depression, although mechanical ventilation may also be required. Vasopressors may be indicated if hypotension fails to respond to conservative measures.

Combinations of TCAs with MAOIs are used in the treatment of resistant depression (Gander, 1965) but their use is regarded as hazardous. The concurrent use of amitriptyline and other secondary amine TCAs and phenelzine has however been shown to reduce the pressor activity of tyramine (Pare *et al.*, 1982). This presumably results from the inhibition of tyramine uptake into the neurone by the TCA. Care should be taken when changing a patient from an MAOI to a TCA, allowing a gap of three weeks between the two drugs. The changeover from a TCA to an MAOI is not such a problem. The adverse interaction between TCAs and MAOIs can be catastrophic, especially adding clomipramine to an MAOI.

Monoamine oxidase inhibitors are also thought to interact with centrally active antihypertensive drugs and neuroleptics. Ashford (1979) in his study of elderly patients found that two of 14 patients treated with MAOIs developed movement disorders when haloperidol was added to their regimen. One, a patient with mild Parkinsonism, developed a moderately severe Parkinsonian bradykinesia which failed to resolve even after treatment was discontinued, and the second developed choreiform movements, which remitted when medications were discontinued. It is unclear as to why this reaction should have occurred since theoretically MAOIs would increase the amount of available dopamine, whilst haloperidol blocks dopaminergic activity. Tranylcypromine and trifluperazine are available as a combination preparation (Parstelin) without apparent hazard. Nevertheless there is a need for caution in combining neuroleptics and MAOIs in the elderly.

12.5.3 Cardiac effects

Orthostatic hypotension is one of the most troublesome side-effects of the MAOIs. It may be particularly hazardous for the elderly patient, whose compromised cardiovascular system is slower to accommodate rapid reductions in blood pressure, especially in those with pre-existing hypertension where the decrease in blood pressure is even more dramatic than in normotensive individuals.

How MAOIs reduce blood pressure is not known. Ganglionic blockade or sympatholytic effects may be involved (Goldman, Alexander and Luchins, 1986). Empirical evidence suggests that phenelzine produces more hypotension than tranylcypromine. Kronig *et al.* (1983), in a study of 14 patients with a mean age of 52 years, showed the mean orthostatic drop increased with time and reached a peak three to four weeks after treatment had been started, contrary to the traditional view that hypotension occurred early in the treatment. The Georgotas study, of nortriptyline and phenelzine (1986), reported orthostatic symptoms with similar frequencies in both groups.

MAOIs have less effects on the resting heart than TCAs (Robinson, Nies and Cencella, 1982). Phenelzine treatment gave a modest six beat per minute reduction of the heart rate after six weeks, and no significant change has been found with tranylcypromine (Razani *et al.*, 1983). In phenelzine-treated patients, orthostatic changes in blood pressure are not accompanied by an increase in heart rate, in contrast to TCAs where significant increases in heart rate occur, presumably as a result of the anticholinergic action of these drugs.

The clinical implications of the orthostatic and heart rate changes are important in the treatment of elderly patients whose cardiac status may already be compromised. The relative lack of significant changes in heart rate with MAOIs may give them a slight advantage over TCAs but the hypotensive effects of both drug classes remain a problem.

Cardiac conduction defects with an increase in the PR interval, prolongation of the QRS complex and the QT segment, are a particular problem of TCAs both in the elderly and younger patients (Reed *et al.*, 1980). MAOIs, although less intensively researched, appear to have negligible effects on cardiac conduction (Robinson, Nies and Cencella, 1982). A slight increase in cardiac conduction has in fact been reported with phenelzine treatment. The decrease in the duration of the QT segment is not related to the degree of platelet MAO inhibition.

Since TCAs are of particular risk in patients with bundle branch disease, MAOIs may well be the drugs of choice for depressed patients with conduction disturbances (Georgotas *et al.*, 1983). MAOIs have no significant effects on cardiac rhythm in contrast to the antiarrhythmic effects of the TCAs, mediated by their quinidine-like action.

12.5.4 Effects on cognitive function

Depressive symptoms may occur together with dementia in the elderly. TCAs can impair memory, presumably because of their anticholinergic effects. Ashford (1979) found that MAOIs were particularly effective in treating depression in patients with senile demetia of Alzheimer's type, but did not improve memory or other cognitive impairments. The effect of MAOIs on cognitive functioning in elderly depressed patients was studied by evaluating the possible pre and post treatment differences on a cognitive test battery. There was no significant change in cognitive functions during a seven-week treatment period. MAOIs were found to be an effective and safe treatment in the depressed elderly and cognitive functioning did not deteriorate during the course of treatment. These findings are of interest since MAOI activity increases with age, and in patients with Alzheimer's disease MAO type B is increased (Georgotas *et al.*, 1983; Robinson, Sourkes and Nies, 1977).

12.5.5 Other side-effects

Dramatic weight gain occurs in some patients treated with MAOIs, although this is not a particular problem of the elderly (Salzman, 1985). Weight gain may contribute to coexisting disease, and should be monitored regularly.

Both insomnia and drowsiness are side-effects of MAOIs. Insomnia can be minimized by giving the medication early in the day, but sedation is more of a problem in the elderly. Georgotas *et al.* (1987) found that phenelzine produced more drowsiness than nortriptyline and both drugs were more sedating than placebo.

Although MAOIs have no anticholinergic action of their own, their sympathomimetic effects can result in autonomic symptoms such as dry mouth and blurred vision (Jenike, 1984). Dry mouth was also the commonest side-effect reported in the Georgotas trial (1986), but less troublesome than with nortriptyline. Other symptoms reported by the phenelzine-treated patients were nasal congestion, urinary symptoms, gastrointestinal upset, skin problems, tremor and jitteriness. Noradrenergic symptoms also occur but respond to propranolol. MAOIs may also interfere with ejaculation and result in anorgasmia in the elderly (Georgotas *et al.*, 1983, 1986). Despite the number of possible side-effects they are for the most part mild and MAOIs were well tolerated in the elderly.

Hepatotoxicity, one of the first complications of MAOIs to be recognized, is very rare. It is an idiosyncratic hypersensitivity reaction. Patients with chronic liver disease may be unable to tolerate MAOIs and serum bilirubin and transaminase activity should be monitored (Halaris, 1986).

12.6 NEW GENERATION MAOIs

Although non-selective MAOIs have been shown to be effective and relatively safe when guidelines are followed, the search for a safer, more effective antidepressant continues.

The hypertensive crises associated with MAO–A inhibition and the recognition that MAO–B is the main brain MAO, has led to interest in the drug L–deprenyl which selectively acts on MAO–B, and has been used to potentiate the action of L–dopa in the treatment of Parkinsonism without the risk of hypertensive crises (Birkmayer *et al.*, 1977; Lees *et al.*, 1977).

L–deprenyl was reported to have antidepressant activity and also to be capable of potentiating the antidepressant activity of 5–hydroxytryptophan (Mann and Gershon, 1980; Mendlewicz and Youdim, 1983). This antidepressant activity was noted in non-endogenous and some bipolar patients. Improvement in mood was also shown to be related to the degree of platelet MAO inhibition (Mann *et al.*, 1982). Mendis *et al.* (1981), on the other hand, failed to demonstrate any antidepressant activity with L–deprenyl, when treating predominantly unipolar depressives.

Mendlewicz and Youdim (1983) in a double-blind placebo-controlled study found L–deprenyl to be significantly better than placebo, and again found a positive relationship between the degree of MAO inhibition and clinical improvement.

A further study (Quitkin *et al.*, 1984) also demonstrated that L–deprenyl was superior to placebo but found that patients with atypical depression required higher doses than the recommended 10–20 mg/day dose. Few side-effects were reported in this short-term study.

None of these studies specifically addresses the problem of elderly depressives, but most have included patients over the age of 50. The apparent safety and low incidence of side-effects would make

L–deprenyl an attractive option for the advanced age group, especially those with co-existing Parkinsonism. Further information is required as to its therapeutic efficacy.

12.7 CONCLUSION

MAOIs are safe, effective drugs for the treatment of depression in the elderly if certain simple precautions are taken. They may well be safer than TCAs under some circumstances. Care should be taken to exclude complicating factors such as cardiovascular or liver disease, and blood pressure should be monitored for the first few weeks of treatment.

MAOIs should be given in small doses which are increased gradually. A therapeutic response may be delayed for up to six or seven weeks, or even longer if small doses are given. A dietary warning is imperative and care should be taken that patients are able to understand this and comply. Drug interactions must also be avoided.

The new generation selective MAOIs may have a particular role in the treatment of the elderly, but this remains to be proven, although it is possible that at doses required to get a therapeutic response, the substrate specificity may be lost and a 'cheese reaction' may still occur.

REFERENCES

Akindele, M.A.O., Evans, J.I. and Oswald, I. (1970) Monoamine oxidase inhibitions, sleep and mood. *Electroencephalography and Clinical Neurophysiol.*, **29**, 45–56.

Ashford, J.W. and Ford, C. (1979) Use of MAO inhibitors in elderly patients, *Am. J. Psych.* **136**(11) 1466–7.

Bevan Jones, A.B., Pare, C.M.B., Nicholson, W.J. *et al.*, (1972) Brain amine concentrations after monamine oxidase inhibitor. *Brit. Med. J.*, **I**, 17–19.

Birkmayer, W., Riedener, P., Ambrou, L. and Youdim, M.B.H. (1977) Implications of combined treatment with 'madopar' and 1–derenyl in Parkinson's disease. A long-term study. *Lancet*, **i**, 434–43.

Blackwell, B. (1963) Hypertensive crisis due to monoamine oxidase inhibitions. *Lancet*, **ii**, 849.

Bosworth, D.M. (1959) Iproniazid, a brief view of its introduction and clinical use. *Ann. N.Y.*, Acad. Sci., **80**, 809.

Browne, B. and Linter, S. (1987) Monoamine oxidase inhibitors and narcotic analgesics. A clinical review of the implications for treatment. *Brit. J. Psych.*, **151**, 210.

Cooper, T.B., Jindal, S.R., Robinson, D.S. and Corcells, J. (1984) Metabolism of phenelzine in man. Lack of evidence for acetylation pathway. Abstract, *Collegium International Neuropsychopharmacologium 14th (CNIP) Congress*, Florence, June 1984.

Costa, E., Pschreidt, G.R., Van Meten, W.G. and Himwich, H.E. (1980) Brain concentrations of biogenic amines and EEG patterns of rabbits. *J. Pharmac. Exp. Ther.*, **130**, 81.

Elsworth, J.D., Glover, V., Reynolds, G.P. *et al.* (1978) Deprenyl administration in man, a selective MAO–B inhibitor without the 'cheese-effect'. *Psychopharmacology*, **57**, 33–8.

Evans, D.A.P. (1968) Genetic variations on the acetylation of isoniazid and related drugs. *Ann. N.Y. Acad. Sci.*, **15**, 723.

Fann, W.E. (1976) Pharmacotherapy in older depressed patients. *J. Gerontol.*, **31**, 304–10.

Fowler, C.J. and Tipton, K.F. (1982) Deamination of 5–hydroxytryptamine by both forms of monoamine oxidase in the rat brain. *J. Neurochem.*, **38**, 733.

Gander, D.R. (1965) Treatment of depressive illness with combined antidepressants. *Lancet*, **ii**, 107.

Georgotas, A., McCue, R., Hapworth, W. *et al.* (1986) Comparative efficacy and safety of MAOIs versus TCAs in treating depression in the elderly. *Biol. Psych.*, **21**, 1155–66.

Georgotas, A., Friedman, E., McCarthy, M. *et al.* (1983) Resistant geriatric depressions and therapeutic response to monoamine oxidase inhibitors. *Biol. Psych.*, **18**(2) 195–205.

Georgotas, A., Mann, J. and Friedman, E. (1981) Platelet monoamine oxidase as a potential indicator of favourable response to MAOIs in geriatric depression. *Biol. Psych.*, **16**, 997.

Georgotas, A., McCue, R., Friedman, E. and Cooper, T. (1987) Reponse of depressive symptoms to nortriptyline, phenelzine and placebo. *Brit. J. Psych.*, **151**, 102–6.

Georgotas, A., Reisberg, B. and Ferris, S. (1983) First results on the effects of MAO inhibition on cognitive functioning in elderly depressed patients. *Arch. Gerontol. Geriatr.*, **2**, 249–54.

Glover, V., Sandler, M., Woen, F. and Riley, G.J. (1977) Dopamine is a monoamine–B substrate in man. *Nature*, **265**, 80–1.

Goldman, C., Alexander, R. and Luchins, D. (1986) Monoamine oxidase inhibitors and tricyclic antidepressants. Comparison of their cardiovascular side-effects. *J. Clin. Psych.*, **47**(5) 255–9.

Goodman, L., Gilman, A., Goodman, L., Theodore, R. and Foriam (1985) Drugs used in the treatment of disorder of mood. In: *The Pharmacological Basis of Therapeutics* (eds. L. Goodman and A. Gilman), 7th edn, MacMillan, New York, p. 424.

Halaris, A. (1986) Antidepressant drug therapy in the elderly. Enhancing safety and compliance. *Intl. J. Psych. Med.*, **16**, 1–19.

Jenike, M.A. (1984) The use of monoamine oxidase inhibitors in the treatment of elderly depressed patients. J. Amer. Geriatr. Soc., **32**, 53–7.

Johnstone, E.C., Marsh, W. (1973) Acetylator status and response to phenelzine. *Lancet*, **i**, 1567–70.

Johnstone, E.C. (1976) The relationship between acetylator status and inhibition of monoamine oxidase, excretion of both drug and antidepressant response in depressed patients on phenelzine. *Psychopharmacol.*, **46**, 289–94.

Johnstone, J.P. (1968) Some observations upon a new inhibitor of monoamine oxidase in brain tissue. *Biochem. Pharmac.*, **17**, 1285–97.

Kronig, M.H., Roose, S.P., Walsh, B.T. *et al.* (1983) Blood pressure effects of phenelzine. *J. Clin. Psychopharmacol.*, **3**, 307–10.

Lees, A.J., Shaw, K.M., Kabout, L.J. *et al.* (1977) Deprenyl in Parkinson's disease. *Lancet*, **i**, 791–5.

Mann, A. and Gershon, S. (1980) 1–Deprenyl, a selective monoamine oxidase type B inhibitor in endogenous depression. *Life Sci.*, **26**, 877–82.

Mann, J.J., Frances, A., Kaplan, R. *et al.* (1982) The relative efficacy of 1–deprenyl, a selective monoamine oxidase type B inhibitor in endogenous and non-endogenous depression. *J. Clin. Psychopharmacol.*, **2**(1) 54–7.

Mendlewicz, J., Youdim, M.B.H. (1983) 1–Deprenyl. A selective monoamine oxidase type–B inhibitor in the treatment of depression. A double-blind evaluation. *Brit. J. Psych.*, **142**, 508.

Mendis, N., Pare, C.M.B., Sandler, M. *et al.* (1981) Is the failure of deprenyl, a selective monoamine oxidase B inhibitor in the treatment of depression, related to freedom from the 'cheese-effect'? *Psychopharmacol.*, **3**, 87–90.

Nies, A. (1984) Differential response to MAO inhibitors and tricyclics. *J. Clinical Psych.*, **45**, 70–77.

Pare, C.M.B. (1964) Side-effects and toxic effects of antidepressants. *Proc. R. Soc. Med.*, **57**, 757.

Pare, C.M.B., Kline, N., Hallstrom, C. and Cooper, T.B. (1982) Will amitriptyline prevent the 'cheese reaction' of monoamine oxidase inhibitors? *Lancet*, **ii**, 183–6.

Pare, C.M. (1985) The present status of monoamine oxidase inhibitors. *Brit. J. Psych.*, **146**, 576–84.

Paykel, E.S., West, P.S., Rowan, P.R. and Parker, R.R. (1982) Influence of acetylator phenotype on antidepressant effects of phenelzine. *Brit. J. Psych.*, **141**, 243.

Quitkin, F., Liebowitz, M., Stewart, J. *et al.* (1984) 1–Deprenyl in atypical depressives. *Arch. Gen. Psych.*, **41**(3) 238.

Ravaris, C.L., Robinson, D.S., Ives, J. *et al.* (1980) Phenelzine and amitriptyline in the treatment of depression. A comparison of present and past studies. *Arch. Gen. Psych.*, **37**(9) 1075–80

Razani, J., White, K.L., White, J. *et al.* (1983) The safety and efficacy of combined amitriptyline and tranylaypromine antidepressant treatment. A controlled trial. *Arch. Gen. Psych.*, **40**, 657–61.

Reed, K., Smith, R.C., Schoolar, J.C. *et al.* (1980) Cardiovascular effects of nortriptyline in geriatric patients. *Am. J. Psych.*, **137**(8) 986–9.

Reigle, T.J., Orsulak, P.J., Avni, J. *et al.* (1980) The effects of trancylcypramine isomers on non-epinephrine H^3 metabolism in rat brain. *Psychopharmacol.*, **69**, 193–9.

Rice, E.D. and Arie, T.H.D. (1981) *Mims Magazine*, **June**, 51–7.

Robinson, D.S., Nies, A., Ravaris, L. *et al.* (1978) Clinical pharmacology of phenelzine. *Arch. Gen. Psych.*, **35**, 629.

Robinson, D.S., Nies, A. and Cencella, J. (1982) Cardiovascular effects of phenelzine and amitriptyline in depressed outpatients. *J. Clin. Psych.*, **43**, 8–15.

Robinson, D.S., Nies, A., Ravaris, C.L. and Lambourn, K.R. (1973) The monoamine oxidase inhibitor phenelzine in the treatment of depresssive anxiety states. *Arch. Gen. Psych.*, **29**, 407.

Robinson, D.S., Sourkes, J.L. and Nies, A. (1977) Monoamine metabolism in human brain. *Arch. Gen. Psych.*, **34**, 89–92.

Sargant, W. and Dally, P.J. (1962) Treatment of anxiety states. *Brit. Med. J.*, **1**, 6.

Salzman, C. (1982) A primer of geriatric psychopharmacology. *Amer. J. Psychiat.*, **139**(1) 67–74.

Salzman, C. (1985) Clinical guidelines for the use of antidepressant drugs in geriatric patients. *J. Clin. Psych.*, **46**(10) 38–44.

Sjoqvist, F. (1965) Interaction between monoamine oxidase inhibitors and other substances. *Proc. R. Soc. Med.*, **58**, 967.

Strolin-Benedetti, M., Dostert, P., Guttray, C. and Tipton, K.F. (1983) Partial or total protection from long-acting monoamine oxidase inhibitors by new short-acting MAOIs of type A MD 780515 and MOA B MD 780236. *Mod. Probl. Pharmacopsychiatry*, **19**, 82.

Tyrer, P., Gardner, M., Lambourn, J. and Whitford, M. (1980) Clinical and pharmacokinetic factors affecting response to phenelzine. *Brit. J. Psych.*, **136**, 359–65.

Tyrer, P., Gardner, M., Lambourn, J. and Whitford, M. (1981) Dosage and acetylator status in clinical response to phenelzine. In: *MAOIs – the state of the art* (eds. M.B.H. Youdim and E.S. Paykel), John Wiley, Chichester.

Van Praag, H.M. (1977) Psychotropic drugs in the aged. *Comprehensive Psychiatry*, **18**(5) 429–42.

West, E.D. and Dally, P.J. (1959) Effect of iproniazid in depressive syndromes. *Brit. Med. J.*, **1**, 1491.

White, H.C. and Stine, D.K. (1982) Monoamine oxidase A and monoamine oxidase B as components of a membrane complex. *J. Neurochem.*, **38**, 1429–36.

Youdim, M.B.H. (1983) *In vivo* noradrenaline is a substance for rat brain monoamine oxidase A and B. *Brit. J. Pharmacol.*, **79**, 477–80.

FIVE

General Management

Chapter Thirteen

Management of acute episodes of depression

HILARY STANDISH–BARRY

CONTENTS

13.1 INTRODUCTION

Depression is a common condition in the elderly. However, reports of its incidence and prevalence have varied, because research workers have different criteria for defining depression. Gurland (1976) pointed out that milder affective disorders have their greatest incidence between the ages of 35 and 45, while psychotic depression presents for the first time most commonly between the ages of 55 and 65. Post (1982) has reported that first episodes of depression become increasingly rare after this age, particularly after the age of 75. Gurland (1976) has suggested that a worldwide prevalence rate for depression of greater than 10% in individuals aged 65 and over is likely. Community survey of an elderly population in Edinburgh (Williamson, 1978) and Newcastle (Kay *et al.*, 1964) reported 'a prevalence of depressive illness in 5.4% and 2.4%

respectively. The prevalence of depression in medically ill elderly patients has been reported as rising to 20–35% in this group (Lancet, 1979; Moffic and Paykel, 1975). Post (1972) in a series of follow-up studies of hospital-treated depressives aged over 60 showed that only 25% of patients failed to have further breakdowns within the next three years. Between 25 and 30% of all suicides occur in those over the age of 65, although this group comprises about 12% of the population (Post, 1982). There are further reports that untreated depression can lower life expectancy (Avery and Winokur, 1976) and is associated with an increased risk of cardiac disease (Tsuang *et al.*, 1980).

Murphy (1983, 1985) has pointed out that depression in the elderly commonly has a very chronic cause, despite vigorous treatment with drugs and electroconvulsive therapy (ECT). In a prognostic study over the course of a year of depressed elderly patients in East London, only 35% had fully recovered by the end of the year. Social factors proved to be very important in influencing outcome. Severe life events were a major contributing factor to an adverse outcome, almost as important in significance as serious physical illness and the initial severity of depression. In another study in East London (Murphy, 1982) the author found that those people who reported having no intimate confiding relationship were much more likely to develop depression than those with such a relationship. However, the author found that once depression had become established, close social support did not necessarily help to alleviate chronicity or prevent relapse, nor was there very convincing evidence that a confidant could buffer the effects of further adverse events or physical health problems (Murphy, 1983).

13.2 DIAGNOSIS

In assessing an elderly depressed patient, the initial purpose is to confirm the existence of major depression. The signs and symptoms of depression in the elderly are very similar to those in the younger age group; depression can be reliably diagnosed in the elderly using DSM–III criteria. In the elderly a frequent complicating factor is the presence of significant physical illness. In this case it has been suggested that the presence of cognitive symptoms such as anhedonia, self-reproach, suicidal ideas and indecisiveness may be useful discriminating factors (Von Ammon and Cavanaugh, 1984). Elderly patients are frequently preoccupied with physical problems and deny low mood (Kayton, 1984). The presence of somatic complaints has correlated highly with risk of attempting suicide in one study (de Alarcon, 1964). Depressive symptoms, secondary to medical disorders, usually have a profile resembling a primary depression. Although one clearly needs to treat the underlying condition, treatment with antidepressants is usually required (Gerner, 1985; Schatsberg *et al.*, 1984).

Another complicating factor is the presence of dementia, which may have signs and symptoms which overlap to such an extent with depression that pseudodementia may be diagnosed (Wills, 1963; Caine, 1981; Gerner, 1985). Not uncommonly, both depression and dementia may co-exist in the same patient, both as discrete entities; the depression being treatable (Ron *et al.*, 1979; McAllister and Price, 1982; Reifler *et al.*, 1982). Unfortunately, biological state markers for depression such as the Dexamethasone Suppression Test are not as useful as discriminators between the two conditions as initially hoped, as abnormal results are found in both dementia and depression (Spar and Gerner, 1982).

Yet another complicating factor in the elderly is the concomitant prescription of large numbers of preparations for physical conditions which may in themselves contribute to the depressive state. If possible, the contributing medications should be discontinued (Jarvik and Perl, 1981).

13.3 DRUG THERAPY

In the management of the acute episode of depression, it is important that drug therapy should be part of a comprehensive treatment programme, which takes account of the presence of any physical illness as mentioned earlier in the chapter and of the patients' social background and network, which may influence the prognosis considerably.

There are other problems of drug therapy in the elderly. As the body ages, it changes its responses to drug therapy in a number of ways. Renal capacity is reduced with increasing age resulting in reduced renal clearance of drugs, even in the presence of a normal serum creatinine. Thus one finds a decreased rate of lithium excretion and also decreased excretion of the tricyclic antidepressants (Lader, 1982; Gerner, 1985; Goff and Jenike, 1986). Metabolism of drugs is mainly carried on by the hepatic microsomal enzymes. Decreased hepatic hydroxylation and demethylation are quite common in the elderly, leading to an increased half-life for the antidepressants. Effect of ageing on pharmacokinetics of antidepressant drugs are discussed in Chapter 8.

Briefly, most elderly patients have an increased sensitivity to anti-depressant medication (Greenblatt *et al.*, 1982) so one must consider using lower doses than in a younger age group. Regrettably, there is a paucity of studies of antidepressant drugs in the elderly population. Protocols for studies of new antidepressant agents tend to exclude patients over 65 years of age. However, a review by Gerner (1985) of some 20 studies of antidepressant efficacy in the elderly concluded that active medication was as effective in treating depression in the elderly as in younger patients.

Generally, one's choice of antidepressant is based on previous treatment response, the patient's symptom profile and the likelihood of the patient developing troublesome side-effects, as discussed in Chapter 9. It is wise to carry out an ECG examination. One begins with a low dose, increasing every few days whilst monitoring clinical efficacy and side-effects. A blood level may be useful in establishing whether a therapeutic level has been reached. A review by Quitkin *et al.* (1984a) suggested that 40% of patients unresponsive to antidepressant therapy at four weeks responded to treatment if the drug trial was extended to six weeks.

13.3.1 Tricyclic and related antidepressants

Anxiety and agitation are common clinical features in the elderly depressive (Kantor and Glassman, 1980; Jacoby, 1981) so the tricyclic antidepressants with sedative effects are often useful. Amitriptyline is useful in this respect but it has pronounced anticholinergic side-effects and can be cardiotoxic. A study by Kretschmar (1980) compared amitriptyline to the tetracyclic mianserin in 37 elderly patients admitted to hospital for treatment of endogenous depression. Both drugs had satisfactory antidepressant activity, but mianserin was reported to be more effective on scales of anxiety and restlessness, whilst having fewer side-effects. Another study by Branconnier *et al.* (1981) compared amitriptyline, mianserin and placebo in the treatment of a group of elderly depressed patients. Both drugs had equivalent antidepressant efficacy but mianserin was slower in therapeutic onset. The study further reported that mianserin produced less cognitive impairment than amitriptyline. Mianserin had no effect on the heart rate, whereas amitriptyline was found to have an effect. A study by Scardigli and Jans (1982) examined the effects of mianserin, trazodone and nomifensine on mood in a group of elderly depressed patients. The three groups showed parallel antidepressant activity, but total side-effects were less with mianserin. A study by Gerner *et al.* (1980) reported that imipramine had no effect on tests of cognitive impairment.

Because of the sensitivity of the elderly to some of the side-effects mentioned above, it is wise to begin treatment with a lower dose than that usually prescribed for the younger patient. On the whole, in the elderly it is best to avoid prescribing the antidepressant in a single dose at night as suggested for younger patients (Ayd, 1974; Lader, 1982) because of an increase in the level of side-effects consequent on a higher peak plasma level. However, insomnia associated with depression can be treated by administering a somewhat higher night-time dose of a sedative antidepressant such as amitriptyline, dothiepin (Ware, 1983), mianserin (Smith *et al.*, 1978; Mendlewicz *et al.*, 1985) and trazodone (Montgomery *et al.*, 1983). So a compromise regimen is to administer the drug in two equal doses morning and night (Lader, 1982). Monitoring of plasma levels of the tricyclic antidepressants can be helpful in adjusting dosages if there are problems with the therapeutic response or with side-effects. The existence of a therapeutic window for nortriptyline between 50 and 150 mg/ml has been suggested by a number of studies (Georgotas *et al.*, 1984). This should be taken into account when adjusting dosage levels.

In the elderly, intolerance to the side-effects of antidepressants often leads to inadequate therapy (Gerner and Jarvik, 1980). One of the most common side-effects is probably orthostatic hypotension which can lead to falls. There is evidence that drug-induced postural blood pressure changes do not improve over time (Roose *et al.*, 1981; Neshkes *et al.*, 1982). Another report by Glassman *et al.* (1979) suggested that pre-treatment postural blood pressure change predicted imipramine-induced orthostatic change. In cases where postural hypotension may be a problem, the use of nortriptyline or trazodone should be considered as both drugs have been shown to have less effect on the blood pressure than imipramine (Gerner *et al.*, 1980; Roose *et al.*, 1981; Thayssen *et al.*, 1981).

It has been shown that the tricyclic antidepressants slow conduction in the bundle of His and in the Purkinje fibres which can prolong ventricular conduction times (Kantor *et al.*, 1975). The elderly are especially susceptible to anticholinergic side-effects. Cardiovascular and anticholinergic side-effects are discussed in detail in Chapters 10 and 11. Clearly, a drug with relatively less cardiovascular and anticholinergic side-effects should be prescribed in elderly patients.

13.3.2 Monoamine oxidase inhibitor antidepressants

It has been shown that monoamine oxidase levels increase in the brain and in platelets in the elderly. This increase is considered to be associated with a decrease in catecholamine levels and that monoamine oxidase inhibitors may thus be especially useful in the elderly (Robinson *et al.*, 1977). A further study suggested that the proportion of depressives responding to monoamine oxidase inhibitors is greater in the elderly than in a younger group, whereas the proportion responding to tricyclic antidepressants decreases with age (Robinson, 1979). Ashford and Ford (1979) and Georgotas (1981) found satisfactory responses to phenelzine in elderly patients resistant to tricyclic antidepressants. A further report (McGrath *et al.*, 1984) suggested that tranylcypramine could be of value in tricyclic-resistant depression. These are summarized in Chapter 12. It should be emphasized that any patient prescribed a monoamine oxidase inhibitor must be able to understand the dietary restrictions associated with these drugs.

13.3.3 Lithium salts

A number of reports have indicated that the addition of lithium carbonate at levels between 0.5 and 1.0 μg may improve the antidepressant activity of both tricyclics and monoamine oxidase inhibitors (Jefferson and Ayd, 1983; de Montigny *et al.*, 1983; Himmelbeck *et al.*, 1972). A further study by Heminger *et al.* (1983) showed a significant reduction of depressive symptoms in a small group of 15 patients when lithium carbonate was added to desipramine, amitriptyline or mianserin. One-third showed a very rapid response within two days of adding lithium, and two-thirds responded within five to eight days of adding lithium. Abou-Saleh and Coppen (1983) have found that lithium maintenance therapy was just as effective in preventing or reducing the severity of depressive episodes in elderly depressives as in a younger age group (Chapter 7). It has been estimated that 1–2% of elderly patients will suffer from bipolar manic-depressive disorder (Gerner, 1985). This group often responds to lithium therapy and develops side-effects at lower blood levels than younger patients (Chapters 6 and 7). The half-life of lithium is considerably increased in the elderly due to decreased renal excretion (Gerner, 1985). In addition to the usual side-effects associated with lithium toxicity, Van der Velde (1971) has reported organic mental syndromes and neuromuscular irritability. In elderly patients maintained on lithium who develop symptoms of depression, lithium-induced hypothyroidism should be considered (Eisderfer and Raskin, 1975; Linstedt *et al.*, 1977).

13.3.4 Other drugs

A review by Baldessarini (1984) has reported that tryptophan potentiated the action of tricyclic antidepressants and monoamine oxidase inhibitors in eight out of 13 studies with appreciable extra side-effects. A study by Goodwin *et al.* (1982) looked at the addition of triiodothyronine (T3) in doses of 25 or 50 μg to 12 patients on imipramine or amitriptyline and reported a significant improvement in three-quarters of the patients, again with few additional side-effects. There is some evidence that carbamazepine, either on its own or in addition to lithium, can be useful in bipolar manic-depressive illness, especially in those patients who cycle rapidly (Post *et al.*, 1983). The combination of a tricyclic antidepressant and a monoamine oxidase inhibitor can be considered if other treatments have not proved successful. It has been suggested that imipramine is best avoided when using this approach. Great care must be taken in starting treatment and in monitoring side-effects (Razani *et al.*, 1983). Although anecdotal reports of its success are plenty (Goff and Jenike, 1986), controlled trials have not demonstrated the efficacy of the combination when compared with either compound used separately.

In the very agitated or psychotically depressed patient, neuroleptics can be useful in combination with a tricyclic antidepressant for a period of up to some weeks (Minter and Mandel, 1979). Care should be exercised, however, as both thioridazine and chlorpromazine have quite marked anticholinergic and hypotensive side-effects, while thioridazine has cardiotoxic side-effects (Heiman, 1977). Again, one should try to avoid long-term use of neuroleptics in the elderly because of the increased risk of developing tardive dyskinesia (Gerner, 1985).

13.4 DURATION OF DRUG THERAPY

There is evidence that the superiority of active drug treatment over a placebo does not become statistically significant until the fifth or sixth week of treatment, suggesting a minimum six-week period of active treatment is indicated (Quitkin *et al.*, 1984a). Quitkin *et al.* (1984b) found in their work that patients receiving placebo were more likely to respond within the first three weeks of treatment and to relapse prior to the fourth week. Klerman and Cole (1965) suggested that superiority of active treatment over placebo begins at around three weeks in controlled drug trials.

13.4.1 Treatment of relapse

There is further evidence that the continued administration of tricyclic antidepressants to patients following recovery from a treatment-responsive depressive illness is of value in reducing the risk of relapse. A number of studies have shown that patients maintained on tricyclic antidepressants for periods between six months and a year following recovery from a depressive episode had a substantially reduced relapse rate (Mindham *et al.*, 1973; Paykel *et al.*, 1975; Coppen *et al.*, 1978; Stein *et al.*, 1980). Those studies where patients were withdrawn from the tricyclic antidepressant found a relapse rate of between 29 and 69%. This relapse rate was halved by continuation of the tricyclic antidepressant. A number of studies suggest that continuation of tricyclic antidepressant medication following ECT reduces the relapse rate (Paykel *et al.*, 1979).

For longer term prophylaxis, there is convincing evidence that lithium carbonate is effective in reducing the relapse rate in bipolar manic depression and unipolar depression (Coppen *et al.*, 1971; Paykel *et al.*, 1979; Kane *et al.*, 1982). Affective disorders tend to be recurrent with a high morbidity (Angst *et al.*, 1973). A study by Coppen *et al.* (1971) confirmed this view as summarized in Chapter 7. Spar *et al.* (1979) have reviewed this area and have described the excellent response to lithium treatment that can occur in the elderly.

Two studies have shown that continuation treatment with tricyclic antidepressants in unipolar depression gives an equally good prophylactic result as treatment with lithium (M.R.C., 1981). However, other studies (Kane *et al.*, 1982; Chapter 7) found continuation therapy with lithium to be superior to continuation with tricyclic antidepressants. All studies agree on the value of continuation of active treatment, whether lithium or tricyclic antidepressant. However, the maintenance studies tend to examine a more severely depressed population.

13.5 ELECTROCONVULSIVE THERAPY

Electroconvulsive therapy (ECT) has been shown to be effective in about half of those patients who do not respond to antidepressants and in about 80% of patients with biological symptoms of depression. Indications and problems of ECT in this age group are extensively reviewed in Chapter 14. Briefly, ECT as a first-line treatment may be indicated in a group of depressed patients with severe psychotic illnesses with features of delusions, psychomotor retardation and food refusal leading to weight loss and a dangerously cachectic state (Post, 1985). Unilateral application of electrodes to the non-dominant hemisphere has been reported to produce fewer cognitive deficits immediately on concluding treatment. A study by Weiner (1982) recommended the use of a brief pulse stimulus, rather than a sine wave stimulus, to minimize side-effects in the elderly. However, an investigation by Calloway *et al.* (1981) showed a significant relationship between the presence of frontal cerebral atrophy on computerized axial tomography and the total number of ECT the patient had received throughout life. Jacoby *et al.* (1980, 1983) have reported increased ventricular size in a subgroup of elderly depressives, but did not relate this to the number of ECT received.

13.6 PSYCHOTHERAPY

Gerner *et al.* (1980) and Jarvik *et al.* (1982) compared psychotherapy, both behavioural and dynamic, against imipramine, trazodone, doxepin and placebo in elderly out-patients suffering from unipolar depression. Those patients who were treated with placebo showed no significant change on depression rating scales. The patients treated with psychotherapy showed a one-third decrease on the Hamilton Depression Scale. However, the patients treated with either trazodone, doxepin or imipramine showed a considerably greater improvement. Total side-effects were reported to be least in the placebo, trazodone and psychotherapy groups and greatest in the imipramine group. In both studies the psychotherapy patients showed a uniform partial response, whereas patients on drug treatment either had no response or a very satisfactory response.

Sloane *et al.* (1984) compared nortriptyline, placebo and interpersonal psychotherapy in the treatment of elderly depressives. At the end of the four-month study period only one patient had responded to placebo but the effects of nortriptyline and psychotherapy were assessed as being equally good. However, psychotherapy alone tends to yield only certain limited benefit in the depressions of old age. In the acute phase of depression, drug treatment should be the treatment of choice. The severely ill depressive will not be able to co-operate with dynamic psychotherapy or the more intensive forms of behavioural psychotherapy.

Quite a large number of patients will suffer from milder depressive mood states. In a survey of nearly 1000 randomly selected elderly people in the community, Blazer and Williams (1980) reported that 4% of the sample reported symptoms consistent with a major depressive episode, while 15% of the sample reported dysphoria. Akiskal (1983) has developed the concept of dysthymia in younger patients. He divides them into three groups. The first group develop a chronic dysthymia following a major depressive episode. They have certain biological features which respond to treatment, but have typical features of passivity, resignation and pessimism. Akiskal describes a second group of chronic dysthymia patients whom he believes have a secondary disorder following on other psychiatric and medical conditions. The third group he describes as 'characterologic'. Here the disorder begins in early life and follows an insidious and fluctuating course. This group he subdivides further into those who have a decreased REM sleep latency similar to those patients with major depressive episodes who respond to antidepressants, and those patients he calls 'character spectrum' who do not respond to antidepressants. A review by Moore (1985) covers the topic of dysthymia in the elderly. Williamson (1978) has described a group of elderly atypical depressives who respond to antidepressants although their symptoms are not typical of depression.

A study by Gillis and Zabow (1982) examined differences between depressed and dysphoric elderly patients. They found that the dysphoric group were very socially isolated with presenting symptoms of dissatisfaction in comparison to the depressed group. The authors felt that the dysphoric group had long-standing difficulties in personal relationships.

Treatment of dysthymia is limited by difficulty in establishing the causes of this condition and the lack of uniform diagnostic criteria (Moore, 1985). Clearly it is important to have a full assessment of all problem areas, including personality and social circumstances, so that an accepting therapeutic relationship can be developed to help minimize the behavioural difficulties (Gillis and Zabow, 1982).

REFERENCES

Abou-Saleh, M.T. and Coppen, A. (1983) The prognosis of depression in old age – The case for lithium therapy. *British Journal of Psychiatry*, **143**, 527–8.

Akiskal, H.S. (1983) Dysthymic disorder. Psychopathology of proposed chronic depressive symptoms. *American Journal of Psychiatry*, **140**, 11–20.

Angst, J., Baastrup, P., Grof, P. *et al.* (1973) The cause of monopolar depression and bipolar psychoses. *Psychiatria Neurologia Neurochinurgia*, **76**, 489–500.

Ashford, J.W. and Ford, C. (1979) Use of MAO inhibitors in elderly patients. *Am. J. Psych.*, **136**(11), 1466–7.

Avery, D. and Winokur, G. (1976) Mortality in depressed patients treated with electro-convulsive therapy and anti-depressants. *Archives of General Psychiatry*, **33**, 1029.

Ayd, F.J. (1974) Single daily dose of anti-depressants. *Journal of the American Medical Association*, **230**, 263–4.

Baldessarini, R.J. (1984) Treatment of depression by altering monoamine metabolism: Precursors and metabolic inhibitors. *Psychopharmacology Bulletin*, **20**, 224.

Blazer, D.G. and Williams, C.A. (1980) The epidemiology of dysphoria and depression in an elderly population. *American Journal of Psychiatry*, **137**, 439–44.

Branconnier, R.J., Cole, J.O., Ghajunian, S. and Rosenthal, S. (1981) Treating the depressed elderly patient – the comparative behavioural pharmacology of mianserin and amitriptyline. In *Typical and atypical anti-depressants advances in Biochemical Psychopharmacology*, **32**, 195–212. Raven Press, New York.

Caine, E.D. (1981) Pseudo dementia: Current concepts and future directions. *Archives of General Psychiatry*, **38**, 1359–64.

Coppen, A., Noguera, R., Bailey, J. *et al.* (1971) Prophylactic lithium in affective disorders: Controlled trial. *Lancet*, **ii**, 275–9.

Coppen, A., Ghose, K., Montgomery, S., Rao, V. and Bailey, J. (1978) Continuation therapy with amitriptyline in depression. *British Journal of Psychiatry*, **133**, 28–33.

de Alarcon, R. (1964) Hypochondriasis and depression in the aged. *Gerontology Clinics*, **6**, 266.

de Montigny, C., Cournoyer, G., Morissette, R. *et al.* (1983) Lithium carbonate addition in tricyclic anti-depressant resistance unipolar depression. *Archives of General Psychiatry*, **40**, 1327.

Eisderfer, C. and Raskin, M.A. (1975) Endocrinologic bases of behaviour in aging. In *Hormonal Correlates of Behaviour* (eds R.L. Sprott and B.E. Eleftherias), Jackson Laboratory, Maine.

Georgotas, A. (1981) Phenelzine in treatment resistive geriatric depression. *World Psychiatric Association Regional Meeting.* New York.

Georgotas, A., Cooper, T., Kim, M. *et al.* (1984) The treatment of affective disorders in the elderly. *Psychopharmacology Bulletin*, **19**, 226.

Gerner, R.H., Estabrook, W., Steiner, J. and Jarvik, L.F. (1980) Treatment of geriatric depression with trazodone, imipramine and placebo – a double blind study. *Journal of Clinical Psychiatry*, **41**(6), 216–20.

Gerner, R.H. and Jarvik, L.F. (1980) Anti-depressant treatment in the elderly. In *Depression and anti-depressants – Implications for cause and treatment* (eds E. Friedman, J. Mann and S. Gershon), Plenum Press, New York.

Gerner, R.H. (1985) Present status of drug therapy of depression in late life. *Journal of Affective Disorders Suppl.*, **1**, 23–32.

Gillis, L.S. and Zabao, A. (1982) Dysphoria in the elderly. *South African Medical Journal*, **62**, 410–13.

Glassman, A.H., Giardina, E.U., Perez, J.M. *et al.* (1979) Clinical characteristics of imipramine induced orthostatic hypotension. *Lancet*, **i**, 468–72.

Goff, D.C. and Jenike, M.A. (1986) Treatment Resistant Depression in the Elderly. *Journal of the American Geriatrics Society*, **34**, 63–79.

Goodwin, F.K., Prange, A.J., Post, R.M. *et al.* (1982) Potentiation of antidepressant effects by L tri-iodothyronine in tricyclic nonresponders. *American Journal of Psychiatry*.

Greenblatt, D.J., Sellers, E.M. and Shader, R.T. (1982) Drug disposition in old age. *New England Journal of Medicine*, **306**, 1081–8.

Gurland, B.J. (1976) The comparative frequency of depression in various adult age groups. *Journal of Gerontology*, **31**, 283–92.

Heiman, E.M. (1977) Cardiac toxicity with thioridazine tricyclic anti-depressant combination. *Journal of Nervous and Mental Disorders*, **165**, 139–43.

Heminger, G.R., Charney, D.J. and Sternberg, D.E. (1983) Lithium carbonate augmentation of anti-depressant treatment. *Archives of General Psychiatry*, **40**, 1335.

Himmelbeck, J.M., Detre, T., Kupfer, J.D. *et al.* (1972) Treatment of previously intractable depressions with tranylcypramine and lithium. *Journal of Nervous and Mental Disorders*, 155–216.

Jacoby, R.J., Levy, R. and Davison, J.M. (1980) Computed tomography in the elderly – affective disorders. *British Journal of Psychiatry*, **136**, 270–5.

Jacoby, R.J. (1981) Depression in the elderly. *British Journal of Hospital Medicine*, **25**, 40–7.

Jacoby, R.J., Dolan, R.J., Levy, R. and Baldy, R. (1983) Quantitative computed tomography in elderly depressed patients. *British Journal of Psychiatry*, **143**, 124–7.

Jarvik, L.F. and Perl, M. (1981) Overview of physiologic dysfunctions related to psychiatric problems in the elderly. in *Psychiatric management of physical disease in the elderly* (eds A. Levenson and R.C.W. Hall) Raven Press, New York.

Jarvik, L.F., Minty, J., Stener, J. and Gerner, R.H. (1982) Treating geriatric depression – a 26 weeks interim analysis. *Journal of the American Geriatric Society*, **30**, 713–17.

Jefferson, J.W. and Ayd, F.J. (1983) Combining lithium and anti-depressants. *Journal of Clinical Psychopharmacology*, **3**, 303.

Kane, J.M., Quitkin, F.M., Rifkin, A. *et al.* (1982) Lithium Carbonate and Imipramine in the prophylaxis of unipolar and bipolar II illness. *Archives of General Psychiatry*, **39**, 1065–9.

Kantor, S.J., Bigger, J., Glassman, A.H., Macken, D.L. and Perez, J.M. (1975) Imipramine induced heart block – a longitudinal case study. *Journal of the American Medical Association*, **231**, 1364–6.

Kantor, S.J. and Glassman, A.H. (1980) The use of tricyclic anti-depressant drugs in geriatric patients. In *Psycho-pharmacology of ageing* (eds C. Eisderfer and W.E. Fann), 99–118. M.T.P. Press, Lancaster.

Kay, D.W.K., Beamish, P. and Roth, M. (1964) Old age mental disorders in Newcastle-upon-Tyne – a study of prevalence. *British Journal of Psychiatry*, **110**, 46–66.

Kayton, W. (1984) Depression: Relationship to somatization and chronic medical illness. *Journal of Clinical Psychiatry*, **45**, 4.

Klerman, G.L. and Cole, J.O. (1965) Clerical Pharmacology of Imipramine and related anti-depressant compounds. *Pharmacology Review*, **17**, 101–41.

Kretschmar, J.H. (1980) Mianserin and amitriptyline in elderly hospitalized patients with depressive illness – a double blind trial. *Current Medical Research Opinion*, **6**(7), 144–50.

Lader, M. (1982) The Psychopharmacology of old age. In *The Psychiatry of Late Life* (eds R. Levy and F. Post), 143–61. Blackwell Scientific Publications, Oxford.

Lancet, **i**, 479 (1979) Editorial: Psychiatric illness among medical patients.

Linstedt, G., Nilsson, L., Walinder, J., Skott, A. and Ohman, R. (1977) On the prevalence, diagnosis and management of lithium induced hypothyroidism in psychiatric patients. *British Journal of Psychiatry*, **139**, 452–8.

Lydiard, R.B., Golenberg, A.J. (1981) Amoxapine: An anti-depressant with some neuroleptic properties? *Pharmacotherapy*, **1**, 163.

McAllister, T.W. and Price, T.P.R. (1982) Severe depressive pseudo-dementia with and without dementia. *American Journal of Psychiatry*, **138**, 626–8.

McGrath, P.S., Quitkin, F.M., Harrison, W. *et al.* (1984) Treatment of melancholia with tranylcypramine. *American Journal of Psychiatry*, **141**, 288.

Medical Research Council (1981) Continuation therapy with lithium and amitriptyline in unipolar depressive illness: A controlled trial. *Psychological Medicine*, **2**, 409–16.

Mendlewicz, J., Dunbar, G.C. and Hoffman, G. (1985) Changes in sleep EEG architecture during the treatment of depressed patients with mianserin. *Acta Psychiatrica Scandinavica*, Suppl. 72, 320–6.

Mindham, R.H.S., Howland, C. and Shephard, M. (1973) An evaluation of continuation therapy with tricyclic anti-depressants in depressive illness. *Psychological Medicine*, **3**, 5–17.

Minter, R.E. and Mandel, M.R. (1979) The treatment of psychotic major depressive disorders with drugs and electroconvulsive therapy. *Journal of Nervous and Mental Disorders*, **67**, 726–33.

Moffic, H.S. and Paykel, E.S. (1975) Depression in medical inpatients. *British Journal of Psychiatry*, **126**, 346.

Montgomery, I., Oswald, I., Morgan, R. and Adam, R. (1983) Trazodone enhances sleep in subjective quality but not in objective duration. *British Journal of Clinical Pharmacology*, **16**, 139.

Moore, J.T. (1985) Dysthymia in the elderly. *Journal of Affective Disorders Suppl.*, **1**, 15–21.

Murphy, E. (1982) Social origins of depression in old age. *British Journal of Psychiatry*, **141**, 135–42.

Murphy, E. (1983) The prognosis of depression in old age. *British Journal of Psychiatry*, **142**, 111–19.

Murphy, E. (1985) General Management of Depression in Late Life. *Journal of Affective Disorders Suppl.*, **1**, 7–10.

Neshkes, R., Gerner R. and Aldrich, J. (1982) A comparison trial of the cardiovascular effects of doxepin and imipramine in elderly depressed outpatients. *Gerontologist*, **22**, 241–5.

Newton, R. (1981) The side effect profile of trazodone in comparison to an active control and placebo. *Journal of Clinical Psychopharmacology*, **1**, 895.

Paykel, E.S., Dimascio A., Haswell, D. and Prusoff, B.A. (1975) Effects of maintenance of amitriptyline and psychotherapy on symptoms of depression. *Psychological Medicine*, **5**, 67–71.

Paykel, E.S., Dimascio, A., Haswell, D. and Prusoff, J.A. (1979) Predictors of treatment response in Psycho-pharmacology of Affective Disorders (eds E.S. Paykel and A. Coppen), Oxford University Press.

Post, F. (1972) The management and nature of depressive illnesses in later life; a follow through study. *British Journal of Psychiatry*, **121**, 393–404.

Post, F. (1982) The Psychiatry of Late Life. Functional Disorders; description, incidence and recognition. 176–96. (eds R. Levy and F. Post), Blackwell Scientific Publications.

Post, F. (1985) Psychotherapy, electro-convulsive treatments and long term management of elderly patients. In Management of depression in late life. *Journal of Affective Disorders Suppl.*, 41–5.

Post, R.M., Uhde, T.W., Ballenger, J.C. *et al.* (1983) Prophylactic efficacy of carbamazepine in manic-depressive illness. *American Journal of Psychiatry*, **140**, 1602.

Quitkin, F.M., Rabkin, J.G., Ross, D. *et al.* (1984b) Duration of anti-depressant drug treatment. *Archives of General Psychiatry*, **41**, 238.

Quitkin, F.M., Rabkin, J.G., Ross, D. and McGrath, P.J. (1984a) Duration of anti-depressant drug treatment. What is an adequate trial? *Archives of General Psychiatry*, **29**, 420–5.

Quitkin, F.M., Rabkin, J.G., Ross, D. and McGrath, P.J. (1984b) Identification of true drug response to anti-depressants, use of pattern analysis. *Archives of General Psychiatry*, **41**, 782–6.

Razani, J., White, K.L., White, J. *et al.* (1983) The safety and efficacy of combined amitriptyline and tranylcypramine anti-depressant treatment. *Archives of General Psychiatry*, **40**, 657.

Reifler, B.V., Lawson, E. and Hanley, R. (1982) Co-existence of cognitive impairment and depression in geriatric outpatients. *American Journal of Psychiatry*, **139**, 5.

Richelsen, E. (1982) Pharmacology of anti-depressants in use in the United States. *Journal of Clinical Psychiatry*, **43**, 4–11.

Robinson, D.S. (1979) Age related factors affecting anti-depressant drug metabolism and clinical response. In Geriatric Psychopharmacology. (ed. K. Vandy) Elsevier North-Holland, New York.

Robinson, P.D., Saurkes, J.L., Nies, A. *et al.* (1977) Monoamine metabolism in the human brain. *Archives of General Psychiatry*, **34**, 89.

Ron, M.A., Toone, B.K., Garralda, M.E. *et al.* (1979) Diagnostic accuracy in pre-senile dementia. *British Journal of Psychiatry*, **134**, 161–8.

Roose, S.P., Glassman, A.H., Siris, S. *et al.* (1981) Comparison of imipramine and nortriptyline induced orthostatic hypotension – a meaningful difference. *Journal of Clinical Psychopharmacology*, **1**, 316–21.

Scardigli, G. and Jans, G. (1982) Comparative double blind study on efficacy and side effects of trazodone, nomifensine and mianserin in elderly patients. *Advances in Biochemistry and Psychopharmacology*, **32**, 229–36.

Schatsberg, A.F., Lipkin, B., Satlin, A. and Cole, J.O. (1984) Diagnosis of affective disorders in the elderly. *Psychosomatics*, **25**, 126–31.

Sloane, R.B., Staples, F., Bender, M., Razani, J. and Schneider, L. (1984) Psychotherapy versus nortriptyline for depression in the elderly. In *Abstracts of the 14th CINP Congress*, Florence, p. 169.

Smith, A.H.W., Naylor, G.S. and Moody, J.P. (1978) Placebo-controlled double blind trial of mianserin hydrochloride. *British Journal of Clinical Pharmacology*, **5**, 675.

Spar, J.E., Ford, C.V. and Liston E.H. (1979) Bipolar affective disorder in aged patients. *Journal of Clinical Psychiatry*, **40**, 504–7.

Spar, J.E. and Gerner, R.H. (1982) Major depression in the elderly: DSM III criteria and the dexamethasone suppression test as predictors of treatment response. *American Journal of Psychiatry*, **140**, 844.

Stein, M.K., Rickels, K. and Weisse, C.C. (1980) Maintenance therapy with amitriptyline: A controlled trial. *American Journal of Psychiatry*, **137**, 370–1.

Thayssen, P., Bjekre, M., Krogh-Sorenson, L. *et al.* (1981) Cardiovascular effects of imipramine and nortriptyline in elderly patients. *Psychopharmacology*, **74**, 360.

Tsuang, M.T., Woolson, R.F. and Fleming, J.A. (1980) Premature deaths in schizophrenia and affective disorders. *Archives of General Psychiatry*, **37**, 979.

Van der Velde, C.D. (1971) Toxicity of Lithium Carbonate in elderly patients. *American Journal of Psychiatry*, **127**, 1075–7.

Von Ammon, K. and Cavanaugh, S. (1984) Diagnosing depression in the hospitalized patient with chronic medical illness. *Journal of Clinical Psychiatry*, **45**, 13.

Ware, J.C. (1983) Tricyclic anti-depressants in the treatment of insomnia. *Journal of Clinical Psychiatry*, **44**, 25.

Weiner, R.D. (1982) The role of electroconvulsive therapy in the treatment of depression in the elderly. *Journal of American Geriatric Society*, **30**, 710–12.

Williamson, J. (1978) Depression in the elderly. *Age and ageing*, **7**, 35–40.

Wills, L.E. (1963) Pseudodementia. *American Journal of Psychiatry*, **120**, 244.

Chapter Fourteen

The use of electroconvulsive therapy in elderly depressive patients

KATY MALCOLM and MALCOLM PEET

CONTENTS

14.1 INTRODUCTION

Though widely used and extensively investigated, electroconvulsive therapy (ECT) remains a controversial treatment. Attitudes to ECT amongst doctors and patients tend to be polarized. Extreme antagonists refer to ECT as 'electrocution' and regard it as a primitive blunderbuss treatment which causes brain damage. This attitude is commoner amongst recipients of ECT than amongst psychiatrists. At the other extreme is the view, held more commonly by psychiatrists than their patients, that ECT is dramatically effective and the treatment of choice in severe depressive illness. These polarized attitudes have led to attempts on the one hand to ban ECT, and on the other hand to the indiscriminate and uncritical overuse of ECT.

The use of ECT in the elderly is particularly emotive. The sight of a frail, emaciated and agitated elderly person being taken to have ECT against her will is one of the most distressing in psychiatry to all but the most dehumanized staff. Nevertheless, there are situations in which ECT is essential and even life-saving. There seems to be no barrier to the age at which ECT may be used. A recent report of ECT given to a 91 year old patient (O'Shea, 1987) was followed by a new 'record' of ECT being given to a 103 year old woman (Bracken, Ryan and Dunne, 1987).

We aim to present a balanced overview of the evidence relating to the use of ECT, particularly in the elderly. The review will focus primarily on the interpretation of available objective data. Evidence relating to the efficacy and safety of ECT will be reviewed, and some current assumptions will be questioned.

14.2 EFFICACY OF ECT

The efficacy of the ECT procedure in relieving symptoms of depressive illness was established in two early influential trials, one conducted in Britain (Medical Research Council, 1965), and one in the United States (Greenblatt, Grosser and Wechler, 1964). Each trial compared the ECT procedure with imipramine, monoamine oxidase inhibitor, and placebo drug treatment. In the MRC study, 71% of patients showed none or slight symptoms after ECT treatment, compared with 52% given imipramine, 30% given phenelzine, and 39% given placebo. In the study of Greenblatt, Grosser and Wechler, marked improvement was found in 76% of ECT-treated patients, 49% of those given imipramine, 50% of patients taking phenelzine, and 46% of placebo-treated patients. Whilst these studies appear at face value to show that ECT is the most effective short-term treatment for severe depressive disorder, there are a number of methodological problems. Not least of these is that ECT is not administered on a double-blind basis. This opens up the possibility not only of bias on the part of the raters but also, more importantly, the likelihood of a strong placebo effect from a procedure which is perceived by patients and psychiatrists to be potent and dramatic.

Subsequent controlled trials have recently been comprehensively reviewed by Crow and Johnstone (1986). A number of these studies have attempted to control the placebo effect by comparing the full ECT procedure with simulated ECT in which the patient is given an anaesthetic only but no convulsive shock. A number of methodologically sophisticated trials have been published in recent years. Two of the more important and representative of these trials are the Northwick Park trial (Johnstone *et al.*, 1980), and the Leicester trial (Brandon *et al.*, 1984).

Johnstone *et al.* (1980) compared real ECT with simulated ECT in 70 patients with endogenous depression defined by research criteria. After eight treatments the patients given real ECT improved significantly more than those given simulated ECT, though the difference was relatively small. After one month and six months follow-up there was no significant difference in outcome between the two groups. In the study of Brandon *et al.* (1984) 96 patients were given up to eight treatments of real ECT or simulated ECT. Again, improvement in depressive symptoms in patients given the real treatment was significantly greater than those given simulated treatment after two and four weeks of treatment. However, at three months and six months follow-up there was no difference in outcome between the two groups. In both studies it was found that the presence of delusions was a predictor of the efficacy of real ECT relative to simulated ECT. Retardation was also found to be a predictor of efficacy, though in the Northwick Park trial (CRC Division of Psychiatry, 1984) it was found that there was an overlap of patients suffering from delusions and retardation and that retardation considered separately from delusions did not significantly predict outcome.

The greater part of the improvement seen after the ECT procedure does not depend upon electrically inducing a seizure. In the Northwick Park trial, only a quarter of the improvement after real ECT was attributable to the shock, the remaining three-quarters occurring also in the simulated ECT group. The authors conclude that 'many depressive illnesses although severe may have a favourable outcome with intensive nursing and medical care even if physical treatments are not given'. Some other studies have shown larger differences between real and simulated ECT. In a meta analysis across a number of studies, but not including more recent trials, Janicak *et al.* (1985) concluded that 40% of patients respond to simulated ECT and 72% to real ECT. They also analysed studies comparing real ECT with tricyclic antidepressants, and found that improvement occurred in 87% of patients given ECT and 67% of patients given tricyclic antidepressants. This overall finding requires qualification. Firstly, the trials were not double-blind with respect to ECT treatment. Secondly, it is now well recognized that patients with delusional depression, who seem to respond particularly favourably to ECT, respond very poorly to tricyclic antidepressants. The combination of a neuroleptic and a tricyclic antidepressant brings a substantially greater response rate (Spiker *et al.*, 1985). It is therefore likely that pharmacological treatment based on current knowledge would bring the response rate up to that of ECT. No adequately-controlled trials have addressed this possibility.

None of the available controlled trials of ECT have been conducted in an elderly population. Indeed, most trials specifically exclude elderly patients. The only available data comes from open uncontrolled studies. Such widely varying response rates have been reported that it is difficult to make any definitive statement about ECT efficacy in this age group. The most optimistic reports indicate short-term response rates of 83% (Fraser and Glass, 1980), 79% (Gaspar and Samarsingh, 1982), 92% (Burke *et al.*, 1985), and 81% (Meyers and Mei-Tal, 1985). Others report less positive experiences. Karlinsky and Shulman (1984) found a short-term response rate of only 42%, but at six months follow-up barely a third of their patients had maintained this improvement. Post (1985) reported a similar experience. These reports of a poor long-term outcome are in keeping with controlled trials in younger patients indicating that ECT has only short-term efficacy.

A number of studies have investigated the relative efficacy of unilateral non-dominant ECT and bilateral ECT. This is particularly pertinent to the elderly because of the lower incidence of memory disturbance induced by unilateral non-dominant ECT. In the meta analysis of Janicak *et al.* (1985), which included ten comparative controlled trials, no overall difference in efficacy was found between unilateral and bilateral ECT. This runs contrary to the commonly held clinical notion that bilateral ECT is more effective than unilateral. However, in some studies which permitted a flexible number of treatments, those given unilateral ECT required one or two more treatments than those given ECT bilaterally in order to produce the same therapeutic effect. This is consistent with evidence that unilateral electrode placement results in significantly more missed seizures than bilateral ECT (Pettinati and Nilsen, 1985). In a study of elderly depressive patients randomly allocated to treatment with bilateral or unilateral ECT, Fraser and Glass (1980) found no significant difference in efficacy.

In summary, the ECT procedure is effective in alleviating symptoms in severe depressive disorder. However, the majority of the improvement does not depend upon electrical induction of a seizure. Unilateral ECT is as effective as bilateral ECT. Electroconvulsive therapy has only a short-term benefit, and the presence of delusions is the only factor which significantly predicts response to real ECT over simulated ECT. There are no adequately designed trials demonstrating that ECT is superior to current pharmacological treatments, including combinations of antidepressant and neuroleptic drugs, in the treatment of severe depressive disorder. Adequately controlled trials of ECT in the treatment of elderly depressive patients are lacking, and data from open studies are inconsistent. The commonly held belief that ECT is a treatment of choice for elderly depressive patients is therefore founded upon clinical experience rather than on sound experimental evidence.

Clinical situations where the short-term benefits of ECT may be desirable include endpoint states of depression, as for example in depressive stupor or in patients who are refusing to eat or drink. In these circumstances ECT can be seen as a short-term expedient to alleviate the emergency situation so that further therapy can be initiated. Another commonly held belief is that ECT should be used preferentially in patients who have immediately active suicidal impulses. However, there is no convincing evidence to support the contention that patients treated with ECT have a lower suicide rate than those given other treatments (Skrabanek, 1986). Treatment-resistant depression – that is, depressive disorder which has not responded to adequate doses of two different antidepressants – is regarded as another indication for ECT. However, the short-term nature of the ECT response necessitates continuation treatment with an effective antidepressant in order to prevent relapse over the subsequent six months. If the clinician recommends ECT rather than seeking an effective antidepressant drug, then there is no way of knowing which drug will be pharmacologically effective during the post-ECT continuation period. Commonly, patients remain on the antidepressant which they have failed to respond to before being given ECT, which must surely be irrational therapy.

In the elderly, a further reason put forward for the use of ECT is the belief that ECT may be safer than antidepressant drugs. It is therefore appropriate to examine this proposition in some detail.

14.3 THE SAFETY OF ECT

ECT is widely considered to be a safe treatment particularly in elderly patients. Moreover it is often held to be safer than antidepressant drugs. Elderly people, with their failing reserve and increased incidence of pre-existing physical illness are prone to adverse side-effects from any biological treatment. It is important, then, to examine the validity of the concept of ECT as a safe treatment, especially in this group of patients.

The principal risks associated with ECT are cardiovascular and neuropyschological. Other risks such as torn muscles and tendons, fractures and cutaneous burns can be prevented or minimized by the use of modified ECT and adequate training in the correct administration of ECT.

The mortality associated with ECT is low. Fink (1979) in a review of studies looking at mortality figures associated with ECT, reports rates of around 0.03%. The commonest time for death to occur is immediately following seizure during the recovery period. Death is usually due to cardiovascular complications – either myocardial infarct or ventricular arrhythmias (Kendell, 1981).

14.3.1 Cardiovascular risks

The cardiovascular changes elicited by ECT are mediated by autonomic nervous system stimulation compounded by increased muscular work and a possible degree of anoxia. Parasympathetic discharge occurring immediately after application of the current results in an initial brady-cardia or even asystole, followed by tachycardia, dysrhythmia and hypertension due to sympathetic stimulation.

Myocardial infarct, cardiac failure and arrhythmias have all been reported as cardiovascular complications of ECT (Fink, 1979). Of these, arrhythmias are the commonest complication. Occurrences have been reported as varying between 8–75% (American Psychiatric Association, 1978). Factors influencing the occurrence of cardiovascular complications include age, pre-existing cardiovascular disease and concomitant pharmacotherapy. Several studies have examined how such factors may affect the risks of ECT. In a study of 293 in-patients, Alexopoulous *et al.* (1984) reported a trend towards more medical complications of ECT in older patients compared with younger. This trend became significant when the problems were cardiovascular in nature; 9% of the elderly patients developed cardiovascular problems compared to 1% of the younger patients. These elderly patients often had a history of pre-existing cardiovascular disease. Gerring and Shields (1982) also found age and pre-existing cardiovascular disease to be associated with car-diovascular complications. A cardiovascular complication rate of 28% was found in their series of 42 patients. All those with cardiovascular complications were over 60 and the rate of cardiovascular complications rose to 70% in those with pre-existng cardiovascular disease. These figures give some cause for concern, particularly in view of the fact that four of the complications were thought to be life-threatening events. Abramczuk and Rose (1979) found 11 of their 367 patients to have had serious complications from ECT. Five of these 11 complications occurred in patients over the age of 75 who had pre-existing cardiovascular disease. However, such high rates of cardiovascular complications may not be typical nor is pre-existing cardiovascular disease always predic-tive of cardiovascular complications. A study by Dec, Stern and Welch (1985) of 26 patients with an average age of 65 revealed no electro-cardiographic or cardiac enzyme abnormalities associated with ECT despite the fact that 24% of their population had pre-existing cardio-vascular disease. Similarly, Burke *et al.* (1985) in a study of 30 patients of average age 72 found that pre-existing cardiovascular disease did not predict subsequent complications although again age was found to correlate significantly with increased cardiovascular complications.

The cardiovascular risks of ECT in the elderly may be compounded if

ECT is given concomitantly with psychotropic drugs. The administration of ECT with simultaneous use of psychotropic drugs is not an uncommon practice. A study by McCleave and Blakemore (1975) showed all ECT patients in their series of 425 to be receiving psychotropic drugs most of which were either tricyclic antidepressants or benzodiazepines. Lithium, monoamine oxidase inhibitors and tricyclic antidepressants can all interact adversely with anaesthetic agents and muscle relaxants as well as having cardiotoxic effects in their own right. These drugs do not appear to improve efficacy when given in combination with ECT (Avery and Winokur, 1977; Barkai, 1985). In view of this, the practice of combining ECT and psychotropic drugs is probably best avoided. However, there has been one study showing that there were no increased cardiovascular abnormalities with a simultaneous administration of tricyclic antidepressants and ECT compared to ECT alone (Azar and Lear, 1984), and some have even suggested that concurrent administration of tricyclic antidepressants may protect against the arrythmias caused by ECT by virtue of their atropinic and antiadrenergic effects (French, 1974).

In summary, the concept of ECT being a safer treatment in the elderly may well rest on its comparison with older tricyclic antidepressants whose cardiovascular risks are well known. However, it is clear that the adverse cardiovascular effects of ECT are not uncommon and are particularly concentrated amongst older patients and probably in those with pre-existing cardiovascular disease. Little work has been done comparing the cardiovascular risks of ECT with the risks of newer tricyclic and tetracyclic antidepressants whose cardiotoxicity is considerably less than the older antidepressants.

14.4 THE EFFECT OF ECT ON COGNITIVE FUNCTION

It is well recognized that a short period of disorientation may occur in the immediate post-ictal period. Also, complaints of persisting memory impairment are common in patients who have received ECT. Thus, Freeman and Kendall (1980) found that 74% of their patients complained of memory disturbances which they associated with ECT and 30% claimed that their memory had never returned to normal following ECT. Because of such complaints from patients, there have been numerous studies of cognitive function following ECT, which have demonstrated impairment of both anterograde and retrograde memory. Such findings are clearly pertinent to the elderly who may have failing memory capacity even before having ECT.

14.4.1 Disorientation

Daniel and Crovitz (1982), in a review of studies looking at recovery of orientation following ECT, suggest that the different components of orientation recover at different rates. The consensus of the studies was that orientation of person returns first, followed by orientation for place and then time. The duration of disorientation was shown to increase across treatment number, and to be worse in bilateral than in unilateral ECT. Post-ictal recovery time is longer in the elderly than in younger patients. Fraser and Glass (1978) treated nine elderly patients with alternate bilateral and unilateral electrode placements during their course of ECT. Post-ictal recovery times were compared for bilateral and unilateral placements, and a comparison made between recovery time in the elderly patients and in the younger patients in the study of Valentine, Keddie and Dunne (1968). Recovery times in the elderly group were five times longer for unilateral and nine times longer for bilateral ECT compared to the younger patients. In a larger series of 29 elderly patients randomly assigned to bilateral or unilateral ECT, Fraser and Glass (1980) again found that bilateral ECT was associated with significantly longer post-ictal recovery times. Recovery times following bilateral ECT were found to be longer when the interval between treatments was diminished, and to show a cumulative effect of lengthening across treatments. Such effects were not shown to operate when unilateral ECT was given. In younger patients, Sackeim *et al.* (1986) used ECT stimulus dosage titrated for each patient to just above seizure threshold, and found that disorientation did not show a cumulative increase across bilateral treatments and indeed showed a cumulative improvement across unilateral treatment. This finding obviously has advantages for the patient, and these advantages may be particularly clear in the elderly patient who may be more vulnerable to the development of a post-ictal confusional state.

14.4.2 Anterograde amnaesia

The anterograde amnaesia associated with ECT diminishes between treatments and accumulates across treatments (Squire, 1986). On completion of the course of ECT, the ability for new learning begins to return. Many attempts have been made to establish the point at which this occurs, and indeed whether there is any permanent impairment of memory function following ECT. Fink (1979) points out the difficulties in reaching conclusions from these numerous studies: comparisons between studies are difficult to make due to differences in selection of patients, modality of treatment (bilateral or unilateral, wave form, brief pulse or sinusoidal), instruments used to test cognitive deficit and the varying time intervals post-treatment at which cognitive performance is tested. Weeks, Freeman and Kendell (1980) reviewed several studies and suggested that return to base-line performance occurred at an average of 72 days. However, there is again a problem of the definition of base-line performance, since depressive illness in itself is often associated with memory deficits (Sternberg and Jarvik, 1976). It may be that depression and ECT affect various components of anterograde memory differently. In one study (Sackeim *et al.*, 1986), of 17 patients who received ECT (10 bilateral, 7 unilateral) compared with a group of 20 normal control patients matched for age, sex, education, socio-economic status, and pre-morbid IQ, a marked deficit in acquisition was shown pre-treatment in the patients compared to controls, whereas disruption in retention of new information was shown post-treatment in the patients relative to controls. These findings are consistent with the study of Cronholm and Ottosson (1961), supporting the claim that depression is associated with deficits in the acquisition of new information, whereas ECT produces a temporary deficit in the retention of new information.

Elderly depressive patients are particularly prone to show memory impairment in association with depressive illness, which may be severe in states of depressive pseudodementia. In the latter patients, the improvement in memory consequent upon recovery from the depressive illness will entirely overshadow any memory impairment caused by the ECT treatment. Objective testing of memory functions in the elderly also indicates that impairment is only temporary (Fraser and Glass, 1980).

Bilateral ECT has consistently been shown to be associated with more severe impairment of memory, both anterograde and retrograde, than unilateral. The difference in favour of unilateral ECT is more clear-cut when verbal memory is tested relative to non-verbal memory. Some have suggested that bilateral ECT affects both non-verbal and verbal memory more severely than unilateral (Squire and Slater, 1978), whilst others appear to show equivalent effects of bilateral and unilateral ECT on non-verbal memory, though bilateral ECT is still shown to produce more impairment of verbal memory (Sackeim *et al.*, 1986). There is also some evidence that brief pulse wave forms produce less amnaesia than sinusoidal wave forms, whilst remaining equally effective therapeutically (Weiner *et al.*, 1986), though the literature is not conclusive (Daniel and Crovitz, 1983). The frequency of seizures affects the extent and rate of development of amnaesia. When frequency of treatment is increased to daily seizures or multiple seizures in one day, memory difficulties become far more severe (Fink, 1979). The duration of seizure has not generally been shown to be related to memory impairment (Weiner *et al.*, 1986), although Miller *et al.* (1985) found a correlation between non-verbal forgetting and seizure duration. Amnaesia appears to increase with total treatment number (Daniel and Crovitz, 1983). There is a certain amount of evidence to suggest that there is an increased incidence, severity and persistence of memory deficits amongst patients receiving prolonged and intensive courses of ECT, such as 50 or 100 applications (American Psychiatric Association, 1978), although prospective controlled studies addressing this issue are not available.

Despite methodological problems and differences in ECT technique, most studies have shown fairly consistent results in that eventually, and certainly by six months after treatment, patients who have received ECT do not show evidence of persisting deficit in new learning ability assessed objectively. However, this is at variance with the frequent complaint by the patients themselves that their memory has never been the same since they received ECT. It therefore remains possible that some aspect of new learning ability which has not been identified by the tests used experimentally, does remain impaired for prolonged periods following ECT.

14.4.3 Retrograde amnaesia

Retrograde amnaesia associated with ECT refers to remote memory of events, either public or personal, which have occurred before treatment. Squire, Slater and Miller (1981) studied remote memory for public events by asking patients to remember facts about television programmes which had been broadcast for one season in the past 15 years. Patients receiving bilateral ECT showed a temporally-limited gradient of impairment in long-term memory, in that they were able to remember programmes broadcast 4 to 17 years previously as well after ECT as before, but showed a marked impairment in recollection of programmes broadcast 1 to 3 years before treatment. However, this impairment diminished in the weeks after treatment and was not in evidence six months later. Patients treated with non-dominant unilateral ECT did not show this impairment in remote memory (Squire, Slater and Chase, 1975). Other studies investigating remote memory have also tended to show no persisting deficit (Weeks, Freeman and Kendell, 1980; Frith *et al.*, 1983) although Weiner (1984) points out that definitive statements regarding this issue cannot yet be made, largely due to methodological difficulties in the studies carried out to date.

Squire, Slater and Miller (1981) also investigated autobiographical retrograde memory by asking patients to give details of their personal history over a period ranging from many years prior to treatment to only a few days prior to treatment. The patients' performance was compared with a group of hospitalized depressed patients who had not received ECT. At seven months retest, the ECT patients still showed occasional failure to recall remote events that they had reported as facts prior to ECT. The memory disturbance was more apparent in the most recent remote events, that is those events occurring immediately before treatment. Control patients, on the other hand, could recall almost as much information at retest as they had reported seven months previously. It therefore appears that autobiographical remote memory shows some long lasting and possibly permanent disruption associated with ECT, particularly for personal events occurring around the time that treatment was given.

In conclusion, elderly patients are more prone than younger patients to suffer cognitive impairment following ECT, particularly in the immediate post-ictal period. Studies conducted primarily in younger patients indicate that anterograde memory, as judged by objective testing, has returned to normal by some months after treatment, though patients commonly complain of persisting subjective memory impairment. There is evidence of persisting retrograde amnaesia, particularly for personal events occurring shortly before commencement of ECT. Because of the particular proneness of the elderly to post-ictal cognitive impairment, which in some cases may compromise an already impaired sensorium, it is of particular importance to use correct techniques when administering ECT to the elderly. This includes the use of unilateral electrode placements, and using the minimum necessary total number of applications of ECT and the lowest effective stimulus dosage.

14.5 PATIENTS' PERCEPTIONS OF ECT

There have been relatively few studies looking at patients' attitudes to, and experience and knowledge of, ECT. None of these have focused on elderly populations in particular. Some studies have selectively examined particular aspects of patients' perceptions of ECT such as subjective side-effects of ECT (Gomez, 1975) or the effect of the media on attitudes towards ECT (Bird, 1979). Other studies have investigated these issues more comprehensively (Freeman and Kendell, 1980; Hughes, Barraclough and Reeve, 1981). Most of these studies were carried out some time after the ECT course had been completed; in some cases over a year had elapsed between the last ECT and interview.

The studies of Freeman and Kendell (1980) and Hughes, Barraclough and Reeve (1981) conclude that patients displayed a lack of knowledge of ECT, and that patients often claimed to have received no explanation of the procedure. The investigators suggest that the explanations were given, but then forgotten. It may be that the patients' perceptions and knowledge of ECT are different before treatment than after treatment. Attitudes and knowledge may also change or fade over time.

A recent study (Malcolm, 1989) chose to examine patients' perceptions and knowledge of ECT both before and after treatment. One hundred patients were interviewed with a semi-structured questionnaire on two occasions; firstly, before treatment but after consent had been sought, and secondly in the week after treatment had been completed. In this way, a comparison of patients' fears or worries before treatment could be made with their actual experiences of treatment, and their general knowledge of what the procedure entailed assessed shortly after it had been explained to them. Of the one hundred patients, 59 were aged 65 or over. These patients displayed a worrying paucity of knowledge about ECT.

Only 2% of patients know that the treatment involved a seizure; some made remarks such as 'they would stop the treatment if you had a seizure', or, 'I am sure the doctors would never do that to me'.

Only 24% knew that electrodes were placed on the head and a current passed through the brain, although most know that electricity was involved in some way during the treatment.

Most patients (84%) understood that they would have a general anaesthetic but only 3% knew the number of proposed treatments and the intervals at which they would be given. Several patients seemed to be under the impression that they would only have one treatment.

Only 27% of patients over 65 thought that they could refuse to have ECT, and they often commented that they would probably be forced to have the treatment anyway. Ten per cent did not know whether they could refuse ECT or not, and the remaining 63% thought they could not refuse ECT.

Despite this lack of knowledge, 68% of patients consented to the procedure, and over half (55%) thought the explanation adequate. Twenty-seven of the 59 patients (46%) said they had received no explanation of the procedure, but only eight of the 27 felt this to be unsatisfactory. The remainder made observations such as: 'I am happy to let the doctor decide what is best for me, it's up to him/her'.

Although the patients were apparently satisfied with the explanation given to them, they still voiced anxieties about the impending treatment, when asked.

Forty-eight per cent said they were frightened or worried about the procedure, 20% said they did not know and only 32% were not worried or frightened.

After treatment the proportions of patients who experienced ECT as frightening or worrying were not very different. Forty-nine per cent found it frightening, 19% did not know and 32% did not find treatment frightening.

The aspect of ECT most commonly feared before treatment was that of brain damage, mentioned by 53%. Thirty-nine per cent feared losing their memory.

After treatment, patients were asked with the use of a checklist if they found particular parts of the procedure frightening or worrying. Waiting for treatment was mentioned by 75% as frightening, followed by injections, mentioned by 41% and being with other patients prior to treatment, mentioned by 34%.

The results show that these patients over 65 displayed a lack of knowledge of ECT. Whether this was due to an inadequate explanation or whether the patients simply failed to retain the information, cannot be ascertained from these data. Patients seemed to have boundless faith in the doctors doing what was in their best interests. Nevertheless, patients did express anxieties before treatment and found some aspects of the treatment unnecessarily unpleasant.

14.6 REASONS FOR HIGH USAGE OF ECT

As there is such a wide variation in the usage of ECT between different clinicians, it is useful to examine some of the possible reasons why ECT is so popular with some psychiatrists.

1. The belief that ECT is the most effective treatment for severe depressive disorder in the elderly. This belief is based upon clinical impression rather than sound evidence. Clinical impression is a notoriously unreliable yardstick, as is shown by the enthusiastic adoption of bleeding and purging in the last century and insulin coma therapy earlier this century. Nevertheless, ECT does appear to be a short-term expedient in endpoint depression, when patients have deteriorated to the point of stupor or severe malnutrition and dehydration.
2. Leaving treatment too late. Endpoint states of depression are not reached suddenly. The great majority of patients receiving ECT have a history of several months of worsening depression. The duration of depressive symptoms is particularly long in the elderly. In traditional psychiatric services patients are treated by their General Practitioners outside hospital, and only those patients who deteriorate into severe depressive states are admitted into hospital by which time ECT may be inevitable. A comprehensive community-based service, which can bring effective pharmacological, psychological and social help at an early stage of the depressive process, is likely to result in

a reduced need for the use of ECT (Peet, 1986). Effective liaison with General Practitioners is particularly important in this respect, as is the provision of good Community Psychiatric Nursing Services and Day Hospital provision.

3. Lack of pharmacological expertise. Antidepressant and other psychotropic drugs are commonly used inexpertly, particularly in the elderly where special knowledge of pharmacokinetic and pharmacodynamic principles is required. In General Practice, the commonest failings are underdosing and too short a duration of treatment (Johnson, 1973). However, psychiatrists are also guilty of misuse of psychotropic drugs. In his illuminating paper '. . . and a small dose of antidepressant might help' Bridges (1983) reported that many patients referred for modified leucotomy have been given inadequate doses of antidepressant drugs, and were often left on these low doses for prolonged periods of time despite an obvious lack of response. This occurred despite the fact that the psychiatrists referring these patients were presumably in favour of a physical approach to treatment. If under-treatment can occur so commonly in patients referred for leucotomy then there can be no doubt that the same has happened to many patients given ECT.

4. The belief that ECT is safer than antidepressants. Whilst ECT is probably safer than the older more toxic antidepressants, there are nevertheless cardiovascular risks with ECT, and newer antidepressants when used properly are much less toxic in the elderly than the older tricyclics (Peet, 1986).

ECT is a treatment of last resort, not first choice. However, in endpoint status of depressive disorder in the elderly this treatment can be markedly effective and indeed life-saving. Nevertheless, it is likely that more effective intervention earlier in the development of the depressive illness would significantly reduce the need to use ECT.

The lack of knowledge which elderly patients display about the treatment they are about to receive is a matter for serious concern and merits further attention.

REFERENCES

Abramczuk, J.A. and Rose, N.M. (1979) Pre-anaesthetic assessment and the prevention of post-ECT morbidity. *Brit. J. Psychiat.*, **134**, 582–7.

Alexopoulos, G.S., Shamoian, C.J., Lucas, J., et al. (1984) Medical problems of geriatric psychiatric patients and younger controls during electroconvulsive therapy. *J. Am. Geriat. Soc.*, 32, 651–4.

American Psychiatric Association (1978) Electroconvulsive therapy: report of the

Task Force on electroconvulsive therapy of the American Psychiatric Association. *Task Force Report 14, Washington D.C.*

Avery, D. and Winokur, D. (1977) The efficacy of ECT and antidepressants in depression. *Biol. Psychiat.*, **12**, 507–23.

Azar, I. and Lear, E. (1982) Cardiovascular effects of electroconvulsive therapy in patients taking tricyclic antidepressants. *Anesth. Analg.*, **63**, 1140.

Barkai, A.I. (1985) Combined electroconvulsive and drug treatment. *Comprehensive Therapy*, **11**, 48–53.

Bird, J.M. (1979) Effect of the media on attitudes to electric convulsion therapy. *Brit. Med. J.*, **2**, 526.

Bracken, P., Ryan, M. and Dunne, D. (1987) Electroconvulsive therapy in the elderly. *Brit. J. Psychiat.*, **150**, 712.

Brandon, S., Cowley, P., McDonald, C. *et al.* (1984) Electroconvulsive therapy: results in depression from the Leicestershire trial. *Brit. Med. J.*, **1**, 22–5.

Bridges, P.K. (1983) '. . . and a small dose of an antidepressant might help'. *Brit. J. Psychiat.*, **142**, 626–8.

Burke, W.J., Rutherford, J.L., Zorumzki, G.F. and Reich, T. (1985) Electroconvulsive therapy and the elderly. *Comprehens. Psychiat.*, **26**, 480–86.

Calloway, S.P., Dolan, R.J., Jacoby, R.J. and Levy, R. (1981) ECT and cerebral atrophy: a computed tomographic study. *Acta Psychiat. Scand.*, **64**, 442–5.

CRC Division of Psychiatry (1984), The Northwick Park ECT trial: predictors of response to real and simulated ECT. *Brit. J. Psychiat.*, **144**, 227–57.

Cronholm, B. and Ottosson, J.O. (1961) Memory functions in endogenous depression before and after electroconvulsive therapy. *Arch. Gen. Psychiat.*, **5**, 193–9.

Crow, T.J. and Johnstone, E. (1986) Controlled trials of electroconvulsive therapy. In: 'Electroconvulsive therapy: Clinical and Basic Research Issues', *Ann. N.Y. Acad. Sci.*, **462** (eds S. Malitz and H.A. Sackeim), p. 12–29.

Daniel, W.F. and Crovitz, H.F. (1983) Acute memory impairment following electroconvulsive therapy. *Acta. Psychiat. Scand.*, **67**, 1–7.

Daniel, W.F. and Crovitz, H.F. (1982) Recovery of orientation after electroconvulsive therapy. *Acta Psychiat. Scand.*, **66**, 421–8.

Dec, G.W., Stern, T.A. and Welch, C. (1985) The effects of electroconvulsive therapy on serial electrocardiograms and serum cardiac enzyme values. *J.A.M.A.*, **253**, 2525–9.

D'Elia, G. and Raotma, H. (1975) Is unilateral ECT less effective than bilateral ECT? *Brit. J. Psychiat.*, **126**, 83–9.

Fink, M. (1979) *Convulsive Therapy: Theory and Practice*. Raven Press, New York.

Fraser, R.M. and Glass, I.B. (1978) Recovery from ECT in elderly patients. *Brit. J. Psychiat.*, **133**, 524–8.

Fraser, R.M. and Glass, I.B. (1980) Unilateral and bilateral ECT in elderly patients. *Acta Psychiat. Scand.*, **62**, 13–31.

Freeman, C.P.L. and Kendell R.E. (1980) ECT: patients' experiences and attitudes. *Brit. J. Psychiat.*, **137**, 8–16.

Freeman, C.P.L., Weeks, D. and Kendell, R.E. (1980) ECT: patients who complain. *Brit. J. Psychiat.*, **137**, 17–25.

French, O. (1974) Electroshock therapy and inadequate ventilation. *Chest*, **66**, 468.

Frith, C.D., Stevens, M., Johnstone, E.C. *et al.* (1983) Effects of ECT and depression on various aspects of memory. *Brit. J. Psychiat.*, **142**, 610–17.

Gaspar, D. and Samarsingh, L.A. (1982) ECT in psychogeriatric practice: a study of risk factors, indications and outcome. *Compr. Psychiat.*, **23**, 170–75.

Gerring, J.P. and Shields, H.M. (1982) The identification and management of patients with a high risk for cardiac arrhythmias during modified ECT. *J. Clin. Psychiat.*, **43**, 140–43.

Gomez, J. (1975) Subjective side-effects of ECT. *Brit. J. Psych.*, **127**, 609–11.

Greenblatt, M., Grosser, G.H. and Wechler, H. (1964) Differential response of hospitalized patients to somatic therapy. *Am. J. Psychiat.*, **120**, 935–43.

Hughes, J., Barraclough, B.M. and Reeve, W. (1981) Are patients shocked by ECT? *J. Roy. Soc. Med.*, **74**, 283–5.

Janicak, P.G., Davis, J.M., Gibbons, R.D. *et al.* (1985) Efficacy of ECT: meta-analysis. *Am. J. Psychiat.*, **142**, 297–302.

Johnstone, E.C., Deakin, J.F.W., Lawler, P. *et al.* (1980) The Northwich Park electroconvulsive therapy trial. *Lancet*, **ii**, 1317–20.

Johnson, D.A.W. (1973) Treatment of depression in general practice. *Brit. Med. J.*, **2**, 18–20.

Karlinsky, H., and Shulman, K.I. (1984) The clinical use of electroconvulsive therapy in old age. *J. Am. Geriat. Soc.*, **32**, 183–6.

Kendell, R.E. (1981) The present status of electroconvulsive therapy. *Brit. J. Psychiat.*, **139**, 265–83.

Malcolm, K. (1989) Patients perceptions and knowledge of electroconvulsive therapy. *Bull. Roy. Coll. Phychiat.* **13**, 161.

McCleave, D.J. and Blackmore, W.B. (1975) Anaesthesia for electroconvulsive therapy. *Anaesth. Intens. Care*, **3**, 250–56.

Medical Research Council (1965) Clinical trial of the treatment of depressive illness. *Brit. Med. J.*, **1**, 881–6.

Meyers, B.S. and Mei-Tal, V. (1985–6) Empirical study on an inpatient psychogeriatric unit: biological treatment in patients with depressive illness. *Int. J. Psych. Med.*, **15**, 111–23.

Miller, A.L., Faber, R., Hatch, J. and Alexander, H. (1985) Factors affecting amnesia, seizure duration and efficacy in ECT. *Am. J. Psychiat.*, **142**, 692–6.

O'Shea, B. (1987) Electroconvulsive therapy and cognitive improvement in a very elderly depressed patient. *Brit. J. Psychiat.*, **150**, 255–7.

Peet, M. (1988) Which antidepressant? Choice of antidepressant for the elderly patient. In: *Antidepressants for the Elderly* (ed. Ghose, K.).

Peet, M. (1986) Network community mental health care in north-west Derbyshire. *Bull. Roy. Coll. Psychiat.*, **10**, 262.

Pettinati, H.M. and Nilsen, S. (1985) Missed and brief seizures during ECT: differential response between unilateral and bilateral electrode placement. *Biol. Psychiat.*, **20**, 506–14.

Post, F. (1985) Psychotherapy, electroconvulsive treatments, and long-term management of elderly depressives. *J. Aff. Dis.* (Suppl 1) 41–5.

Sackeim, H.A., Portnoy, S., Neeley, P. *et al.* (1986) Cognitive consequences of low dosage electroconvulsive therapy. In Electroconvulsive therapy: Clinical and Basic Research Issues. *Ann. N.Y. Acad. Sci.*, **462** (eds S. Malitz and H. A. Sackeim), 326–40.

Skrabanek, P. (1986) Convulsive therapy: a critical appraisal of its origins and value. *Int. Med. J.*, **79**, 157–65.

Spiker, D.G., Weiss, J.C., Dealy, R.S. *et al.* (1985) The pharmacological treatment of delusional depression. *Am. J. Psychiat.*, **142**, 430–36.

Squire, L.R. (1986) Memory functions as affected by electroconvulsive therapy. In Electroconvulsive therapy: Clinical and Basic Research Issues. *Ann. N.Y. Acad. Sci.*, **462** (eds S. Malitz and H.A. Sackeim), 307–14.

Squire, L.R., Slater, P.C. and Miller, P.L. (1981) Retrograde amnesia and bilateral electroconvulsive therapy; long-term follow-up. *Arch. Gen. Psychiat.*, **38**, 89–95.

Squire, L.R., Slater, P.G. and Chace, P.M. (1975) Retrograde amnesia: temporal gradient in very long-term memory following electroconvulsive therapy. *Science*, **187**, 77–9.

Squire, L.R. and Slater, P.C. (1978) Bilateral and unilateral ECT: effects on verbal and non-verbal memory. *Am. J. Psychiat.*, **11**, 1316–20.

Sternberg, D.E. and Jarvik, M.E. (1976) Memory functions in depression. *Arch. Gen. Psychiat.*, **33**, 219–24.

Valentine, M., Keddie, K.M.G. and Dunne, D. (1986) A comparison of techniques in electroconvulsive therapy. *Brit. J. Psychiat.*, **149**, 494.

Weeks, D., Freeman, C.P.L. and Kendell, R.E. (1980) ECT: enduring cognitive deficits? *Brit. J. Psychiat.*, **137**, 26–37.

Weiner, R.D. (1984) Does electroconvulsive therapy cause brain damage? *Behav. Brain Sci.*, **7**, 1–53.

Weiner, R.D., Rogers, H.J., Davidson, J.R.T. and Squire, L.R. (1986) Effects of stimulus parameters on cognitive side effects. In Electroconvulsive therapy: Clinical and Basic Research Issues. *Ann. N.Y. Acad. Sci.*, **462** (eds S. Malitz and H.A. Sackeim), 315.

Chapter Fifteen

Drug therapy in the management of treatment-resistant depression in elderly people

DAVID M. SHAW

CONTENTS

15.1 INTRODUCTION

As a working definition, treatment-resistant depression has been considered as a major depressive illness (DSM-III) which has failed to respond to two families of antidepressant therapy given for sufficient time and in adequate dosage (or number in the case of ECT) for that individual. The phrase 'two families of antidepressant therapy' in this context implies that, for instance, drugs presumably acting mostly via presynaptic re-uptake blockade of serotoninergic or noradrenergic neurones might be considered as one family, and monoamine oxidase inhibitors would belong to another. This is not an ideal definition because there are areas of pharmacological overlap, and it does not fit with all clinical situations. Treatment resistance is a difficult subject to research in any age group, and while there are areas of expansion in the field of the elderly, at the present time by necessity there has to be some degree of inappropriate reliance on data from younger patients. Some useful reviews on the subject have appeared recently, e.g. those of Goff and Jenike (1986) and by Borson and Raskind (1986), to which the present author is indebted.

15.2 APPARENT RESISTANCE TO ANTIDEPRESSANT TREATMENT

A number of patients presenting with apparent treatment resistance prove not to fulfil the criteria in that they have not received or taken two adequate courses of therapy matched to their needs. Individuals with psychiatric illnesses are well known for their non-compliance. Looked at from the other perspective, people who are feeling miserable, desperate, despondent, physically ill and distressed and puzzled by what is happening to them are expected to take drugs which often produce unpleasant side-effects and do not give instant magical relief of symptoms. The patient may have been given the information, but may not have 'heard' or has 'forgotten' the explanation they have received that a drug may act slowly, or unevenly and incompletely, and is successful in only a percentage of individuals.

Understandably many do not take the tablets, or take them inconsistently – frequently only at times when they feel particularly unwell, or they terminate treatment early.

This situation does not constitute true 'treatment-resistance'. Non-compliance in the sense of missing doses or terminating treatment early is not all that happens. In the report entitled *Medication for the Elderly* (Royal College of Physicians, 1984) it was stated that as many as three-quarters of elderly patients make errors in their compliance to prescriptions, a quarter of which are potentially serious.

So it can be expected that a large proportion of the older group of depressed patients will fail to take drugs, others will take them chaotically and yet others perhaps will combine them with drugs prescribed elsewhere or previously for the same or other conditions (Table 15.1).

As the prescribers of these drugs, we have a responsibility to make sure that the chosen drug is the most appropriate one, that the dosage should be increased gradually to what is a suitable level for the patient

Table 15.1 Possible reasons for poor compliance

General
Poor memory worsened by cognitive disturbances, agitation, and loss of drive associated with depression
Selective attention/inattention, e.g. preoccupation with pain of arthritis
Too complicated a regime
Inadequate, unclear labelling, failing eyesight
Poor grip and/or coordination for small bottles

Motivation/attitude
Low motivation because of side-effects
Belief in instant action of drugs
Dislike of or disbelief in efficacy drugs: experience of therapy failure
Insufficient explanation to patient or relatives, lack of written instructions, failure of doctors and others to establish rapport
Low acceptance of drugs because of personality (e.g. the person seeing drugs as loss of autonomy) or because of depressive overvalued ideas (self blaming/ punishing, persecutory, catastrophic, nihilistic, etc.)

Misunderstandings/errors
Cessation therapy at first sign of recovery
Using hoarded drugs, drug 'swapping' or sharing
Failure of patient/relative to understand nature of depressive illness and the need for continuous prolonged therapy

Support/checking
Inadequate support services
Failure to follow up lack of attendance
Lack of checks on following the regime and tablet counts

and that, if no response is forthcoming in six to eight weeks, some other treatment will be given.

As doctors we may succumb to therapeutic nihilism with the depressed elderly – to accept that depression is the natural course of events in the old – their expected lot, something to be comprehended. With this attitude, and realistic anxiety about the complications and difficulties of giving antidepressant drugs to people in this age band, patients can be left untreated, or maintained long-term on ineffective regimes.

Prescribing for the old is not an easy task. If the pharmacokinetics of drugs are variable in the young, this is nothing compared with the range seen in the old. Some old people seem to tolerate drugs in a way comparable to that seen in young adults, while the majority have a wide spectrum of decreasing tolerance, so that what is an inadequate level of therapy to one is a toxic insult to another. Again, careful selection of drug and dosage is of particular relevance to treatment resistance or apparent resistance in the aged.

One of our tasks may be to try to ensure maximum compliance, and the following measures may be helpful in achieving this:

1. Simplifying drug programmes and using once a day treatments (this may not be possible in this group).
2. Providing written instructions about the times to take drugs, the nature and the timing of a response if it occurs, anticipated side-effects, etc.
3. Packaging drugs by dose. Calendar packs are a way of dispensing drugs for the elderly but have limited applicability because most patients require a more flexible scheme. Some elderly individuals can use 'Dosett boxes' which can be loaded with a week's supply of drugs separated into its various doses. The filling of these boxes is time-consuming but of value to those patients who can manage them.
4. Reducing or discounting other drugs whenever possible.
5. Trying to get other drug supplies returned or destroyed.
6. Where necessary, invoking the aid of relatives, community nurses, etc.
7. Careful monitoring of patient's visits and arranging contact with those who fail to keep follow-up appointments.
8. Having drug containers brought back to the clinic/out-patients, etc. for tablet counts.
9. Having frequent follow-up for support, to check the way the patient is managing the regime and to observe side-effects (especially central and cardiovascular).
10. If available, assaying blood levels (indeed some, such as lithium, must be assayed).
11. When possible, arranging for the patient to attend a group or have brief psychotherapy. This has been shown to markedly reduce drop-out (DiMascio *et al.*, 1979) and the education and information given will also enhance compliance considerably (Blackwell, 1982).

15.3 FACTORS CONTRIBUTING TO TREATMENT RESISTANCE

There are factors contributing to treatment resistance of which we are ignorant, others are suspect and seem to occur in individuals but are difficult to substantiate statistically in groups, which anyway are particularly heterogenous in the elderly. Some however, like phsyical illness, are common, but there is sometimes uncertainty as to which is primary – the affective illness or the physical diseases.

As compared with younger patients, prognosis for depression is poor in the elderly (Post, 1962, 1972; Murphy, 1983) although some of this poor outlook is because of the tendency to relapse which is discussed in Chapter 13.

Unlike younger individuals, the more severely depressed are the ones least likely to recover and severe life events and problems of physical health go with a poor outcome (Murphy, 1983). Untreated depression and decreased life expectancy are associated (e.g. Sendbuehler and Goldstein, 1977; Resnick and Cantor, 1967; Rabins, Harvis and Koven, 1985; Kukull *et al.*, 1986). The concurrence of a relationship between cardiovascular disease and depression (Kay and Bergman, 1966; Dreyfuss, Dashberg and Assall, 1969) is unclear as regards cause and effect, but appears to be independent of the introduction of antidepressant drugs in that it was observed before their time (Fuller, 1935; Malzburg, 1937).

Table 15.2 Causes of depression

Physical causes of depression
    Parkinson's disease
    Multiple sclerosis
    Dementia
    CNS tumours
    Trauma to CNS
    Epilepsy
    Stroke

Metabolic/endocrine
    Hyperthyroidism, hypothyroidism
    Cushings and Addison's disease
    Hypoglycaemia
    Hyperkalcaemia
    Hypokalaemia
    Porphyria

Nutritional
    Iron
    B_{12}
    Folate

Other
    Cardiovascular disease?
    Obstructive airway disease?
    Malignancy
    Viral infections

Table 15.3 Drugs reported as causing depression

Alcohol
Amantadine
Antihypertensive drugs (clonidine, guanethidine, methyldopa, pindolol,
                              propanolol, reserpine)
Chloroquine
Cimetidine
Corticosteroids
Cytotoxic agents
Digoxin
Flufluramine (rebound)
Immunosuppressive drugs
Indomethacin
Minor tranquillizers (rebound)
Phenobarbitone
Phenytonin
Theophylline

Endocrine disorders and other causes of treatment resistance have been studied in recent years mostly in relationship to rapidly cycling bipolar illness (Cowdry *et al.*, 1983; Roy-Byrne *et al.*, 1984) rather than in 'fixed' treatment-resistant episodes of illness, but thyroid abnormalities and other physical contributors to depression may need to be investigated (Gerner, 1984; Goff and Jenike, 1986) (Table 15.2). Similarly, some drugs have been reported to provoke depression (King, 1986; Goff and Jenike, 1986; Gerner, 1984) (Table 15.3).

Depression-provoking factors and therefore those leading some to treatment resistance tend to be multiple in the aged and may include poor physical health, new physical illness, losses and other traumatic life events, diminishments, and also malnutrition, marginal endocrine dysfunction, depressogenic drugs, and damage to, disease of, or deterioration in the central nervous system.

In summary, the clinician is faced with the dilemma that an elderly treatment-resistant patient, particularly if severely ill, is likely to have poor prognosis, with an associated enhanced mortality. There may be multiple contributing factors and the person to be treated may have low tolerance to and acceptance of drugs (Table 15.4).

Suggested principles behind the treatment programme include:

1. Treatment is preceded by detailed reassessment.
2. Treatment resistance requires an active flexible approach.
3. Polypharmacy may be a necessary evil but the risk of using potentiating or adjuvant agents as well as the main drug themselves must

Table 15.4   Some putative causes of treatment resistance

Psychosocial stress – traumatic life events including bereavement, other losses and diminishments
Ageing itself – does this predispose to treatment resistance?
Physical disabilities, handicaps
Physical illnesses especially 'new' superadded ones
Endocrine dysfunction
Malnutrition
Depression-inducing drugs
Difficulty in achieving therapeutic drug levels in patients with low tolerance
Damage to central nervous system
Failure to use flexible drug regimes tailored to patients' metabolism

be weighed against the consequences of the patient failing to recover.
4. Attention must be paid to compliance.

15.4 ASSESSMENT AND MANAGEMENT

Any elderly patient provisionally considered as being 'treatment-resistant' needs complete reassessment of diagnosis, contributory factors and previous drug history. The individual is considered as a new patient, the history is retaken together with a reappraisal of the mental state, a repeat physical examination and laboratory tests. Any further physical investigations indicated can be pursued.

The phenomenology may seem blurred. With all chronically or subacutely depressed patients, symptoms become difficult to evaluate, but it is usually possible to discern the characteristics of major depressive illness in what by now will be a very distressed person. The key features of affective illness may be but small signals amongst a growing background, but it is vital to confirm or refute the diagnosis. If it is confirmed, then its treatment is amongst the priorities of management.

Assuming it is confirmed, the team can seek out ways of treating whatever areas are amendable to action. This is a point at which colleagues may be requested to consider altering their treatments of physical disease or perhaps to discontinue any drug suspected of potentiating the depressed state.

15.5 CHOICE OF ANTIDEPRESSANTS

This topic has been dealt with in Chapters 9 and 13, and by various authors elsewhere (Gerner, 1985). A few extra points are necessary to explain aspects of the flow diagrams (pp. 263–5).

259

15.5.1 Monoamine oxidase inhibitors and the elderly treatment-resistant patient

One of the views being discussed currently is that the efficacy of tricyclic antidepressants may tend to decline with age, and that of the monoamine oxidase inhibitors (MAOI) increases (Robinson, 1979). There have been a number of studies of MAOI in the elderly and elderly resistant groups using the range of drugs available (Jenike, 1984; Georgotas *et al.*, 1983; McGrath *et al.*, 1984; Lazarus *et al.*, 1986; Ashford and Ford, 1979) with favourable results not only in these patients but in individuals with dementia (Jenike, 1985, 1986).

Obviously with MAOIs, either the person concerned or someone in the environment must be able to take the dietary precautions and be aware of the dangers of drug interactions.

15.5.2 Mianserin

It may be a surprise to some that mianserin has been included in the flow diagrams in view of the reports on the proportion of individuals developing blood dyscrasias. Some people may prefer trazodone (Cole *et al.*, 1981) and the format suggested may or may not become obsolete when the selective 5–HT re-uptake blockers have been in wide use for a few years.

The reasons for keeping it in the armamentarium is the balance of risks, the fact that mianserin has a wide therapeutic margin, and in other respects is one of the safer drugs to use in patients with doubtful or erratic compliance. The rate of fatal adverse reactions is two to three per million prescriptions for mianserin compared with one to two for imipramine and nortriptyline, less than one for amitriptyline, dothiepin, doxepin, protriptyline and trimipramine, and five for clomipramine (CSM Update, 1985).

15.5.3 Lithium

Lithium and the growing literature on its use, and mode of employment in the elderly as a prophylactic agent is discussed in Chapter 7. It has been introduced here only in so far as it has a possible role as an adjuvant or potentiating agent for antidepressant therapy (Fig. 15.3).

15.5.4 Matching and adjustment of dosage

With most antidepressant drugs and with the 'elderly old' matching of dosage involves caution and a gradual progressive increment in amounts given. These can be increased further if no clinical benefit is obtained, sometimes going near to the point of tolerance.

For the young old, and those who have remained relatively robust biochemically and physiologically, some drugs can be pushed gradually to an endpoint determined by the characteristics of that drug. In other words, side-effects can be used to determine what may be the optimum level for that individual. This stance is taken because for most tricyclic drugs, plasma levels have not proved to be outstandingly useful in predicting response, and assays of platelet MAO inhibition as a means of determining how much MAOI to give (Georgotas *et al.*, 1983) will not be available in most centres.

The following means, to be introduced mostly in the robust elderly, are proposed tentatively, and with awareness of the risks which will be run unless the process is carefully monitored.

There are two limiting factors to the amount of phenelzine which can be given – postural hypotension and a sedative/anxiolytic activity. The predominance of one over the other differs from patient to patient. Assuming that the dose is increased gradually (and its formulation of 15 mg tablets is too large to allow fine adjustments) then the endpoint is either the presence of slight sedation which does not habituate after five or six days at that dosage level, or the beginnings of early postural/ effort hypotension, the effects of which can still be controlled by being slow about changes in posture, and careful about making muscular efforts.

The dose of mianserin can be monitored upwards using its sedative action in a way similar to those employed with phenelzine. The dosage of tranylcypromine, clomipramine* and amitriptyline may be assessed as for the effect of phenelzine in its production of orthostatic hypotension.

For the majority of other antidepressant drugs currently available these means of monitoring therapy are not available. For these drugs and for the less robust elderly we are left with the policy of cautious increments, and observing clinical effects while being watchful for side-effects.

15.6 ADJUVANTS OR POTENTIATING AGENTS

By potentiating agent or adjuvant is meant those drugs which either enhance the activity of an antidepressant drug synergetically, or alternatively have some additive effect. Which of these two is operating with a particular additional treatment is irrelevant here.

The main agents reported to have this type of activity are:

1. Lithium (Jefferson and Ayd, 1983; deMontigny *et al.*, 1983; Heninger,

* Not available in USA.

Charney and Sternberg, 1983; Nelson and Mazure, 1986; Himmelhoch *et al.*, 1972; deMontigny *et al.*, 1983, 1985; Price, Charney and Heninger, 1985; Kushnir, 1986);
2. Triodothyronine (Goodwin *et al.*, 1982); and
3. Tryptophan (Baldessarini, 1984; Walinder, Carlsson and Persson, 1981; Coppen, Shaw and Farrell, 1963; Pare, 1963; Glassman and Platman, 1969; Walinder *et al.*, 1976).

Of these three, there has been most controversy about the usefulness of tryptophan. Tryptophan is non-toxic in the doses recommended and, in the author's opinion, its place cannot be evaluated further in this role until trials have been done in which it has been given in doses below those likely to induce hepatic tryptophan pyrrolase. For this reason it has been included in the flow diagrams.

Other putative adjuvants for tricyclic antidepressants are reserpine (Hopkinson and Kenny, 1975) and methylphenidate and similar drugs (Katon and Raskind, 1980; Klein *et al.*, 1980; Kaufman, Murray and Cassem, 1982; Drimmer, Gitlin and Guirtsman, 1983).

15.7 FLOW CHARTS

These are illustrated in Figs. 1–3.

It has been assumed that treatment periods are in the 6–8 week region allowing within that some time for achieving the final dose level. 'Exit points' have not been given – in other words, it has been taken for granted that when a treatment has been successful it will be continued, and that for many, maintenance therapy (Cook *et al.*, 1986) or prophylactic therapy will be started. Only failure of therapy is followed through in the flow charts.

It is appreciated that doctors have their preferences and that no flow chart can cover even a fraction of the contingencies of everyday clinical practice.

REFERENCES

Ashford, J.W. and Ford, V.C. (1979) Use of MAO inhibitors in elderly patients. *Am. J. Psychiat.*, **136**, 1466–7.

Avery, D. and Winokur, G. (1976) Mortality in depressed patients treated with electroconvulsive therapy and antidepressants. *Arch. Gen. Psychiat.*, **33**, 1029–37.

Baldessarini, R.T.J. (1984) Treatment of depression by altering monoamine metabolism: precursors and metabolic inhibitors. *Psychopharmacol. Bull.*, **20**, 224–39.

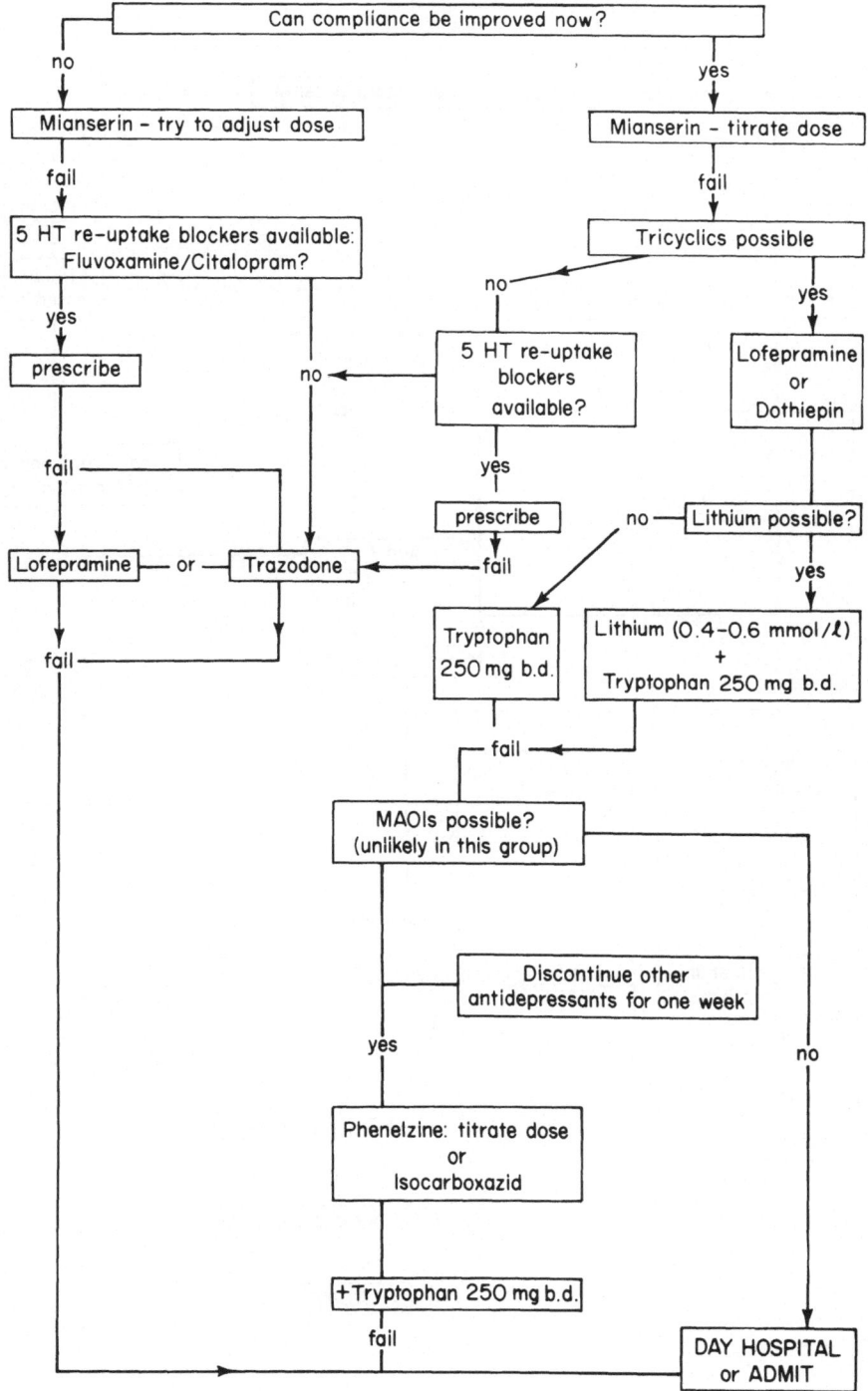

Fig. 15.1 Mild/moderate depression: poor compliance/cooperation: out-patient.

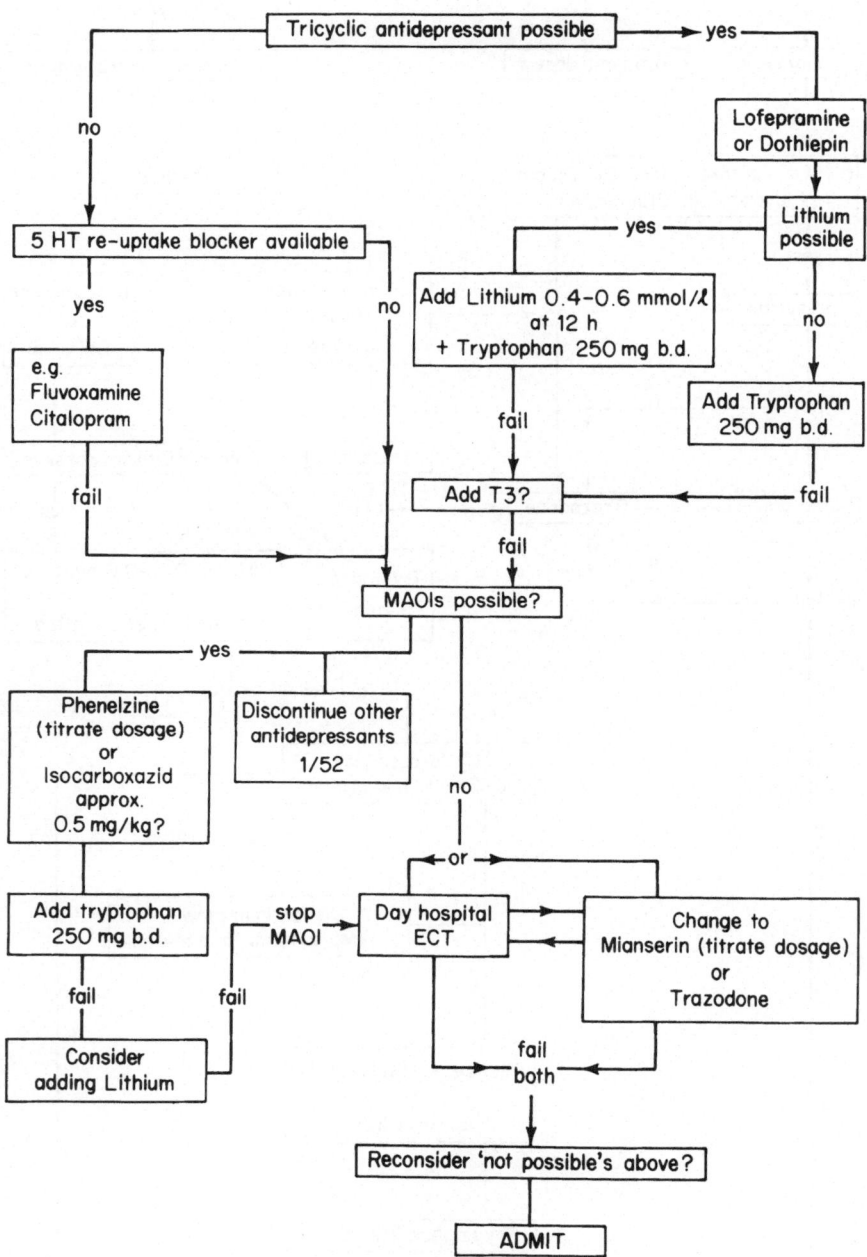

Fig. 15.2 Moderately ill: good compliance: out-patient.

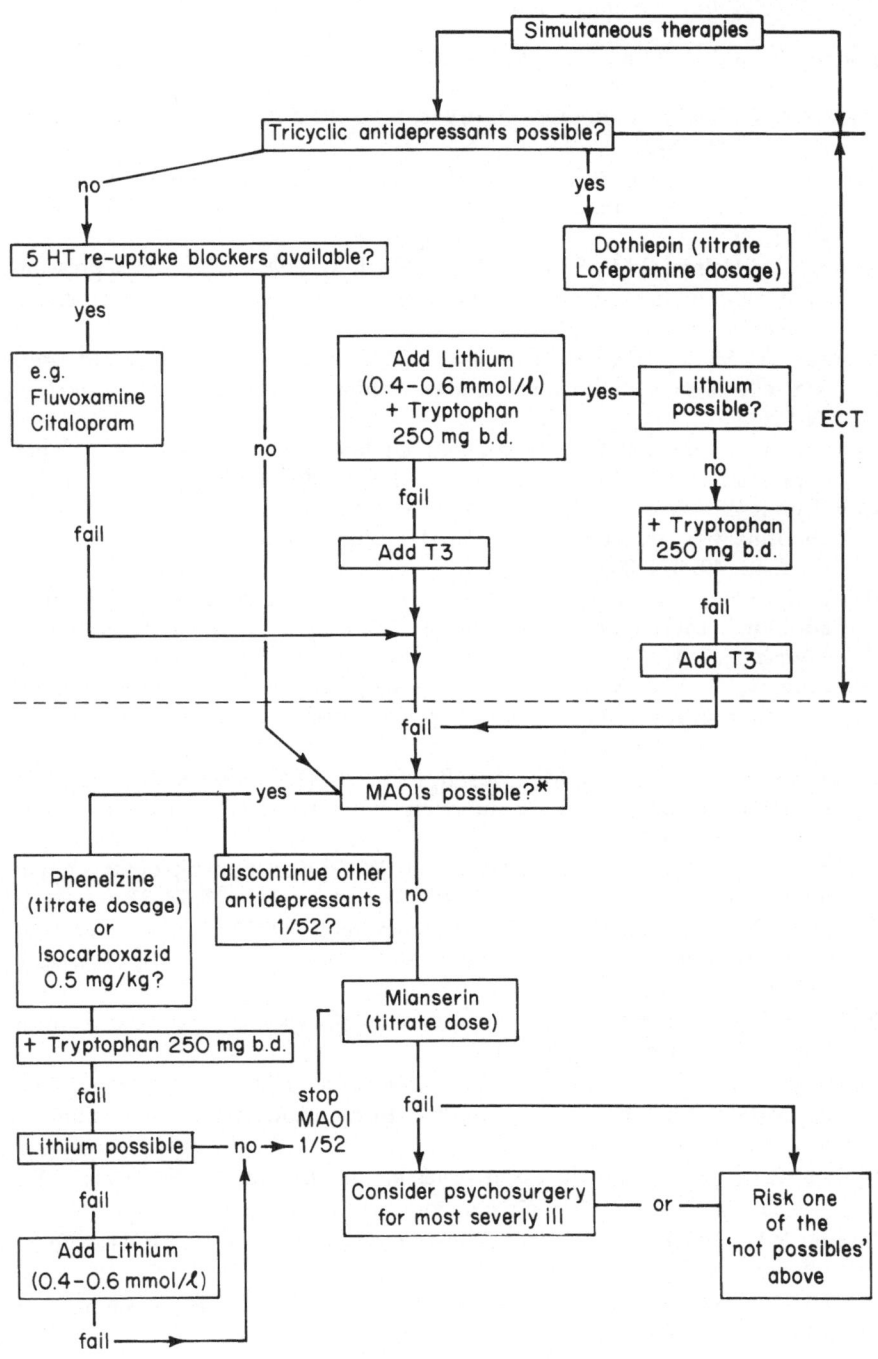

* There are very few contraindications to MAOIs.

Fig. 15.3 Severely depressed in-patients.

Borson, S. and Raskind, M. (1986) Antidepressant-resistant depression in the elderly. *J. Am. Geriatr. Soc.*, **34**, 245–7.

Blackwell, B. (1982) Antidepressant drugs. Side-effects and compliance. *J. Clin. Psychiat.* **43**, 14–21.

Cole, J.O., Schatzberg, A.F., Sniffin, C. *et al.* (1981) Trazodone in treatment-resistant depression: an open study. *J. Clin. Psychopharmacol.*, **1** (Suppl. 49S–54S).

Cook, B.L., Helms, P.M., Smith, R.E. and Tsai, M. (1986) Unipolar depression in the elderly. Reoccurrence on discontinuation of tricyclic antidepressants. *J. Affective Disord.*, **10**, 91–4.

Coppen, A., Shaw, D.M., and Farrell, J.P. (1963) Potentiation of the antidepressive effects of a monoamine oxidase inhibitor by tryptophan. *Lancet*, **i**, 79–81.

Committee for the Safety of Medicines Update: Adverse reactions to antidepressants (1985) (Anonymous). *Br. Med. J.*, **291**, 1636.

Cowdry, R.W., Wehr, T.A., Zis, A.P. and Goodwin, F.K. (1983) Thyroid abnormalities associated with rapid cycling bipolar illness. *Arch. Gen. Psychiat.*, **40**, 414–20.

deMontigny, C., Cournoyer, G., Morissette, R. *et al.* (1983) Lithium carbonate addition in tricyclic antidepressant-resistant unipolar depression. *Arch. Gen. Psychiat.*, **40**, 1327–34.

deMontigny, C., Elie, R. and Caille, G. (1985) Rapid response to the addition of lithium in Iprindole-resistant unipolar depression: a pilot study. *Am. J. Psychiat.*, **142**, 220–23.

DiMascio, A., Weissman, M.M., Pousoff, B.A. *et al.* (1979) Differential symptom reduction by drugs and psychotherapy in acute depression. *Arch. Gen. Psychiat.*, **36**, 1450–56.

Dreyfuss, F., Dashberg, H. and Assall, M.I. (1969) The relationship of myocardial infarction to depressive illness. *Psychother. Psychosom.*, **17**, 73–81.

Drimmer, E.J., Gitlin, M.J. and Guirtsman, H.E. (1983) Desipramine and methylphenidate combination treatment for depression. *Am. J. Psychiat.*, **140**, 241–2.

Fuller, R.G. (1935) What happens to mental patients after discharge from hospital? *Psychiat. Q.*, **9**, 95–104.

Georgotas, A., Friedman, E., McCarthy, M. *et al.* (1983) Resistant geriatric depressions and therapeutic response to monoamine oxidase inhibitors. *Biol. Psychiat.*, **18**, 195–205.

Gerner, R.H. (1984) Antidepressant selection in the elderly. *Psychosom.*, **25**, 528–35.

Gerner, R.H. (1985) Present status of drug therapy of depression in late life. *J. Affective Disord.* (Suppl. 1) S23–S31.

Glassman, A.H. and Platman, S.R. (1969) Potentiation of a monoamine oxidase inhibitor by tryptophan. *J. Psychiat. Res.*, **7**, 83–8.

Goff, D.C. and Jenike, M.A. (1986) Treatment-resistant depression in the elderly. *J. Am. Geriat. Soc.*, **34**, 63–70.

Goodwin, F.K., Prange, A.J., Post, R.M. *et al.* (1982) Potentiation of antidepressant effects by 1–triiodothyronine in tricyclic non-responders. *Am. J. Psychiat.*, **139**, 34–8.

Heoninger, G.R., Charney, D.S. and Sternberg, D.E. (1983) Lithium carbonate augmentation of antidepressant treatment. *Arch. Gen. Psychiat.*, **40**, 1335–42.

Himmelhoch, J.M., Detre, T., Kupfer, J.D. *et al.* (1972) Treatment of previously intractible depressions with tranylcypromine and lithium. *J. Nerv. Ment. Dis.*, **155**, 216–20.

Hopkinson, G. and Kenny, F. (1975) Treatment with reserpine of patients resistant to tricyclic antidepressants. *Psychiat. Clin.*, **8**, 109–14.

Jefferson, J.W. and Ayd, F.J. (1983) Combining lithium and antidepressants. *J. Clin. Psychopharmacol.*, **3**, 303–7.

Jenike, M.A. (1984) The use of monoamine oxidase inhibitors in elderly depressed patients. *J. Am. Geriatr. Soc.*, **32**, 571–5.

Jenike, J.A. (1985) MAO inhibitors as treatment for depressed patients with primary degenerative dementia (Alzheimer's Disease). *Am. J. Psychiat.*, **142**, 763–4.

Jenike, M.A. (1986) Use of MAOIs for demented depressed patients. *Am. J. Psychiat.*, **143**, 254–5.

Katon, W. and Raskind, M. (1980) Treatment of depression in the medically ill elderly with methylphenidate. *Am. J. Psychiat.*, **137**, 963–5.

Kaufmann, M.W., Murray, G.B. and Cassem, N.H. (1982) Use of psycho-stimulants in medically ill patients in *Psychosomatics.*, **23**, 817–19.

Kay, D.W.K. and Bergman, K. (1966) Physical disability and mental health in old age. *J. Psychosom. Res.*, **10**, 3–12.

King, D.J. (1986) Drug-induced psychiatric syndromes. *Prescriber's Journal*, **26**, 50–58.

Klein, D.E., Gittelman, R., Quitkin, F. and Rifkin, A. (1980) Clinical management of affective disorders. In: *Diagnosis and Drug Treatment of Psychiatric Disorders – Adults and Children*, 2nd ed, Williams and Wilkins, Baltimore, pp. 409–48.

Kukull, W.A., Koepsell, T.S., Inui, T.S. *et al.* (1986) Depression and physical illness among elderly medical clinic patients. *J. Affective Disord.*, **10**, 153–62.

Kushnir, S.L. (1986) Lithium-antidepressant combinations in the treatment of depressed, phsically ill geriatric patients. *Am. J. Psychiat.*, **143**, 378–9.

Lazarus, L.W., Groves, L. Gierl, B. *et al.* (1986) Efficacy of phenelzine in geriatric depression. *Biol. Psychiat.*, **21**, 699–701.

McGrath, P.J., Quitkin, F.M., Harrison, W. *et al.* (1984) Treatment of melan-cholia with tranylcypromine. *Am. J. Psychiat.*, **141**, 288–9.

Malzburg, B. (1937) Mortality among patients with involutional melancholia. *Am. J. Psychiat.*, **93**, 1231–38.

Murphy, E. (1983) The prognosis of depression in old age. *Br. J. Psychiat.*, **142**, 111–19.

Nelson, J.C. and Mazure, C.M. (1986) Lithium augmentation in psychotic depression refractory to combined drug treatment. *Am. J. Psychiat.*, **143**, 363–6.

Pare, C.M.B. (1963) Potentiation of a monoamine oxidase inhibitor by trypto-phan. *Lancet*, **ii**, 527–8.

Post, F. (1962) *The Significance of Affective Symptoms in Old Age*, Oxford University Press, London.

Post, F. (1972) The management and nature of depressive illness in late life – a follow-through study. *Br. J. Psychiat.*, **121**, 393–404.

Price, L.H., Charney, D.S. and Heninger, G.R. (1985) Efficacy of lithium-tranylcypromine treatment in refractory depression. *Am. J. Psychiat.*, **142**, 619–23.

Rabins, P.V., Harvis, K. and Koven, S. (1985) High fatality rates of late-life depression associated with cardiovascular disease. *J. Affective Disord.*, **9**, 165–7.

Resnick, H. and Cantor, J. (1967) Gerifacts. *Geriatrics*, **22**(12), 68.

Robinson, D.S. (1979) Age-related factors affecting antidepressant drug metabolism and clinical response. In: *Geriatric Psychopharmacol.* (ed. K. Nandy) Elsevier/North-Holland, New York, 17–29.

Roy-Byrne, P.P., Joffe, R.T., Uhde, T.W. and Post, R.M. (1984) Approaches to the elevation and treatment of rapidly cycling affective illness. *Br. J. Psychiat.*, **145**, 543–550.

Royal College of Physicians (1984) Report: Medication for the elderly. *J. R. Coll. Physicians*, **18** (1), 7–17.

Sendbuehler, J.M. and Goldstein, S. (1977) Attempted suicide among the aged. *J. Am. Geriatr. Soc.*, **25**, 245–8.

Walinder, J., Carlsson, A. and Persson, R. (1981) 5–HT re-uptake inhibitors plus tryptophan in endogenous depression. *Acta. Psychiat. Scand.*, **63** (Suppl. 290), 179–90.

Walinder, J., Skott, A., Carlsson, A. *et al.* (1976) Potentiation of the antidepressant action of clomipramine by tryptophan. *Arch. Gen. Psychiat.*, **33**, 1384–9.

Chapter Sixteen

Long-term antidepressant treatment in old age

I.C.A. MOYES

CONTENTS

16.1 INTRODUCTION

Management of depressive illness in old age presents a challenge to the clinician. Depression in the elderly tends to be different in presentation and form from that usually found in younger people. In contrast to younger patients, diagnostic groups tend to be less clear-cut and many patients may go undiagnozed and untreated either because their presentation is at first sight not characteristic of the condition or because it is masked by physical illness. Depression in this group may also be characterized by a state of apathy in which the person appears to lack drive and to be uninterested in his or her normal activities. Unfortunately, this may be accepted by some observers as an unavoidable part of an ageing process and this behaviour has sometimes been interpreted as a form of 'disengagement' rather than as a symptom of depression. This can result in specific treatment for depressive illness being withheld.

16.2 PRESENTATION AND PROGNOSIS OF DEPRESSION

16.2.1 Epidemiological studies

Post in 1972 assessed 92 consecutively admitted depressed patients who were aged over 65. These patients were followed up for three years after discharge from in-patient treatment. When seen initially, 37% were severely ill with retardation, agitation, and perplexity, 24% were less severely depressed but still showed delusions of guilt or high levels of self-reproach together with paranoid ideas. Thirty-nine per cent could be considered to be neurotic depressives where the illness was accompanied by anxiety with little overt sadness. In spite of these striking differences in symptomatology no correlation could be found with aetiology, response to treatment or long-term outcome. The other surprising finding was that only a third of the patients maintained a consistent recovery. Seventeen percent remained markedly ill and the rest had either frequent relapses or sank into a kind of chronic invalidism with moodiness and anxiety.

A number of investigators, including Kay (1959), Hopkinson (1964) and Post (1972) have shown that late-onset depressives have significantly less family history of affective disorder. The suggestion was made that older people had undergone longer periods of stress than younger ones and that this had eventually taken its toll. In 1982 Murphy reported a study which had looked more closely at life events in a group of depressed elderly patients. Essentially the same results were found as in Post's work. However, she paid particular attention to the importance of adverse emotional experiences and the factors associated with a good outcome. Surprisingly there was little evidence to support the widely held view that decreasing isolation and encouraging attendance at day centres, together with other appropriate psychotherapeutic measures were beneficial in refractory cases. Even close relationships were not markedly protective against depression.

16.2.2 Relationship with organic brain disorders

The possibility that failure to improve in late-onset depressive illness might be related to minor degrees of brain damage is an interesting one. Post investigated this between 1962 and 1972 and reported that although a proportion of patients went on to develop either multi-infarct or senile dementia of Alzheimer type (SDAT), this did not exceed the number which might be expected in the age-matched general population.

In 1980 Jacoby and Levy published a clinical, psychometric, and computer assisted tomographic (CAT) scan investigation of three groups of elderly subjects. There were 50 normals, 40 patients with senile dementia, and 41 suffering from affective disorder. In both the normal group and those suffering from affective disorder ventricular size increased with age. The prevalence of cerebrovascular disease was 12% in the patient group. A subgroup of patients emerged who showed evidence of enlarged ventricles and whose first depression began later in life. At the time of the study they were in the higher age range and showed more endogenous features. The authors felt that it was therefore likely that organic factors had contributed to the depression. The brain density obtained from computerized tomographic scans of 37 elderly depressed patients was compared with that of 23 patients suffering from senile dementia and 36 healthy controls. As a group the depressed patients resembled the dements more than the controls. In the depressed group ventricular dilation, which in the earlier work had been shown to be correlated with increased mortality, was also associated with lower brain density.

In a similar study reported in 1985 in Baltimore, Rabins showed that when elderly patients with recurrent depressive illness were compared with normals and dements there was a consistent change in ventricular brain ratio (VBR) from normals through depressed subjects to those with dementia. Those who were depressed, in whom there was objective evidence of slight cognitive impairment, occupied an intermediate position between those with depression and those with dementia.

Robinson in 1984 reported on a series of patients who had suffered from strokes in whom depressive symptomatology was common. He correlated this with the location and size of the lesion as seen on a computerized tomographic scan. In general left-sided anterior lesions were the most highly correlated with depression. He also found that these patients responded well to antidepressant medication and he considered that early intervention with amitriptyline was of value.

This group of studies lends support to the idea that recurrent depressive illness may well represent the unmasking of a subtle brain problem in some cases while in others it may accompany major physical illness. The long-established view that patients with endogenous features respond best to antidepressant medication and electroconvulsive therapy (ECT) has been linked to the idea that such episodes of depression may be associated with brain neurotransmitter changes. Where there is organic brain damage, from whatever cause, it seems reasonable to postulate that there could be associated neurotransmitter changes. As the brain may never recover full normal function the likelihood of long-term medication being required is therefore greater.

16.3 NEED FOR LONG-TERM THERAPY

The finding that amelioration of environmental and social conditions alone may not be effective reinforces the need for specific investigations of the most effective therapy in old age. Indeed, Post in his chapter on functional psychoses in *Studies in Geriatric Psychiatry*, published in 1978, states 'the management of elderly patients with affective disorders should be planned on the assumption that one will have to work with the patient and his family not just during the present attack but for many years to come'. He suggested that the first therapeutic approach in the psychotic depressive should continue to be ECT but that many patients benefited from antidepressants. He also noted that in a three year follow-up study of depressed elderly patients it had been possible to discontinue treatment permanently in only 18%. In 75% relapse occurred when dosages were lowered after three months or when supervision had been discontinued. Thirty-eight percent of cases had needed tricyclics intermittently or continuously. Others had been given lithium or had had a further course of ECT.

In view of this it is surprising that relatively little work appears to have been done on investigating the effect of long-term treatment in old age nor even upon establishing for how long patients identified by General Practitioners as suffering from depression are treated. However, in 1985 about eight million prescriptions were written in Great Britain for antidepressants and of these 1.6 million were for 55 to 64 year olds and 2.4 million for those aged over 65.

Most studies have been carried out using younger age groups. In 1968 Pare pointed out that it was becoming increasingly common for antide-pressant drugs to be given concomitantly with ECT and afterwards continued in the hope of preventing relapse, although at that time there were only two reports on long-term treatment.

16.4 TRIALS OF LONG-TERM THERAPY

Seager and Bird (1962) selected a series of 43 depressed patients who were suitable for ECT. They were allocated either to imipramine 50 mg three times daily or placebo. After a week on this regime they were given a course of ECT until adequate clinical response had been obtained. Seven days later patients were discharged on their earlier regime. They were seen at monthly intervals for six months. Of the 28 patients who completed the follow-up period, relapse was recorded in two of the 12 patients receiving imipramine but in 11 of the 16 on placebo. Imlah, Ryan and Harrington (1965) described a study in which the treatment of depression by ECT was combined with imipramine, phenelzine or placebo, administered on a random allocation basis. At the time of discharge those on placebo were given no medication while those on drugs continued. Assessment of progress, however, was not made without knowledge of the regime. In this study also the relapse rate amongst those on medication was significantly less than those on placebo.

Kay, Fahy and Garside (1970) reported a study in which depressed patients were given ECT and either diazepam or amitriptyline. After recovery the patients continued on the same regime for seven months. They were assessed at one month, four months and seven months. Although a number of patients were lost to follow-up, again the relapse rate was least on amitriptyline.

Mindham, Howland and Shepherd (1973) reported on a study designed to assess whether a six month course of continuation therapy would prevent a recurrence of symptoms in patients successfully treated for a depressive episode with either imipramine or amitriptyline. Mindham pointed out that the earlier studies had not, strictly speaking, been studies of continuation therapy as the original response may have been due to the ECT rather than the drug treatment. The trial by Mindham and his co-workers was therefore confined to patients whose depressive episodes had shown good improvement on tricyclic anti-depressant medication. In addition, the investigation attempted to answer the question as to whether there is any advantage, after the episode has settled, in continuation of therapy with the same drug at a lower dosage.

Ninety-two patients entered the trial and of those 22% relapsed compared with 50% of those receiving placebo. Patients with residual symptoms on entry to the trial responded better to continuation therapy than those who appeared to have made a complete recovery. The dose of medication given during the continuation phase was lower than the initial one. An interesting feature of this trial was the finding that the patients on amitriptyline showed a relapse rate of 24% compared with 19% on imipramine.

16.5 PROBLEMS OF LONG-TERM THERAPY

16.5.1 Compliance

One of the problems of long-term therapy is that of compliance. Many patients treated for an extended period are likely after the first few weeks to be returned to the care of their General Practitioner even if they are being followed up by a consultant psychiatrist at intervals. A study by Johnson (1973) showed that the drop-out rate from a group of 73 depressed patients treated in General Practice increased from 16% at the end of the first week to 68% at the end of one month. The poor compliance was not due primarily to side-effects as this accounted for only 7% of the dropouts. Twenty-one percent were doubtful about the potential benefit of any sort of medication.

This highlights a problem raised by Blackwell in 1982. He discussed the findings that, in a 16-week study comparing antidepressant treatment with psychotherapy alone, combined treatment or medication only on demand, as many as 17% refused to enter when they realized they might have medication only. Fifty percent of those receiving antidepressants only dropped out as compared with 29% given combined treatment. Blackwell suggests that treatment should be related to patients' expectations and take account of their belief in the importance of communication between doctor and patient in therapy and of fears about possible dangers in medication. Anxiety about side-effects may be more likely when patients are told to take the treatment for an extended period.

A more recent double-blind study using placebo (unpublished) carried out in 1984/85 by a group of psychiatrists including the author, involved a 13-week observation period of a group of 100 patients aged over 65. Only 30% completed. The completers were almost equally divided amongst those taking a lower drug dose, a higher drug dose and placebo. The reasons for poor compliance are clearly complex and there appears to be little work concerned specifically with the expectations of elderly patients in respect of medication or other forms of therapy for depression. Most clinicians working in this field give anecdotal reports of patients who are resistant to the idea of taking medication. Some fear that they will become dependent and be unable to give it up, while some think it may interact badly with other treatment they are having. In addition some elderly people appear pessimistic in general about the likelihood of ever being fully well in old age and cannot see any point in taking an antidepressant. Thus, any extended course of treatment seems likely to be unsuccessful unless reassurance and encouragement to continue are given. This is an area which requires further investigation.

16.5.2 Unwanted effects

The issue of unwanted effects is also of interest in this group. It is possible that long-term treatment might result in accumulation of the drug and especially in older people, whose metabolism may be less rapid, produce dangerously high plasma levels of a drug or its metabolites.

Kragh-Sorensen and his co-workers in 1974 posed the question whether long-term treatment with nortriptyline would result in accumulation. The study showed that this did not occur. However only three of the twenty-two patients taking part were over 65 years of age. In the study by Coppen and his colleagues in 1978, thirty-two patients taking 150 mg of amitriptyline daily were reported upon. Their ages ranged from 33 to 70 years. A small but progressive rise in the mean plasma concentrations of parent drug and its metabolite nortriptyline was observed.

A small study was carried out in East Yorkshire by the authoress in 1982 to investigate whether long-term treatment produced side-effects or resulted in abnormal plasma levels of the drug.

The first enquiry compared (without the investigators' knowledge of the medication regime) a group of 34 patients whose General Practitioner had continued them on the same prescription they had been given at an out-patient clinic. Patients had been receiving either 30 mg daily of nortriptyline and 1.5 mg of fluphenazine as 'Motipress', clomipramine 75 mg daily or amitriptyline 75 mg daily (Table 16.1). Side-effects were measured on a 23-point questionnaire and dyskinetic movements on the Abnormal Involuntary Movements Scale (AIMS). The possibility of dyskinesia was considered because fluphenazine is a neuroleptic drug although here given at very low dosage. The age range was from 35 to 83 years.

Table 16.1 Details of patients studied

Drug	Patient no.	Daily dose	Weeks on drug Mean ± SD	Range
Motipress	18		30 ± 8	22–48
Fluphenazine		1.5 mg		
Nortriptylene		30 mg		
Clomipramine	6	75 mg	38 ± 32	21–104
Amitriptyline	10	75 mg	26 ± 4	19–34

Side-effects were negligible with all three types of medicine as shown in Table 16.2. No patient achieved a score on AIMS of 12 or more which is regarded as indicating dyskinesia. Two female patients aged 71 and 63 years taking Motipress showed a Parkinsonian tremor of the upper limbs but this may have been associated with unusually high plasma levels (nortriptyline 234 and 80 ng/ml, fluphenazine 4.0 and 1.84 ng/ml respectively).

Table 16.2 Incidence of side-effects during long-term antidepressant therapy

Drug	Mean side-effects score ± SD	Mean AIMS score ± SD
Motipress	3.9 ± 1.99	0.17 ± 0.37
Clomipramine	2.8 ± 1.57	1.00 ± 1.16
Amitriptyline	4.3 ± 2.80	0.70 ± 1.8

The plasma levels were compared with a similar group of patients who had taken medication for less than three months (Table 16.3).

Table 16.3 Plasma drug levels during short-term and long-term medication

Parent drug	Drug metabolite	Short-term ng/ml Mean ± SD	Long-term ng/ml Mean ± SD
Motipress →	Nortriptyline	60.91 ± 48.40	58.30 ± 45.40
	Fluphenazine	1.18 ± 0.92	1.35 ± 0.72
Clomipramine →	Clomipramine	108.0 ± 13.6	78.0 ± 106.0
	Desmethyl metabolite	163.0 ± 16.3	125.0 ± 209.0
Amitriptyline →	Amitriptyline	67.2 ± 42.0	73.4 ± 101.0
	Nortriptyline metabolite	57.8 ± 55.0	34.3 ± 56.0

It was also noted that there was no correlation between plasma levels on Motipress and time on the drug or between plasma level and age if the two patients with idiosyncratically high levels were excluded. From this type of retrospective study few firm conclusions can be drawn as no internal checks on compliance were used so the plasma levels might reflect occasional forgetting of medication after a long period of treatment. However, specific studies on side-effects in elderly patients on long-term medication would clearly be of value as information in this area is sparse.

16.6 CONCLUSION

In conclusion it appears that there is a dearth of evidence about the value of long-term medication with antidepressants in old age. Investigation of compliance, unwanted or adverse effects, plasma levels and patient expectations about the value of treatment and the likelihood of improvement is required.

The fact that depressive illness is a treatable condition with potentially a good prognosis in many patients, even in old age, needs to be recognized and understood by both physician and patient.

REFERENCES

Blackwell, B. (1982) Antidepressant drugs: side-effects and compliance. *J. Clin. Psychiatry*, **43**:II: 14–18.

Coppen, A., Ghose, K., Montgomery, S., *et al.* (1978) Amitriptylene plasma concentration and clinical effect. *Lancet*, **i**, 63–6.

Hopkinson, F.J. (1964) A general study of affective illness in patients over 50. *Brit. J. Psychiat.*, **116**, 244–54.

Imlah, N.W., Ryan, E. and Harrington, J.A. (1965) The influence of antidepressant drugs on the response to electroconvulsive therapy and on subsequent relapse rates. *J. Neuropsychopharm.*, **4**, 439–42.

Jacoby, R.J. and Levy, R. (1980) Computed tomography in the elderly III: affective disorders. *Brit. J. Psychiat.*, **136**, 270–6.

Johnson, D.A.W. (1973) Treatment of depression in General Practice. *Brit. Med. J.*, **2**, 18–20.

Kay, D.W., (1959) Observations on the natural history of affective illness in patients over 50. *Proc. Roy. Soc. Med.*, **52**, 791–7.

Kay, D.W.K., Fahy, T. and Garside, R.F. (1970) A seven month double-blind trial of amitriptyline and diazepam in ECT-treated depressed patients. *Brit. J. Psychiat.*, **117**, 667–73.

Kragh-Sorensen, P., Hansen, C.E., Larsen, N.E. *et al.* (1974) Longterm treatment of endogenous depression with nortriptylene with control of plasma levels. *Psychol. Med.*, **4**, 174–80.

Mindham, R.H.S., Howland, C. and Shepherd, N. (1973) An evaluation of continuous therapy with tricyclic drugs in depressive illness. *Psychological Medicine*, **3**, 5–17.

Murphy, E. (1982) Social origins of depression in old age. *Brit. J. Psychiat.*, **141**, 135–42.

Pare, B.M. (1968) Recent advances in the treatment of depression. In: *Recent Advances in Affective Disorders* (eds A. Coppen and A. Walk), *British Journal of Psychiatry*, Special Publications No. 2, London.

Post, F. (1978) *Studies in Geriatric Psychiatry*, (eds F. Post and A.B. Isaacs), Wiley, Chichester.

Post, F. (1972) The management and nature of depressive illness in late life: a follow-through study. *Brit. J. Psychiat.*, **121**, 393–404.

Rabins, P. (1985) Cortical studies in depressive illness in old age. *Communication at Psychogeriatric Meeting, Baltimore.*

Robinson, R.G., Starr, L.B. and Price, T.R. (1984) A two-year longitudinal study of mood disorder following stroke. *Brit. J. Psychiat.*, **144**, 256–62.

Seager, C.B. and Bird, R.L. (1962) Imipramine with electrical treatment depression: a controlled trial. *J. Ment. Sci.*, **10**, 704–7.

Chapter Seventeen

Factors influencing the outcome of treatment

KLAUS P. EBMEIER and GEORGE W. ASHCROFT

CONTENTS

17.1 THE PROGNOSIS OF DEPRESSION IN OLD AGE

While the prognosis of depression in old age is not directly equivalent to the outcome of controlled trials of treatment, it is closer to clinical reality and has been researched in more detail. It is likely to be affected by current clinical practice. Factors like concurrent physical illness, preoccupation with bodily symptoms and neurotic presentation can lead to underdiagnozing depression in the elderly (Baldwin, 1988), and there is some evidence that General Practitioners (MacDonald, 1986) and even psychogeriatric services (Baldwin, 1988) do not treat depression effectively. At the same time elderly depressed patients require one and a half times as many bed days as their younger counterparts and use a quarter of all acute bed days in a general psychiatric hospital (Murphy and Grundy, 1984). Meanwhile a controversy about whether to stress the hopeful or the gloomy aspects of outcome studies (Murphy, 1987; Baldwin and Jolley, 1987) may reflect a degree of helplessness in the face of a puzzling array of outcome data.

There have so far been seven studies of elderly patients with depres-

Factors influencing the outcome of treatment

Table 17.1 Clinical status at follow-up and between index admission and follow-up

Study	Age	n	Follow-up time	Well %	Relapsed %	Residual symptoms or continuing depression %
Post, 1962[b,d]	>60	81	6 years	31	28	41
Post, 1972[b,d]	>60	92	3 years	26	37	37
Whitehead and Hunt, 1982[a,d]	>60	47	5 years	33	66*	
Murphy, 1983[a,c]	>65	103	1 year	43	22	35
Cole, 1983[b,c]	>65	38	1 year	41	25	22
Baldwin and Jolley, 1986[a,c]	>65	90	1 year	63	17	21
Baldwin and Jolley, 1986[b,d]	>65	96	3–8 years	22	39	40
Godber et al., 1987[b,d,e]	>65	163	3 years	33	28	34

a = demented and dead patients excluded
b = including demented and dead patients
c = clinical status at follow-up
d = clinical outcome during observation period
e = only patients treated with ECT
* = this includes relapsed and residual symptoms or continuing depression

sion who were followed up beyond the first episode of their illness (Post, 1962; 1972; Whitehead and Hunt, 1982; Murphy, 1983; Cole, 1983; Baldwin and Jolley, 1986; Godber et al., 1987) (see Table 17.1). In comparing the results of these studies it is important to keep in mind that some were only including patients admitted to psychiatric beds (Post, 1962, 1972; Whitehead and Hunt, 1982; Baldwin and Jolley, 1986), whilst another was examining all referrals to a psychogeriatric service from the community (Murphy, 1983). The age and sex distributions differed between studies as did the follow-up intervals. While some studies compared cross-sectional outcome data at one year (Murphy, 1983; Baldwin and Jolley, 1986) others examined retrospective information from index contact to date of follow-up (Post, 1962, 1972; Whitehead and Hunt, 1982; Baldwin and Jolley, 1986). While an approach using standardized methods and a prospective design has obvious advantages (Murphy, 1987), the assessment of the clinical course between index contact and follow-up requires some retrospective enquiry which is likely to produce more robust and valid results than a pinpoint cross-sectional approach (Baldwin and Jolley, 1986). This is most obvious for the patients classified as 'well' at follow-up. In Baldwin and Jolley's study (1986) only 20 of 57 patients well at one year had been continuously well over the 42 to 104 months' follow-up period, 28 suffered relapses with full recovery, and nine showed depressive invalidism. It is therefore not surprising that follow-through studies have resulted in a very stable ratio of about one-third recovery, one-third relapsing course (intermittent episodes of depression) and one-third residual states and continuous depressive symptoms (Post, 1978), whereas the cross-sectional studies show wider variations in outcome.

17.1.1 Mortality

While patients with depression have a significantly higher risk of death, this is additionally increased over a 20 year follow-up period to a rate twice the expected level in depressives with first admission after the age of 70 (Kay, 1962). Murphy (1983) found a four-year death rate of 37% amongst her cohort, while Baldwin and Jolley's (1987) result of 26% is closer to the expected rate of 20% for this age group.

17.1.2 Risk of suicide

There is good evidence that, in western societies, suicide rates rise with increasing age, and even rise within birth cohorts as they grow older (Post and Shulman, 1985). As the ratio between parasuicides and suicides shifts towards suicides in the elderly, any suicidal gesture or ideation must be taken as a serious prognostic sign which is – more often than with the young – associated with a depressive illness (Post and Shulman, 1985).

17.1.3 Progression to dementia

Dementia in patients with a history of depression is as common as expected in the general population (Post, 1986). While mild disorders of memory and orientation in depressed patients over 70 were shown to be associated with a poorer social adjustment but did not lead to dementia and increased mortality (Cole and Hickie, 1976), a recent follow-up of 22 cases of depressive pseudodementia over an average of eight years found only two patients well. Sixteen patients had developed a progressive dementia, confirmed as Alzheimer's disease at post-mortem in 11 (Kral, 1983). Jacoby and co-workers (1980,1981) found a subgroup of hospitalized depressed elderly patients to have enlarged cerebral ventricles. On follow-up two years later ventricular enlargement predicted increased mortality, albeit from extra-cerebral causes.

281

Accepting the heterogeneity of different samples of patients examined as the cause of observed differences, there seems to be a subgroup of patients in whom depression is associated with organic changes and increased mortality. However, preliminary results from an open trial of nortriptyline ($n=22$) or ECT ($n=10$) suggest that elderly patients with mixed depression and cognitive impairment show improvement of depressive symptoms (and cognitive performance) similar to that observed in cognitively intact depressives (Reynolds *et al.*, 1987). Depression, therefore, warrants a trial of treatment, even in the presence of dementia.

17.2 FACTORS AFFECTING LONG-TERM PROGNOSIS

17.2.1 Age and sex

Most studies find sex to be irrelevant for the prediction of outcome in old age depression (Post, 1986). An exception is Baldwin and Jolley's study (1986) which found a significant effect for sex ($p<0.05$) due to only one male in the lasting recovery group and four males in the continuously ill group of seven, with women outnumbering men by almost four to one in the whole study.

The evidence for the influence of age on outcome is contradictory. Earlier studies found a poor prognosis for depressed patients older than 60 years in a General Practice setting (Watts, 1956) and for psychiatric in-patients older than 70 years (Post, 1972). Baldwin and Jolley (1986) found no relationship to age at admission and Cole (1983) and Murphy (1983) found no age effect after controlling for the effect of ill health.

17.2.2 Age of onset

Similarly, the effect of age of onset of the depressive illness is unclear. While Post (1972) found late-onset depression to have a trend towards a poor prognosis, Winokur *et al.* (1980) and Murphy (1983) found no effect, and Cole (1983) and Whitehead and Hunt (1982) found later-onset depression to actually have a better prognosis.

17.2.2 Family history

A better prognosis in the late-onset group might be related to the fact that late-onset depressives have less of a family history than earlier onset depressives (Mendlewicz, 1976; Cole, 1983). However, neither Post (1972) nor Baldwin and Jolley (1986) found an effect of family history on prognosis.

17.2.4 Symptom pattern of depressive illness

The majority of studies find previous episodes of depressive illness of no import for prognosis (Murphy, 1983; Baldwin and Jolley, 1986), but Whitehead and Hunt (1982) found that many previous admissions augured badly. Those who had been ill continuously for a long time did worse than patients with short-lived illnesses (Whitehead and Hunt, 1982; Murphy, 1983; Post 1986), but Baldwin and Jolley (1986) could not replicate these results. In their study, illness lasting longer than 12 months did not have a significantly worse prognosis. Suicide attempts seem not to be associated with a poorer prognosis (Baldwin and Jolley, 1986). Severity of symptoms, whether measured with the Present State Examination (Murphy, 1983) or with the Hamilton Rating Scale for Depression (Baldwin and Jolley, 1986), appears to be an important predictor of poor outcome. While there is no difference between neurotic and psychotic patients in outcome (Post, 1972; Murphy, 1983), Murphy found a core group of depressives with biological features but without delusions and hallucinations to have a good recovery in 70% after one year, while the presence of typical depressive delusions and hallucinations predicted a very poor outcome (10% recovery after one year). This latter result could not be confirmed by Baldwin and Jolley (1986).

17.2.5 Physical illness

Chronic physical ill-health (Roth, 1983; Murphy, 1983), as well as acute health problems and changes in health during the follow-up period (Murphy, 1983; Baldwin and Jolley, 1986) are associated with a poor prognosis. Baldwin and Jolley (1986) found no link of poor prognosis to illness affecting any particular one of six body systems. This suggests that the meaning of the particular illness played perhaps as significant a role as the direct impact of the illness on brain function. In particular, if acute health problems and changes in health during follow-up assumed the significance of life events, they were related to poor outcome (Murphy, 1983; Baldwin and Jolley, 1986).

17.2.6 Premorbid personality

The assessment of premorbid personality in depression is fraught with the problems of retrospective research as well as the dearth of instruments especially validated for use with elderly populations (Burvill, Stampfer and Hall, 1986). There can, consequently, only be impressionistic findings, relating good outcome to euthymic and extrovert premorbid personality and poor outcome to longstanding dysthymic and introvert traits (Post, 1986).

17.2.7 Social factors

While Murphy (1983) found a trend towards poor prognosis in lower social classes, which was confirmed by significant differences in out-come between homeowners and patients in rented accommodation, she concluded that this might be accounted for by the preponderance of major social difficulties and life events in the lower social classes. Murphy (1983) elicited life events and social difficulties during the (structured) follow-up interview. A retrospective case-note analysis by Baldwin and Jolley (1986) did not produce any particular associations between major adverse life events and outcome. Earlier studies by Post did not produce effects of social factors on outcome, probably due to the higher social class of the sample (Post, 1986).

17.2.8 Social support

In contrast to studies in a General Practice sample (Mann, Jenkins and Belsey, 1981) and in depressed patients faced with social adversity (Surtees, 1980), Murphy (1983) did not find a protective effect of social support structures, including the presence of a spouse, living in company, and the presence of a confiding relationship. These results were confirmed by Baldwin and Jolley (1986) who found no statistically significant difference between patients living alone or in company, and between patients of different marital status.

There is a peculiar dissonance between the findings that life events and social difficulties predict poor outcome but that a close social support system does *not* protect against this effect. This might be explained by a greater sensitivity of the elderly to adverse events and difficulties – particularly since certain life events may be unique to the elderly (Blazer, 1982). Alternatively, the elderly may be more unresponsive to interpersonal support, just as they seem to be relatively insensitive to bereavements (Neugarten, 1970).

17.2.9 Differences in treatment

Inadequate doses of treatment (Burvill, Stampfer and Hall, 1986; Baldwin and Jolley, 1986) as well as overcautious use of ECT (Baldwin and Jolley, 1986) might be responsible for insufficient treatment response and consequently poor longer term outcome in elderly depressives. There seem to be no differences between hospital follow-up and community surveillance as regards the course of the illness and the length of further treatment episodes (Post, 1972).

17.3 FACTORS INFLUENCING THE SHORT-TERM OUTCOME OF ANTIDEPRESSANT TREATMENT

Although there seems to be a certain symmetry in prognostic factors between younger (Anonymous, 1986) and older depressives (see 17.2), predictors of treatment outcome should not be uncritically accepted if only documented in younger patients. Because of the scarcity of outcome research in elderly depressives, some results from research in younger patients will be discussed below, but identified accordingly. Factors predicting treatment response have been subdivided into illness-related and non illness-related factors. Taking one step further, one could assume a continuum from specific factors, which are related to the pathophysiology of the illness or the mechanism of action of treatment, to non-specific factors. A similar dichotomy is that of static versus dynamic factors proposed by Fähndrich (1984). He argues that static factors like symptom pattern, sex, or age of first onset of the illness are unlikely to make useful predictors of outcome, while dynamic variables, i.e. course of episode, short-term response to therapeutic interventions like drugs, sleep deprivation and ECT, are more closely related to the disease process of the current episode and, therefore, make better predictors. There is, as yet, little good evidence in favour of this hypothesis. The classification of predictors will, therefore, be descriptive. Patient characteristics will be discussed first, followed by treatment factors like type and dose of drug. Finally, interaction effects will be examined for their prognostic value.

17.3.1 Patient characteristics

While age does not appear to be a relevant factor for the prediction of treatment outcome in most studies (Bielski and Friedel, 1976), no direct conclusions can be drawn for depression in the elderly. The age range in most drug trials is usually too narrow, and other exclusion criteria, like physical illness, eliminate a further proportion of elderly patients from trials. For this reason, usually-accepted predictors of a good treatment response, like anorexia and weight loss; psychomotor retardation or agitation; middle and late insomnia; and first episode illness without delusions, neurotic, hypochondriacal or hysterical traits (Bielski and Friedel 1976) can only be accepted with caution for elderly patients. The same is true for the prediction of the response to lithium treatment. Predictors of successful prophylaxis in bipolar patients like family history, histocompatibility antigens other than HLA–A3 and high mean red blood cell-plasma ratio of lithium, as well as predictors in unipolar patients like low neuroticism (Eysenck Personality Inventory) and anxiety/phobic scores (Middlesex Hospital Questionnaire), high levels of psychomotor retardation and other biological symptoms of melan-cholia (Maj *et al.*, 1984, 1985) have only been established for, at best, mixed populations of younger and elderly patients.

Doctors' (Downing and Rickels, 1983) and patients' (Priebe, 1987) expectations of improvement and their relevance for treatment outcome have only been examined in younger age groups. The same is true for biological markers, like tryptophan and tyrosine availability (Møller and Larsen, 1984), monoamine neurotransmitter concentrations and interac-tions (Hsiao *et al.*, 1987) and a blunted TSH response to TRH challenge (Loosen and Prange, 1982). Studies of the dexamethasone suppression test (DST) in elderly depressed patients confirm the finding in younger patients that DST does not predict treatment response (Young *et al.*, 1984; Georgotas *et al.*, 1986).

A recent report by Jarvik *et al.* (1983) that a pretreatment orthostatic blood pressure change of more than 10 mmHg in patients older than 55 years predicted a good treatment response to imipramine and doxepin, deserves replication.

17.3.2 Treatment factors

Evidence from drug trials in the elderly points towards the superiority of tricyclics over placebo. However, other antidepressant drugs, includ-ing monoaminoxidase inhibitors (Georgotas *et al.*, 1987) which might have fewer side-effects, have been evaluated less thoroughly (Jarvik and Gerson, 1985). In clinical practice the presence of side-effects is likely both to decrease patient compliance with treatment and General Prac-titioners' readiness to prescribe adequate doses of medication.

17.3.3 Interaction between treatment and patient

In clinical practice a symptomatic response to treatment is used as an indicator of continued response and, conversely, a lack of improvement within a limited period is used as an indication for alternative treatment. This is borne out by controlled studies of treatment response which suggest that improvement of symptoms after three weeks (Möller, Fischer and v. Zerssen, 1987) or even one week (Katz *et al.*, 1987) predicts recovery. However, not all studies have shown this pattern (Coryell *et al.*, 1982).

Instead of clinical symptomatic response, alternative measures can be used. For example, the failure of DST non-suppression to normalize within seven weeks predicted a lack of clinical response to nortriptyline or phenelzine in the elderly (Georgotas *et al.*, 1986). Similarly, the failure to establish plasma nortriptyline levels between 50 and 150 ng/ml at week 4 predicted a poor treatment response in a group of elderly depressives (Young *et al.*, 1984).

The response to one night's sleep deprivation has been used for the prediction of treatment outcome, albeit only in younger patients (Fähndrich, 1983; Joffe *et al.*, 1984).

While studies trying to establish prognostically relevant factors have been of some considerable theoretical interest, the proportion of variance explained by these factors or their combination remains fairly modest (Möller, Fischer and v. Zerssen, 1987). In clinical practice the best strategy remains empirical, trying alternative treatments if there is no treatment response. This should be done in a systematic and vigorous fashion (Baldwin and Jolley, 1987) to improve at least the short-term prognosis of depressed elderly patients.

REFERENCES

Anonymous (1986) Predicting chronicity in depression (leading article). *The Lancet*, **ii**, 897–8.

Baldwin, R.C. (1988) Late life depression: undertreated? *Brit. Med. J.*, **296**, 519.

Baldwin, R.C. and Jolley, D.J. (1986) The prognosis of depression in old age. *Brit. J. Psychiat.*, **149**, 574–83.

Baldwin, R.C. and Jolley, D.J. (1987) Prognosis of depression in old age (letter). *Brit. J. Psychiat.*, **151**, 129.

Bielski, R.J. and Friedel, O. (1976) Prediction of tricyclic antidepressant response. A critical review. *Arch. Gen. Psychiat.*, **33**, 1479–89.

Blazer, D.G. (1982) *Depression in Late Life*, C.V. Mosby, St. Louis.

Burvill, P.W., Stampfer, H. and Hall, W. (1986) Does depressive illness in the elderly have a poor prognosis? *Austr. N.Z. J. Psychiatry*, **20**, 422–7.

Cole, M. and Hickie, R.N. (1976) Frequency and significance of minor organic signs in elderly depressives. *Can. Psychiat. Ass. J.*, **21**, 7–12.

Cole, M.G. (1983) Age, age of onset and course of primary depressive illness in the elderly. *Can. J. Psychiatry*, **28**, 102–4.

Coryell, W., Coppen, A., Zeigler, V.E. and Briggs, J.T. (1982) Early improvement as a predictor of response to amitriptyline and nortriptyline: a comparison of two patient samples. *Psychol. Med.*, **12**(1), 135–9.

Downing, R.W. and Rickels, K. (1983) Physician prognosis in relationship to drug and placebo response in anxious and depressed psychiatric outpatients. *J. Nerv. Mental Dis.*, **171**(37), 182–5.

Fähndrich, E. (1983) Clinical and biological parameters as predictors for antidepressant drug responses in depressed patients. *Pharmacopsychiat.*, **16**, 179–85.

Factors influencing the outcome of treatment

Fähndrich, E. (1984) Wann gebe ich im Einzelfall welches Antidepressivum? *Nervenarzt*, **55**, 477–82.

Georgotas, A., McCue, R.E., Friedman, E. and Cooper, T.B. (1987) Response of depressive symptoms to nortriptyline, phenelzine and placebo. *Brit. J. Psychiat.*, **151**, 102–6.

Georgotas, A., Stokes, P., McCue, R.E. *et al.* (1986) The usefulness of DST in predicting response to antidepressants: a placebo-controlled study. *J. Affect. Disord.*, **11**, 21–8.

Godber, C., Rosenwinge, H., Wilkinson, D. and Smithies, J. (1987) Depression in old age: prognosis after ECT. *Internat. J. Geriat. Psychiatry*, **2**, 19–24.

Hsiao, J.K., Agren, H., Bartko, J.J. *et al.* (1987) Monoamine neurotransmitter interactions and the prediction of antidepressant response. *Arch. Gen. Psychiat.*, **44**, 1078–83.

Jacoby, R.J., Levy, R. and Bird, J.M. (1981) Computerized tomography and the outcome of affective disorder: a follow-up study of elderly patients. *Brit. J. Psychiat.*, **139**, 288–92.

Jacoby, R.J., Levy, R. and Dawson, J.M. (1980) Computerized tomography in the elderly: 3. Affective disorder. *Brit. J. Psychiat.*, **136**, 270–5.

Jarvik, L.F. and Gerson, S. (1985) Outcome of drug treatment in depressed patients over the age of fifty. In: *Treatment of Affective Disorders in the Elderly* (ed. C.A. Shanovian), American Psychiatric Press, Washington, D.C.

Jarvik, L.F., Read, S.L., Mintz, Z. and Neshkes, R.E. (1983) Pretreatment orthostatic hypotension in geriatric depression: predictor of response to imipramine and doxepin. *J. Clin. Psychopharmacol.*, **3**(6), 368–72.

Joffe, R., Brown, P., Bienenstock, A. and Mitton, J. (1984) Neuroendocrine predictors of the antidepressant effect of partial sleep deprivation. *Biol. Psychiat.*, **19**(3), 347–52.

Katz, M.M., Koslow, S.H., Maas, J.W. *et al.* (1987) The timing, specificity and clinical prediction of tricyclic drug effects in depression. *Psychol. Med.*, **17**, 297–309.

Kay, D.W.K. (1962) Outcome and cause of death in mental disorders of old age: a long-term follow-up of functional and organic psychoses. *Act. Psychiat. Scand.*, **38**, 249–76.

Kral, V.A. (1983) The relationship between senile dementia (Alzheimer type) and depression. *Can. J. Psychiatry*, **28**, 304–6.

Loosen, P.T. and Prange, A.Z. (1982) Serum thyrotropin response to thyrotropin releasing hormone in psychiatric patients: a review. *Am. J. Psychiat.*, **139**, 405–16.

MacDonald, A.J.D. (1986) Do General Practitioners 'miss' depression in elderly patients? *Brit. Med. J.*, **292**, 1365–7.

Maj, M., Arena, F., Lovero, N. *et al.* (1985) Factors associated with response to lithium prophylaxis in DSM–III major depression and bipolar disorder. *Pharmacopsychiat.*, **18**, 309–13.

Maj, M., Del Vechio, M., Starace, *et al.* (1984) Prediction of affective psychoses response to lithium prophylaxis. The role of socio-demographic, clinical, psychological and biological variables. *Acta. Psychiat. Scand.*, **69**, 37–44.

Mann, A.H., Jenkins, R. and Belsey, E. (1981) The twelve month outcome of patients with neurotic illness in General Practice. *Psychol. Med.*, **11**, 535–50.

Mendlewicz, J. (1976) The age factor in depressive illness: some genetic considerations. *J. of Gerontol.*, **31**, 300–3.

Möller, H.J., Fischer, G. and v. Zerssen, D. (1987) Prediction of therapeutic response in acute treatment with antidepressants. *Eur. Arch. Psychiatr. Neurol. Sci.*, **236**, 349–57.

Møller, S.E. and Larsen, O.B. (1984) Tryptophan and tyrosine availability: relation to clinical response to antidepressive pharmacotherapy. In: *Frontiers in Biochemical and Pharmacological Research in Depression* (ed. E. Usdin), Raven Press, New York.

Murphy, E. (1983) The prognosis of depression in old age, *Brit. J. Psychiat.*, **142**, 111–19.

Murphy, E. (1987) The prognosis of depression in old age (letter). *British J. Psychiat.*, **150**, 268.

Murphy, E. and Grundy, E. (1984) A comparative study of bed usage by younger and older patients with depression. *Psychol. Med.*, **14**(2), 445–50.

Neugarten, B.Z. (1970) Adaptation and life cycle. *J. Geriatric Psychol.*, **4**, 71.

Post, F. (1962) *The Significance of Affective Symptoms in Old Age*, Maudsley Monograph 10, Oxford University Press, London.

Post, F. (1972) The management and nature of depressive illness in late life: a follow-through study. *Brit. J. Psychiat.*, **121**, 393–404.

Post, F. (1978) The functional psychoses. In: *Studies in Geriatric Psychiatry* (eds A.D. Isaacs and F. Post), John Wiley, Chichester.

Post, F. (1986) Course and outcome of depression in the elderly. In: *Affective Disorders in the Elderly* (ed. E. Murphy), Churchill Livingstone, Edinburgh.

Post, F. and Shulman, K. (1985) New views on old age affective disorders. In: *Recent Advances in Psychogeriatrics* (ed. T. Arie), Churchill Livingstone, Edinburgh.

Priebe, S. (1987) Early subjective reactions predicting the outcome of hospital treatment in depressive patients. *Acta. Psychiat. Scand.*, **76**(2), 134–8.

Reynolds, C.F. Perel, J.M., Kupfer, D.J. *et al.* (1987) Open-trial response to antidepressant treatment in elderly patients with mixed depression and cognitive impairment. *Psychiatry Res.*, **21**, 111–22.

Roth, M. (1983) Depression and affective disorder in late life. In: *The Origins of Depression: Current Concepts and Approaches* (ed. J. Angst), Springer, Heidelberg.

Surtees, P.G. (1980) Social support, residual adversity and depressive outcome. *Social Psychiatry*, **15**, 71–80.

Watts, C.A.H. (1956) The incidence and prognosis of endogenous depression. *Brit. Med. J.*, **1**, 1392–7.

Whitehead, A. and Hunt, D. (1982) Elderly psychiatric patients: a five year prospective study. *Psychol. Med.*, **12**, 149–57.

Winokur, G., Behar, D. and Schlesser, M. (1980) Clinical and biological aspects of depression in the elderly. In: *Psychopathology in the Aged* (eds J.D. Cole and J.E. Barrett), Raven Press, New York.

Young, R.C., Alexopoulos, G.S., Manley, M.L. *et al.* (1984) Treatment outcome in elderly depressives: plasma nortriptyline concentration and pretreatment dexamethasone suppression test. In: *Frontiers in Biochemical and Pharmacological Research in Depression* (ed. E. Usdin), Raven Press, New York.

Subject index

Pharmacological and therapeutic agents index